Narrative Medicine

Trauma and Ethics

Edited by

Anders Juhl Rasmussen
University of Copenhagen, Denmark

Morten Sodemann
University Hospital Odense and University of Southern Denmark, Denmark

Cognitive Science and Psychology

VERNON PRESS

www.vernonpress.com

In the Americas:
Vernon Press
1000 N West Street, Suite 1200,
Wilmington, Delaware 19801
United States

In the rest of the world:
Vernon Press
C/Sancti Espiritu 17,
Malaga, 29006
Spain

Cognitive Science and Psychology

Library of Congress Control Number: 2023952289

ISBN: 978-1-64889-845-7

Cover design by Vernon Press.

Cover image by Jesper Skytte Sodemann.

Table of Contents

Acknowledgment

We extend our heartfelt thanks to photographer Jesper Skytte Sodemann for providing the cover image, a vital part of the book's presentation.

We are deeply indebted to the extraordinary editorial support from Tine Birkebæk. Tine handled the communication with the authors and the review process with elegance and respect for the significance of each author's contribution. She made the process a pleasant and professional editorial experience, and her input was a major factor in the high quality of this anthology.

List of Figures

Foreword

Rishi Goyal
Columbia University, US

With the generous invitation to write a foreword for this volume, I would like to offer a few words on the oscillating nature of trauma as it relates to my dual disciplinary frameworks, Emergency and trauma care and Narrative medicine or medical humanities. The vernacular usage and field of intelligibility for trauma has expanded considerably, but as Rasmussen and Sodemann note in their excellent introduction, it is rooted in a wound or injury. The spectrum of trauma that I encounter in the hospital on a daily basis is wide. On the one hand, I care for patients with serious injuries to their bodies: a man with a bleeding chest wound from a gunshot; an older woman with a scalp laceration and internal hemorrhage after a trip and fall; a youth with a cervical bone fracture following a diving accident. On the other hand, sometimes related to these and other physical insults, trauma also captures the psychological distress and emotional responses associated with life threatening, terrible or emotionally charged events. I have cared for patients with traumatic reactions to car accidents, lightning strikes, stabbings and rape but also to police brutality, racism, transphobia and even slower forms of violence like poverty, neglect, and daily low levels of stress. Trauma is a heuristic that highlights embodied cognition and permits us to perceive the entanglements of psyche and soma.

Trauma's purview and compass are not limited to the individual, the event or the clinical encounter. Trauma echoes and expands to incriminate, diagnose and explain cultural, historical, and institutional forces. In my related work as a medical humanities and narrative medicine scholar, I often read literature, philosophy, medical memoirs, and histories to account for collective, cultural and intergenerational trauma. In *Reading Capital,* Louis Althusser defines a practice of reading he labels as symptomatic reading. This reading is not limited to the surface, superficial meaning of a text, but uncovers and unearths what a text represses as a condition of its possibility. This kind of symptomatic reading is an interpretive act that frames the boundaries of ideology and reveals invisible but present forces that structure our ways of knowing, being and, relating to one another. Like a physician listening for symptoms of trauma in our patients, a symptomatic reading of the many kinds of texts discussed in this volume like Sarah Manguso's poetic memoir *Two Kinds of Decay,* reveals trauma as pervasive and constitutive of contemporary sociopolitical relations.

Through a symptomatic reading of cultural documents, we can reconnect individual stories and experiences of physical and mental traumas with historical and collective traumas.

One of the important outstanding questions in the etiology of post-traumatic stress disorder is why some people experience it and others do not. Given similar or comparable circumstances, the common assumption is that some people become "traumatized" and others do not. But as traumatic reactions have gained in visibility and cultural acceptance, we might say that we are all traumatized. Living in the twenty-first century, under the constant threat of war, climate catastrophe, and infectious apocalypse, we exist proximate to traumatic experience. What unites all traumatic experience is a combination of vulnerability, precarity, and exploitation. This risk is unevenly distributed, no doubt. Peoples of the Global South and former Anglo-European colonies, brown and black people all over the world, the impoverished, the incarcerated, the undomiciled, women and trans people, all certainly experience more vulnerability, precarity, and exploitation. Nor do I want to diminish the specificity of a clinical trauma that can cause debilitating nightmares, anxiety, exhaustion, and isolation. I'm only suggesting that the widespread discussion and experience of trauma have given us a valuable framework with which to understand our shared and collective experiences and to guide a symptomatic reading of cultural texts.

If the movements in clinical medicine are the organization of symptoms, diagnosis and diagnostic thinking, and therapeutics, then while I have touched on the first two, I have not mentioned the last. And here again this volume makes an important contribution. Trauma's force seems to be the way in which it blurs boundaries, leaps time and space, and diffuses through experience. While it may sometimes have a clear beginning and signify a discrete event, trauma often outpaces the moment. It ripples and repeats even as repetition is one of its defining symptoms. From Freud's "talking cure" to narrative medicine's insistence on the importance of storytelling, narrativity, narratability and the telling of one's story have been seen as central to a *therapeutic* practice in medicine, not just a diagnostic one. This volume extends that insight through chapters on trauma-informed practice, narrative-based practice, critical race theory, and expressive and creative writing. While telling one's story of trauma can be a powerful way of mitigating the persisting effects of trauma, it can sometimes also be re-traumatizing. By framing trauma in the context of narrative medicine and ethics, we can develop new research and models to understand and dismantle power relations between tellers and listeners that might adversely the therapeutic power of storytelling. Not everyone is allowed to tell their story and not everyone is heard. We might call the complex of what stories get heard and what can be told, *narrative audibility*. Ideology, institutional racism, and histories of sexism prevent many traumatic stories from being told or heard in the medical context. We must learn how to create empathic and safe spaces to allow the telling of stories of trauma to be therapeutic and to not be unwitting perpetrators of new traumatic experiences.

Almost every day I have to tell someone that their loved one has died. This can be a traumatizing experience for the family member, and the emergency room is a particularly difficult place to create a safe space. But it can be done and if we can do it here, we should be able to do it everywhere in medicine. By avoiding assumptions, by staying sensitive to cultural, racial, and social difference, by minimizing hierarchy and approaching the moment with narrative humility, we must prevent the formation of new traumatic experiences and support the healing power of storytelling. But we must also recognize that stories and individuals do not exist in a vacuum. They exist in an expanded cultural, social, economic and historical matrix that is sometimes traumatizing, but that can also be therapeutic.

Reference List

Althusser, L. (2015 [1965]) *Reading capital.* Translated from the French by Ben Brewster and David Fernbach. New York: Verso Books.

Manguso, S. (2008) *The two kinds of decay.* London: Granta Books.

Introduction

Anders Juhl Rasmussen

University of Copenhagen, Denmark

Morten Sodemann

University Hospital Odense and University of Southern Denmark, Denmark

The present volume repositions narrative medicine with trauma studies and ethics in a global context. Trauma is a rapidly growing field of especially literary and cultural studies, perhaps because we tend to label more and more events ranging from the casual to the catastrophic as traumatic. Ethics has, since the invention of narrative ethics in the medical humanities, a permanent and significant relevance for the interpretation of these events and their medical treatment. The ways in which the phenomenon and the concept of trauma have asserted its relevance across disciplines, intersecting with narrative medicine and ethics, and how it has widened the scope of narrative research and medical practice constitute the principal concerns of this edited volume.

This collection brings together contributions from established and emerging scholars coming from a wide range of academic fields within the faculty of humanities and of health care, and this crossing of disciplines is also represented by the collaboration between the two editors. We have accepted in our volume 20 chapters from disciplines that include ethnography, literary and media studies, psychology, philosophy, and history as well as medical education and health care studies. Although with a weight on the Euro-American academy, the scholars cover—in geographical affiliations—most of the world: Europe (8), US (6), Asia (3), Canada (1), Middle East (1) and Australia (1). If trauma studies with ethical orientation have been accused of prevailing a bias stemming from the Western perspective, then this book contributes to a global, and yet locally differentiated, understanding of narratives in medicine.

This book had its inception at the final *Uses of Literature* conference (held online) organized by University of Southern Denmark to honor Rita Felski's collective research project. One panel in the conference entitled "Narrative Medicine: Trauma and Ethics" brought together scholars from various countries and disciplines to engage with the topic. Since 2017 narrative medicine has been integrated into this university's medical and health care education, and several research interventions testing writing and reading with patients has been evaluated (Rasmussen, Mai and Hansen, 2022). The overwhelming interest generated by the following call for chapters highlighted the urgency to follow up on the panel with a volume to fill this gap in interdisciplinary research.

The Invention of Narrative Medicine

Narrative medicine was given its name and has had its methodology established since the beginning of this century by Rita Charon, a medical doctor, and professor of internal medicine with a PhD in English literature at Columbia University in New York (2001, 2006). Through the creation of the interdisciplinary field of narrative medicine, she extended her scope to include narratives and aspects of narrative in all medical practice, with a particular focus on the value of empathy and ethics. With the aim of promoting clinicians' understanding of patients' narratives of illness, Charon and her colleagues at Columbia University brought to bear methods from literary studies of close reading and creative writing. The result is that these have been adapted and integrated into the teaching of physicians and other health professionals at Columbia and elsewhere. Close reading is used to designate an exploratory reading of a shorter text, often carried out in plenum, where every word acquires meaning in an interplay with the whole, while creative writing is regarded as a means by which to examine one's thoughts in the aftermath of a shared close reading. The hypothesis is that the clinician's skills in receiving, interpreting, understanding, and acting on patients' stories can be trained by methodically working with literary texts or other similar forms of artistic expression.

In an anthology on narrative medicine and medical ethics, Charon argued convincingly that although illness is a biological phenomenon, the human response to it is neither biologically determined nor arithmetical. She continued:

> In extending help to a sick person, one not only determines what the matter might be; one also by the necessity of illness determines what its meanings might be. Such a search requires the narrative competence to follow the patient's narrative thread, to make sense of his or her figural language, to grasp the significance of stories told, and to imagine the illness from its conflicting perspectives. Narrative approaches to ethics recognize that the singular case emerges only in the act of narrating it and that duties are incurred in the act of hearing it. (Charon and Montello, 2002, p. 1)

How the patient tells of illness, how the doctor represents it in words, who listens as the intern presents at rounds, what the audience is being moved to think—all these narrative dimensions of health care are of defining importance in medical ethics. A literary, critical ear focuses on the narrator's reliability, on whose voice is being heard, the motives, attributes, and tactics of the main characters of a case, and on moral and human differences between alternative outcomes under consideration.

Through the discipline of narrative medicine, Charon brought together her own passion for literature, an extensive tradition of courses in literature and medicine taught in American medical programs, and a broader epistemological orientation toward the exploration of the significance of narratives that cut across academic subject areas in the humanities, sometimes called the "narrative turn." In this, Charon and her colleagues have been extending the tradition of investigating the significance of narratives in health care. This tradition was established by researchers with an interest in ill people's stories rather than their bodily data such as anthropologist and physician Arthur Kleinman (1988) and sociologist Arthur W. Frank (1995). Frank has over the years developed his own parallel research area to narrative medicine, exploring the significance of oral and written illness narratives, most recently how a reading of Shakespeare's dramas can help vulnerable people find consolation (2022).

Charon consolidated the innovative methodology combining close reading and creative writing in her monograph *Narrative Medicine: Honoring the Stories of Illness* (2006). Recently, she has further expanded its theoretical and, not least, didactic range in the collective book *The Principles and Practice of Narrative Medicine* (2016), of which she was one of eight co-authors from Columbia University. Although the methodology is relatively sharply restricted to reading and writing, to creative and reflective processes, the breadth of theory in narrative medicine is suggested by the fact that, among Columbia's researchers and teachers, there are specialists in film studies, oral storytelling, creative writing, philosophy, psychoanalysis, and qualitative evaluation. However broad in its theoretical foundation, narrative medicine is defined as centered on three significant elements of the health professional's encounter with patients:

> We early recognized attention, representation, and affiliation" as the three movements of narrative medicine that emerged from our commitment to skilled listening, the power of representation to perceive the other, and the value of the partnerships that result from narrative contact. (Charon et al., 2016, p. 3)

Narrative medicine attempts thereby to develop physicians' skills in creating a trusting relation between physician and patient by paying careful attention to what patients say about their illness and suffering or to what they hesitate to say or partially omit. This is, obviously, of particular interest for the phenomenon of trauma understood as an unspeakable or untellable event. Not all messages from patients to physicians are, strictly speaking, narratives, but from relatively few signals, the health professional can co-create a story of a social, cultural, or family situation that the patient will often be able to collaborate on, and this reciprocity can lead to empathetic and ethically contact. According to the hypothesis of narrative medicine, the ability to produce such co-created narratives can be stimulated by close acquaintance with aesthetic narratives in literature and other art forms. In one article published in the literary journal *Narrative*, Charon directly linked narrative medicine to trauma studies, and yet this coupling of narrative and trauma is still rather unexplored in research (West, 2021), when not considered as narrative therapy as developed by Michael White and David Epston:

> We are also turning toward the work of oral historians and those who work in trauma studies and testimony to learn how they equip themselves as witnesses to others' suffering. The oral historian or the interviewer in testimony archives is positioned to encourage the telling, to enable the teller to hear himself or herself speak. If the telling cannot go on without a listener, those listeners know that they become themselves implicated, traumatized in their acts of listening. (Charon, 2005, p. 264)

It has been stated that narrative itself embodies the traumatic problem, in that it represents through its narration of past events a ceaseless and obsessive return to the site of trauma (Kurtz, 2018, p. 4). At the same time, it can be argued that narratives offer an expressive mechanism that might potentially offer a solution to the problem as argued in Narrative Exposure Therapy or Trauma Informed Care. Neither of these dynamics is, as you will see in the following chapters, straightforward or simple.

Most of the authors in our volume use "narrative medicine" to refer to the methodology pioneered by Charon and her colleagues at Columbia University, but in some chapters, the authors use it to refer to other methodologies and pedagogies using that descriptor. That is for example the case in the chapter of John Launer, who has been part of the development of narrative-based medicine in England beginning with Trisha Greenhalgh and Brian Hurwitz's edited volume *Narrative-Based Medicine: Dialogue and Discourse in Clinical Practice* from 1998. Some contributors also refer to the critique of narrative medicine formulated in various degrees from absolute rejection (Woods, 2011; O'Mahony, 2013) to constructive revision (Wear and Aultman, 2005; Kalitzkus and Matthiesen, 2009). One shortcoming of narrative medicine may be that it relies almost exclusively on exchanges between individual entities—listeners and patients—and not on social structures. As argued in the chapters of both Brooke Covington and Victoria Simpson, counterstorytelling provides a new tool to enrich the practice of narrative medicine by enabling practitioners to attend to the social, historical, and structural contexts from which these narratives of emerge.

Despite all criticism, narrative medicine and ethics seem to evolve in new, unpredictable directions. Recently, the narratologist James Phelan has contributed to the field with a book, *Narrative Medicine: A Rhetorical Rx* (2023), grounded in the rhetorical theory of narrative. This contribution from a Professor of English and leading specialist in narrative theory and ethics demonstrates and expands the interdisciplinary range of Charon's invention.

Aesthetic, Cultural, Psychological and Historical Trauma Studies

Fundamentally, trauma is a wound. This, at least, is its Greek origin, where it denotes a physical injury from an external cause. Yet today, we more frequently use the term trauma to describe emotional or psychological injury, as opposed to bodily harm. The first modern theory of trauma was defined by physician and inventor of psychoanalysis Sigmund Freud more than hundred years ago. In *Beyond the Pleasure Principle* (1920) Freud emphasized the overwhelming nature of trauma, the fact that traumatic events act like a breach in the psyche's defensive wall, so that it represents "excitations from outside which are powerful enough to break through the protective shield" (1953, p. 29). Freud based his research partly on people with memories of childhood abuse, and partly on soldiers with traumatic experience from World War I. More than 50 years later in the century, in 1980, based on American soldiers' experiences from the Vietnam War, trauma became defined as a diagnosis when the American Psychiatric Association included a description of what it termed Post-Traumatic Stress Disorder (PTSD) in the third edition of its influential *Diagnostic and Statistical Manual of Mental Disorders* (DSM). The medicalization with antidepressants in the treatment of the phenomenon was, and still is, a debated invention.

In literary trauma theory, the perhaps most cited definition is formulated by American literary scholar Cathy Caruth in her introduction to the edited collection *Trauma: Explorations in Memory* (1995). The psychoanalytical-inspired claim is that trauma consists "in the structure of its experience or reception: the event is not assimilated fully at the time, but only belatedly, in its repeated possession of the one who experiences it" (ibid., pp. 4-5). Later in the famous *Unclaimed Experience: Trauma, Narrative and History* (1996), Caruth elaborated her theory that literary language, by its very nature, offers a uniquely effective vehicle for representing the experience of trauma in ways that ordinary language cannot. An idea, once again reflected in *Literature in the Ashes of History* (2013).

From the perspective of another discipline, namely modern history and memory studies, the American scholar Dominick LaCapra has written over a life course about how trauma theory engages with the representation of Holocaust during World War II, and how this still might be productive for today's reflection and analysis. LaCapra pointed out the paradoxical relation between trauma and emotions in his canonical *Writing History, Writing Trauma*: "Trauma brings about a dissociation of affect and representation: one disorienting feels what one cannot represent; one numbingly represents what one cannot feel" (2001, p. 42). As a historian, LaCapra is concerned with traumas that are both personal and collective at the same time.

In the past twenty years, the field of trauma studies has almost exploded combining history, culture, politics, medicine, and geography. The terrorist attack September 11, 2001, and its coverage in the media provoked Ann Kaplan to study trauma and its cultural politics in *Trauma Culture: The Politics of Terror and Loss in Media and Literature* (2005). More specifically attuned to literature, Anne Whitehead in *Trauma Fiction* (2004) focuses on the ways in which contemporary novelists explore the theme of trauma and incorporate its structure into their writing. British literary scholar Roger Luckhurst has traced the ways in which ideas of trauma have become a major element in contemporary Western conceptions of the self in *The Trauma Question* (2008). Belgian literary scholar Stef Craps' aimed at widening the political-geographical perspective to non-Western and minority groups in *Postcolonial Witnessing: Trauma out of Bounds* (2013), and most recently he wrote, with Lucy Bond, an updated introduction to the field, *Trauma* (2020). From an interdisciplinary perspective, Didier Fassin and Richard Rechtman, both anthropologists and physicians, revealed how trauma has come to authenticate the suffering of victims in *The Empire of Trauma: An Inquiry into the Condition of Victimhood* (2009). From Fassin and Rechtman we learn about the historical construction and the political uses of trauma. Comparable to this approach is literary scholar Shoshana Felman and psychiatrist Dori Laub's almost classical *Testimony": Crises of Witnessing in Literature, Psychoanalysis and History* (1992) in which they investigate the relation between knowledge and event, literature and evidence, speech and survival, witnessing and ethics.

Also, numerous anthologies about cultural trauma theory have been published in the recent years: *Trauma Narratives and Herstory* (Andermahr and Pellicer-Ortin, 2013), *Trauma in Contemporary Literature* (Nadal and Calvo, 2014), *The Future of Trauma Theory* (Buelens, Durrant and Eaglestone, 2014), *Trauma and Literature* (Kurtz, 2018), *The Routledge Companion to Literature and Trauma* (Davis and Meretoja, 2020), *Terrorizing Images: Trauma and Ekphrasis in Contemporary Literature*, (Armstrong and Langås, 2020), and *Trauma and Motherhood in Contemporary Literature and Culture* (Lazzari and Ségeral,

2021). No doubt, trauma has become a catchword of our time and a central category in contemporary cultural studies. Trauma is now understood both in the restricted, clinical sense in which it is used in the mental health field, and in its more widespread, popular usage. This edited collection aspires to prolong, deepen, and advance the area of narrative medicine, trauma, and ethics in especially two important aspects: by bringing together both the cultural and the clinical side of trauma and ethics, and by opening the investigation to a truly global horizon.

Clinical Perspectives on Trauma and Ethics

What is a dangerous experience for a human being? You can survive a cut from a sword but a mosquito bite can kill you. Similarly, a dance floor for a spider can be a killing field for a fly. Context as well as perspective matter in the definition of trauma and its consequences. Traditionally, it has been a condition for the diagnosis that symptoms were present within 6 months of the trauma-eliciting experience, which meant that individual variations in context could exclude some patients from the diagnosis. There are several types of trauma; some have clinical consequences while others have non-clinical cognitive, perceptive or emotional consequences. As a reflection of the historical development of understanding trauma, the WHO has introduced a new approach in its latest version of the International Classification of Diseases (ICD-11) by including broader concepts such as a violent or terrifying incident as trauma exposures, which opens the way for psychological violence, bullying, or a doctor's unexpected experience of a patient's sudden death to result in PTSD. Some of the chapters in this volume are in line with this new paradigm.

Trauma presents diagnostic and ethical challenges to clinicians, something particularly evident in the Migrant Health Clinic at Odense University Hospital in Denmark: exactly what constitutes trauma, and who has the authority (and competence) to decide? Often the definition of psychological trauma collides with the individual patient experience. In modern clinical medicine, clinicians are obliged to involve patients, share decisions and co-create solutions. To adhere strictly to narrow definitions of clinical trauma and related clinical syndromes would therefore be unethical as humans experiencing violence, extreme helplessness or disasters tend to have distinct and individual experiences with their own unique consequences. If the patient feels exposed to a severe trauma that has caused an alteration or disturbance in their mental and/or physical body functions, this has to be the starting point for conversation. The carefully determined co-creation process to establish the patient's perception and the narrative surrounding it requires active deep listening by the clinician with a sense for hints, analogies and metaphors—a sort of pre-diagnostic deep reading of the patient's mindset and how the trauma has marked the patient's self-perception, memory and agency.

Traumatic experiences may have a disturbing impact on our lives, but they can nonetheless help us evolve as individuals, bringing us forward in a realization, providing insights into our relationships with others, or lead to personal growth in the face of illness. Other traumas lead to a disruption that leaves the biophysical body and soul in a different state, slows it down, blocks normal flow of thought, brings the person into a constant state of alertness resulting in a chronic personal derailment that limits or stops options for action and aspirations. Trauma can focus (retain) memory in certain violent or extremely helpless experiences or they can disrupt memory so that the structures for recollection and remembrance fundamentally changes and becomes erroneous, unpredictable and chaotic. Trauma can happen repeatedly during the course of life since early childhood years resulting in a complex PTSD condition when a child is exposed to repeated constant abuse and physical/psychological violence. These childhood traumas can later create challenges in contact with adults because the personality has developed in a dysregulated way—and thus more frequently as an adult encounters new traumas (violence in relationships, rape, fights, and exclusion). Trauma can be infectious: trauma causing trauma in oneself or it can be transmitted from parents to offspring and even to grandchildren as has been documented among Jewish and Japanese communities (Kellermann, 2013). There are traumas that settle in the body while others settle in the soul and others that do both. The Palestinian American Hala Alyan's 2017 novel *Salt Houses* describes how nightmares and traumatic events can be transmitted to future Palestinian generations and define their transnational identity in diaspora (Salam and Mahfouz, 2020). The burden of inherited trauma has also been described in Nicole Kraus' novel *Great house* from 2010 (Berger and Milbauer, 2013). There is biomedical science describing morphological changes in the brain following violent assaults, disasters, violent accidents, torture, rape, confinement, bomb shelling, etc. (Sherin and Nemeroff, 2011). Trauma can result in brain damage and disturbance of stress hormones and increase the risk of chronic diseases. Psychological violence in intimate relationships is repeated acts that demean, humiliate, violate, manipulate, threaten or isolate. The actions can be done out of emotion or be planned and have the purpose of controlling or limiting the life expression of the victim of violence. Therefore, a general trauma definition emphasizes that there has been a life-threatening situation with a risk of death or injury or sexual violence (DSM).

To sum up, trauma can manifest itself as either physical or psychological distress. Often physical and psychological symptoms can undergo a metamorphosis where one leads to the other. With increasing interaction, they become indistinguishable ending up as a complex fusion of anxiety, alertness, altered body awareness, and unfamiliar pain sensations. The psychiatrist and trauma researcher Bessel van der Kolk has described these processes in his for all clinicians' famous textbook *The Body Keeps the Score* (2015), which is now translated into 38 languages. In the case of forced and traumatized refugees, not only are they often displaced and alienated either within their own country or in a foreign country, they are also mentally and physically displaced and alienated from their normal state of equilibrium between physical sensations and psychological processes. This reinforces the ongoing dissolvent by trauma of memory, language, self-perceptions and interpretations of feelings and symptoms. Trauma survivors have different and unique experiences of the mutuality of mental and bodily trauma, but they circle around the same implicit experience of body affecting mind affecting body in a constant pattern. Here are some patient quotes illustrating this metamorphosis from the Migrant Health Clinic at Odense University Hospital:

> If life shouldn't settle in my bones, where else should it?
>
> I have lived an unlivable life. My body is open 24-7 and my mind keeps having these fights with my body. My body and I are not on friendly terms.
>
> I am 42 years old, but I feel like I'm 80 years old because I have seen too much blood and it wears out your body. (Sodemann, 2022, pp. 230-238)

Normally, we interact with friends and relatives about our everyday experiences. We describe what we saw, and how we felt about it, and we expect to be met by recognition and feedback to help us mentalize the experience by adding meaning and placing it somewhere on a scale of significance and consequences. Trauma survivors often lose the ability to describe what they experienced because trauma is characterized by an unexpected event of extreme helplessness, near death or violent assault—an event that forever makes the borderline between "I" and "Other" permeable and vague. Body and mind are on constant alert and will never forget. A constantly overworked alarm system reacts indiscriminately to any kind of body sensation with intense fear and any change in routines and traditions evokes uncontrollable anxiety. Trauma is not experienced in a vacuum, is it observed based on previous life experiences, and the subsequent developments are formed by interactions with society norms, social networks, and relatives. The path a trauma takes with each individual trauma survivor is unique and depends on the survivors' preexisting psychological characteristics, resilience, and vulnerability factors and how they are received by the community, friends, and family as well as by health professionals in somatic and psychiatric health care.

Hopefully, the contributions in this edited collection will increase the global, clinical understanding of how the life history and the social context of trauma forms the extent and consequences of the trauma together with the effects of the reception and interaction with health care professionals, psychologist, social norms, social networks, and relatives.

The Structure and Content of This Volume

With this book we seek to explore broad questions about how traumas are narrated and witnessed, how they are conceived through artworks and treated in the health care systems by narrative methods. Kinds of trauma and ethical orientation investigated in the chapters vary from adverse childhood events, sexual abuse, violence and war, to trauma related to experiences of parents dying, severe illness, disability, etc. To ensure coherence and clarity, we have structured the 20 chapters into three parts:

1. Autoethnographical Research
2. Narrative Methods and Ethics in Trauma Care
3. Studies of Aesthetic Trauma Narratives

Chapters dealing with autoethnographical stories are related to lived experiences of trauma, but not necessarily restricted to that experience. We believe that reading these chapters up front can help our readers to realize how pervasive trauma is in our world, and how we can understand our responsibilities in the fact of trauma. The following two parts are larger, and these parts are again divided into two sections each depending on the perspectives of the narrative methods and ethics in trauma care and on the objectives of the studies of aesthetic narratives. The perspective is either health care- or patient-centered, the objective either therapeutic or analytical. Of course, most chapters have more than one aim and are affiliated with other sections in this provisional genre system, yet we believe that a systematic ordering contributes to clarification of this heterogeneous material. Ordered in this way, we also intend to illuminate how the book covers not only many dimensions of narratives on trauma and ethics in society, culture, and health care, but also many fields, disciplines, and methodologies.

The first part, "Autoethnographical stories of trauma," consists of three chapters which include voices of people living with disability and traumatized cancer patients. These voices are often excluded from strict academic research. Annmaree Watharow, Sue Joseph, and Georgia Fagan's chapter explores how people living with disability can experience trauma any day through oppressive events and discriminatory treatment. Inventing an "ethical" storytelling space for these people might be a way to improve accessibility needs, equality, and inclusion. Sarah Pini and Lillian Wilde's draws from one of the authors' lived experiences of cancer, and they discuss how sharing the experience of trauma and recovery contributes to a re-constitution of a sense of belonging in the world. The chapter by Astrid Joutseno suggests that a critical narrative medicine should develop approaches to the grief of the dying as an everyday trauma. It is written by an author with experience of living with metastatic cancer.

In the second part, "Narrative methods and ethics in trauma care," we begin with the "health care-centered" perspective on the applied methods. A chapter by John Launer deriving from the field of narrative-based practice presents a training method called "Conversations Inviting Change," which is multi-professional supervision groups attended by experienced practitioners sharing narratives of encounters in their work that may have been traumatic. The focus is on the medical and ethical dilemmas. On the opposite end of the scale, the following chapter by Colleen McMillan and Aaron Smith explores the impact of "small trauma" occurrences; how collecting stories of trauma over a health care professional's career impacts the sense of self and capabilities. Elizabeth Lanphier's chapter focuses on reading and writing in the narrative medicine workshop and argues that such practices can—and should—be complemented and deepened by Trauma Informed Practice. Finally, Mark Celinscak's chapter takes a historical view and explores the narratives of the Allied medical personnel who worked at the Bergen-Belsen concentration camp at the end of the Second World War.

In the following section with a "patient-centered perspective" on the methods, we find a chapter by Oddgeir Synnes and Hilde Bondevik where creative and expressive writing are used in an intervention with cancer patients at Oslo University Hospital. It is argued that writing can open towards repair, finding a voice, and re-connecting to the world and others. Jacob Y. Stein and Rivka Tuval-Mashiach have a chapter on how narrative methods guided by hermeneutics and phenomenology may present suitable solutions to diminish the loneliness that may consolidate after trauma. This part of the book is closed by a chapter by Emma McKenzie reflecting on how creative writing and storytelling can be used to highlight the need for humanity as a central focal point of the delivery of mental health care.

In the third part, "Studies of aesthetic trauma narratives," here with a "therapeutic objective," we open with Ssanyu Birigwa and Molly Lindberg's chapter which examines sexual assault in a TV-series centering on the challenges of how to tell one's trauma story. They argue that healing for the individual and community relies on a survivor's choice to tell their story. Ricardo Rato Rodrigues' chapter examines a series of cases narrated by an American psychiatrist in a British novel, and it argues on a general level for the therapeutic role of literary narratives. The cultural, political, and medical aspects of cancer are explored by T.S. Kavitha and Mahesh Sharma in the reading of an illness memoir. They apply the model of Levinasian ethics injected as a rhetoric of care and responsibility in the medical practitioner when listening and responding to the patient. Cancer is considered an incomprehensible event in life, and narrative medicine might be a holistic form of healing. Finally, an illustrated chapter by Preeti Puri and Shefali investigates how verbo-visual modes of storytelling support a novel about a pregnant mother's psychological trauma. The argument is that a close reading of the narrative can help trauma patients in psychiatric treatment to overcome their isolation.

In the second section of aesthetic studies, here with an "analytical objective," a chapter by Mona Baie looks at a recent American illness memoir where a rare neurological disease is experienced as traumatic. Brooke Covington examines the effects of storytelling and counterstorytelling as a praxis for negotiating meaning and identity of Black women with physical dismemberment caused by trauma. Similarly, the chapter by Victoria Simpson is rooted in critical race theory and presents an interdisciplinary methodology that draws attention to the dominant narratives that circulate about health and trauma while also bringing attention to the stories that run "counter" to those dominant interpretations. A chapter by Margaux Danby discusses through the lens of narrative ethics a tv-series for its ability to function in society as both witness and metabolization of racially charged traumas. Nora Simonhjell explores the role of next of kin in Norwegian literature, and how a parent's chronic illness can create traumatic experiences in their children's life. In the end, Hannah Ming Yit Ho analyzes the curative impulse of storytelling in a novel, which offers ways to make sense of alternative medicine practices in the community-oriented Malay Muslim nation Brunei.

Wrapped around all those tightly edited chapters, the editors have asked Rishi Goyal to open the whole book with a foreword and Arthur W. Frank to close the book again with an afterword. Goyal is educated in narrative medicine by Charon from Columbia University, he is now the director of a Medical Humanities program at the Institute of Comparative Literature and Society, and he serves as a physician in the Emergency clinic of New York-Presbyterian hospital. In his foreword, he reflects on trauma as a heuristic that highlights embodied cognition and permits us to perceive the entanglements of psyche and soma. Frank is former professor of Sociology at Calgary University and author of widely known books on narrative ethics. He is meditating on how severe illness can be a traumatic event, how people come to terms with it in the present healthcare system, and what counts as *medicine* in the term narrative medicine. With a clinical-based foreword and a culturally grounded afterword spinning around narrative medicine, trauma, and ethics, we hope to present a coherent and cross-disciplinary volume.

Reference List

American Psychiatric Association (1987) *Diagnostic and statistical manual of mental disorders*, 3rd edn., revised (DSM-III-R), Washington DC: American Psychiatric Press.

Andermahr, S. and Pellicer-Ortin, S. (eds.) (2013) *Trauma narratives and Herstory*. London: Palgrave Macmillan.

Armstrong, C.L. and Langaas, U. (eds.) (2020) *Terrorizing images: trauma and ekphrasis in contemporary literature*. Berlin/Boston: De Gruyter.

Berger, A.L. and Milbauer, A.Z. (2013) 'The burden of inheritance,' *Shofar: An Interdisciplinary Journal of Jewish Studies*, 31(3), pp. 64-85. doi: https://doi.org/10.1353/sho.2013.0050

Bond, L. and Craps, S. (2019) *Trauma*. Abingdon: Routledge.

Buelens, G., Durrant, S. and Eaglestone, R. (eds.) (2014) *The future of trauma theory: contemporary literary and cultural criticism*. London: Routledge.

Caruth, C. (ed.) (1995) *Trauma: explorations in memory*. Baltimore: John Hopkins University Press.

Caruth, C. (1996) *Unclaimed experience: trauma, narrative, and history*. Baltimore: John Hopkins University Press.

Caruth, C. (2013) *Literature in the ashes of history*. Baltimore: Johns Hopkins University Press.

Charon, R. (2001) 'Narrative medicine: a model for empathy, reflection, profession, and trust,' *JAMA: Journal of the American Medical Association*, 286(15), pp. 1897-1902. doi: http://dx.doi.org/10.1001/jama.286.15.1897

Charon, R. and Montello, M. (eds.) (2002) *Narratives matter. The role of narrative in medical ethics*. New York, London: Routledge.

Charon, R. (2005) 'Narrative medicine: attention, representation, affiliation,' *Narrative*, 13(3), pp. 261-270. doi: https://doi.org/10.1353/nar.2005.0017

Charon, R. (2006) *Narrative medicine: honoring the stories of illness*. New York: Oxford University Press.

Charon, R. et al. (2016) *The principles and practice of narrative medicine*. New York: Oxford University Press. doi: https://doi.org/10.1093/med/9780199360192.001.0001

Craps, S. (2013) *Postcolonial witnessing: trauma out of bounds*. Basingstoke: Palgrave Macmillan.

Davis, C. and Meretoja, H. (eds.) (2020) *The Routledge Companion to literature and trauma*. London: Routledge.

Fassin, D. and Rechtman, R. (2009) *The empire of trauma: an inquiry into the condition of victimhood*. Translated from the French by Rachel Gomme. Princeton and Oxford: Princeton University Press.

Felman, S. and Laub, D. (1992) *Testimony: crises of witnessing in literature, psychoanalysis and history*. New York and London: Routledge.

Frank, A.W. (1995) *The wounded storyteller: body, illness, and ethic.* Chicago: University of Chicago Press.

Frank, A.W. (2022) *King Lear: Shakespeare's dark consolations.* Oxford: Oxford University Press.

Freud, S. (1953) 'Beyond the Pleasure Principle,' in Strachey, J. (ed.) *The standard edition of the complete psychological works of Sigmund Freud (1920-1922).* Translated from the German under the general editorship of James Strachey in collaboration with Anna Freud, London: The Hogarth Press.

Greenhalgh, T. and Hurwitz, B. (eds.) (1998) *Narrative-based medicine: dialogue and discourse in clinical practice.* London: BMJ Books.

Kalitzkus, V. and Matthiesen, P.F. (2009) 'Narrative-based medicine: potential, pitfalls, and practice,' *The Permanente Journal* 13(1), pp. 80-86. doi: http://doi.org/10.7812/TPP/09.996

Kaplan, A.E. (2005) *Trauma culture: the politics of terror and loss in media and literature.* New Brunswick: Rutgers University Press.

Kellermann, N.P.F. (2013) 'Epigenetic transmission of holocaust trauma: can nightmares be inherited,' *The Israel Journal of Psychiatry and Related Sciences,* 50(1), pp. 33-39. PMID: 24029109.

Kleinman, A. (1988) *The illness narratives: suffering, healing, and the human condition.* New York: Basic Books.

Kurtz, J. R. (ed.) (2018) *Trauma and literature.* Cambridge: Cambridge University Press.

LaCapra, D. (2001) *Writing history, writing trauma.* Baltimore: Johns Hopkins University Press.

Lazzari, L. and Ségeral, N. (eds.) (2021) *Trauma and motherhood in contemporary literature and culture.* London: Palgrave Macmillan.

Luckhurst, R. (2008) *The trauma question.* New York and London: Routledge.

Nadal, M. and Calvo, M. (eds.) (2014) *Trauma in contemporary literature. Narrative and representation.* New York and London: Routledge.

O'Mahony, S. (2013) 'Against narrative medicine,' *Perspectives in Biology and Medicine,* 56(4), pp. 611-619. PMID: 24769751. doi: https://doi.org/10.1353/pbm.2013.0032

Phelan, J. (2023) *Narrative medicine: a rhetorical rx.* New York: Routledge.

Rasmussen, A.J., Mai, A.-M. and Hansen, H.P. (eds.) (2022) *Narrative medicine in education, practice, and interventions.* London: Anthem Press.

Salam, W.J. and Mahfouz, S.M. (2020) 'Claims of memory: transgenerational traumas, fluid identities, and resistance in Hala Alyan's Salt Houses,' *Journal of Postcolonial Writing,* 56(3), pp. 296-309. doi: https://doi.org/10.1080/17449855.2020.1755718

Sherin, J.E. and Nemeroff, C.B. (2011) 'Post-traumatic stress disorder: the neurobiological impact of psychological trauma,' *Dialogues in Clinical Neuroscience,* 13(3), pp. 263-78. PMID: 22034143; PMCID: PMC3182008. doi: https://doi.org/10.31887/dcns.2011.13.2/jsherin

Sodemann, M. (2022) *What you don't know will hurt the patient.* Odense: Own Publisher. Available at: www.ouh.dk/textbook (Accessed: 8 March 2023).

van der Kolk, B.A. (2015) *The body keeps the score: brain, mind, and body in the healing of trauma.* London: Penguin Books, Limited.

Wear, D. and Aultman, J.M. (2005) 'The limits of narrative: medical student resistance to confronting inequality and oppression in literature and beyond,' *Medical Education*, 39(10), pp. 1056-1065. doi: http://dx.doi.org/10.1111/j.1365-2929.2005.02270.x

West, J.D. (ed.) (2021) *Using image and narrative in therapy for trauma, addiction and recovery.* London: Jessica Kingsley Publishers, Ltd.

Whitehead, A. (2004) *Trauma fiction.* Edinburgh: Edinburgh University Press.

Woods, A. (2011) 'The limits of narrative: provocations for the medical humanities,' *Medical Humanities* 37(2), pp. 73-78. doi: http://dx.doi.org/10.1136/medhum-2011-010045

Part 1: Autoethnographic Research

1.1.1

Creating Ethical Storytelling Spaces, in Research and Beyond, for People Living with Disability and Trauma

Annmaree Watharow

University of Sydney, Australia

Sue Joseph

Central Queensland University, Australia

Georgia Fagan

University of Sydney, Australia

Abstract

People living with disability (PLWD) can experience trauma any day, even every day, through oppressive events, discriminatory treatment and ableist attitudes. PLWD are disproportionately disadvantaged through the social determinants of wellbeing and workplace adaptations during and post disasters, as evidenced through the COVID pandemic and natural disasters. PLWD are more likely than others to experience instances of violence, and those living with communication disabilities may not be able to tell their stories in conventional ways. Subsequently, their experiences are not heard, counted, valued, or made visible.

This chapter explores how this deficit can be rectified through a discussion of three distinct yet interrelated elements. We first explicate the necessary features of an "ethical" storytelling space; then we engage with how these features can be practically employed as a means to establish safe and effective story relaying and receiving spaces. We conclude with a roadmap to guide seekers of stories to create ethical and safe narrative spaces, using the lived experience and research of Author 1. Unmet accessibility needs equal unvoiced stories and exclusion. Open dialog, inclusive practices and accessibility provision are therefore key to narrative engagement for PLWD.

***

People living with disability (PLWD) comprise just under 20% of the population, are found everywhere, in known and general populations, and may be visible or invisible (Australian Bureau of Statistics, 2018). The world of disability is vastly heterogeneous and comprises people with diverse residual functions, specific physical access needs, hundreds of different communication methods, a multitude of environmental adaptations as well as differences in social functioning; sometimes, often even, multiple disability considerations are necessary.

They want to participate in qualitative research and tell their stories. PLWD, however, are often disproportionately disadvantaged compared to those without disability when it comes to sharing experiences of disability, trauma and living realities. Research is often rife with sins of omission due to the often unacknowledged ableist presuppositions and methodologies that underlie disability and its discourse in academia. Qualitative research is traditionally built on storied data and can be ableist in both visible and invisible ways (Watharow and Wayland, 2022).

Despite many PLWD wanting to participate in the research process, particularly when the research pertains to them, PLWD frequently face systematic disadvantages in sharing their experiences—in many instances, these barriers are sufficient to silence their voices outright. All too often, this silencing of PLWD leaves the narrative and academic discourse *de facto* regarding their disability, voiced by those without disability. As one of the early social modelists writes:

> [It is] society which disables physically impaired people. Disability is something imposed on top of our impairments by the way we are unnecessarily isolated and excluded from full participation in society. Disabled people are therefore an oppressed group in society. (Oliver, 1996, p. 22)

We see disability as layered and contingent. Individuals will have many diverse impairments, impairment effects, experiences, characteristics, intersections and socially determined influences. This chapter takes therefore, a social relational understanding of disability (Shakespeare 2013, Shakespeare and Watson 2001, Thomas 2004, Reindal 2008). This means disability is both the lived experience (body and psycho-emotional) and the barriers in society that disadvantage, harm and exclude. Furthermore, the moral responsibility is on society to support PLWD, remove barriers and promote participation.

Just as in wider society, many research practices and paradigms exclude PLWD, the roll-on effect is that story and data invisibility then mean that society, services, supports, and policies are not fully inclusive of all, and never have been. We need to hear more stories (and stories of stories by researchers) so that society is more understanding and inclusive of diverse ways of being, doing and telling. As Damian Mellifont and colleagues urge: "Universities need to end the idea that the able-bodied or neurotypical ways are the more 'rigorous' ways and the conception that methods cannot be adjusted and still yield valuable, rich data" (2023, forthcoming). We believe this applies to all research, whether conducted from within the university space, or external to it.

We explore here the concept of epistemic injustice, the theoretical ethics of safe storytelling in narrative inquiry spaces, and the practicalities of co-creating ethically safe narrative spaces for PLWD. Giving voice to all in the room is not a conceptually difficult task but it can be complex in its execution. We offer a roadmap for readers and researchers to learn, adjust and innovate so that storytelling is part of emancipatory research and that all voices are included.

Epistemic Injustice

In order to construct bodies of knowledge that serve communities, such as health institutions, disaster preparedness schemes, and social support systems, we should require that the processes of their construction are informed by, and co-produced by, those they work to serve. Given this, the capacity to absorb and subsequently learn from, and alongside, the testimonies of individuals within our communities determines the extent to which these community-serving systems are indeed capable of *successfully* serving those who comprise them. As Miranda Fricker suggests, an epistemic injustice occurs when agents are wronged in their capacities as knowers (2007). PLWD are the expert-knowers of their own conditions and experiences, even if these are not sought, counted, or valued. When the testimonies of particular individuals are unheard, or altogether not sought, an epistemic injustice is made against both those individuals and any who stand to be benefactors of those individuals' testimonies.

PLWD are disproportionately disadvantaged in social systems of health and wellbeing, and in community participation more broadly. This disadvantage equips PLWD, and other marginalized persons, with unique epistemic insights into the nature of their own exclusion. Given this, any project which aims to mitigate instances of disadvantage and discrimination needs to avoid committing epistemic injustices against these populations. Failing to do so constitutes both an act of injustice against knowers with epistemic insight but just as crucially, directly weakens the capacity for any such project to realize its stated goals.

Fricker's establishment and subsequent exploration of the notion of epistemic injustice helpfully contributes to the possibility of undertaking more comprehensive discourses on matters of injustice, exclusion, and silencing, and is employed in this chapter (2007). We believe those who solicit stories must collaborate with PLWD as they are the expert-knowers in the construction of knowledge of stories about their own lives, conditions, and experiences. "No research about us, without us" to rephrase the activist mantra. "No storytelling about us, without us." This means creating ethical storytelling spaces, valuing lived experience researchers and challenging old assumptions and ableist methodologies.

What Constitutes Ethical Storytelling Spaces?

Storytelling spaces can in part be understood as spaces in which those with epistemic insight of their particular experiences of social exclusion or trauma, for example, can share their understandings and engage in dialog with individuals or groups who are interested in utilizing these insights in myriad ways. Socially just research operatives ordain that such uses must benefit the community they arise from. Principles of ethical and emancipatory research seek to restore parity of power to the qualitative narrative inquiry space by prioritizing the voices of marginalized groups, skill development and ownership of the knowledge produced (Biggeri and Ciani, 2019). Mellifont and colleagues note that it is not enough to have PLWD as participants in order to be inclusive; the project must have "a design which prioritizes the voice of people with disability through all phases of the research and focuses on eliminating disabling barriers in society" (2023, forthcoming).

The inclusion of PLWD in knowledge production about disability and other domains necessitates providing a climate of safety in which these stories are told and heard, disseminated, and acted upon. Giving voice to stories in a safe, ethical storytelling space allows the hearing of individual experiences, and the garnering of collective commonalities for social, and political change (Stone and Priestley, 1996). The establishment of storytelling spaces that permit the successful transmission of testimonies is subsequently methodologically central to the avoidance of incurring epistemic injustices by individuals and groups that aim to utilize participant testimony.

As we understand it, storytelling spaces predominately aim to construct a place in which knowers are not harmed, constrained, or silenced in their capacity as knowers. In its positive articulation, this requires that knowers' testimonies are made legible, and communicable beyond the spaces in which they are uttered. In other words, ethical storytelling spaces are ones where the risk of epistemic injustice is comprehensively assessed and mitigated; that individual accessibility made through adjustments and accommodations is both inextricable and imperative to the ethical status of that space.

The diverse needs of PLWD exceeds the borders of what a person without disability would consider the domain of research and budgets. For instance, environments require consideration and modifications to allow storytellers with physical and/or sensory disabilities. While the post-pandemic pre-eminence of the "virtual space" revolutionized storytelling spaces and access for many PLWD, these now ubiquitous virtual spaces are not necessarily accessible to all; this is especially the case for some PLWD or those who are culturally and linguistically diverse (CALD).

If no heed is paid to the diverse (and sometimes complex) needs of PLWD then the research undertaken fails to elicit testimonies and thus harms occur by this negligence. An example is participant choice and control over interpreter provision for Deaf, Deafblind and/or CALD participants. If this is missing, epistemic injustice occurs. As Annmaree Watharow and Sarah Wayland write: "The use of known, trusted interpreters enhance inclusion, because interpreters have knowledge of idiosyncrasies, personal styles, preferences, and meanings, while also providing a safeguard against inappropriate touch and communication failure" (2022, p. 6).

Neglect, Silence and Erasure

The neglect of the testimonies of marginalized voices is an engrained tenet in much contemporary research and public policy (Mellifont et al., 2023, forthcoming). So-called "vulnerable" populations are "too hard" to include in qualitative or narrative inquiry study populations because most qualitative methodologies are inherently ableist. For example, the use of an online survey excludes those without devices, internet access, skills, lingua franca proficiency, or CALD people. Alternatively, the requirement to travel to a focus group may exclude others such as those living with neurodiversity, psychosocial, or physical disability.

This exclusionary tradition is posited as emerging from two distinct, yet interrelated causes. The first is that silenced voices, those which suffer epistemic injustices, run counter to dominant narratives which work to assert that current schemes, such as public welfare systems, are functionally competent regarding their recognition of diverse needs and commitment to equality more broadly. Due to the ongoing disenfranchisement experienced in their interactions with such systems, PLWD possess insights that have the capacity to challenge the integrity of such narratives. Their testimonies, if ever comprehensively absorbed, can effectively destabilize assertions of egalitarianism made by systems of social care.

When storytelling spaces are not made safe and ethical, or if they are produced without the expert-knowers themselves, they perpetuate old epistemic injustices, as well as create new ones. In the absence of safe storytelling or "yarning" space for First Nations stories of disability, post-colonial legacies of silence and erasure persist (Avery, 2018). Through yarning with lived experience First Nations researchers, however, Avery captures experiences of disability, trauma and double disadvantage that dispels notions of equality and equity in contemporary Australia.

PLWD are constrained by more than their impairments, often with other intersectional influences (Moodley and Graham, 2015) such as ageism, racism, and gender discrimination. For many PLWD, intersectional influences (race, indigeneity, socioeconomic status, gender, gender identity, sexual orientation, age, disability, spirituality, immigration, refugee status, language and education), shape not only their life course but also their access to research and storytelling that is cognizant of these contingencies and willing to adapt the storytelling spaces.

The second, perhaps less contemptuous causes of ongoing epistemic disenfranchisements of contemporary research processes, and their subsequent outputs, are the intellectual descendants of historic exclusionary norms. These propagate exclusionary epistemic injustice through inherited a priori beliefs about the roles of the researcher and the researched. Safety and trust in the research process and its spaces are critical to truthful knowledge building. Potential participants who foresee a minimal chance of benefitting from research or who feel explicitly unsafe may choose to self-exclude. Comparatively, to their research subjects, researchers emerge as disproportionately powerful figures who disregard the needs of those who should be prioritized (Scheman, 2011). Researcher power imbalances are amplified when accessibility, accommodations and adjustments are not provided or withheld.

Subsequently, systems of research and research-based policy are formed and ongoingly reinforced as sites of epistemic injustice, where the insights of those who are excluded are inadequately heard or made legible. Narrative inquiry, therefore, necessitates an approach that seeks to provide safe and accessible storytelling spaces, implemented by trustworthy researchers on topics important to PLWD and their communities. This collaboratively located knowledge is then disseminated and translated into a tangible benefit for the community.

Further confounding these two notions is the parlous position in traditional academia of lived experience researchers (Mellifont et al., 2019; Mellifont et al., 2023, forthcoming). Lived-experience researchers bring their own expert knowledge to the research table, coming closer to the insider position of the expert-knower participants, thus reducing the likelihood of instances of epistemic injustices. However, they do so in the face of traditionalist academics who cite the loss of academic rigor by the methodological adjustments, accommodations, and accessibility provisions as undermining the validity of lived researchers' insights. We contend that, far from a loss of rigor, the imbuement of lived experience researchers into research spaces enables the narrative space to be closer to the experiential reality of the participant group. This reduces the risk of epistemic injustices, and while admittedly does involve methodological challenges, they are far from insurmountable and pale in comparison to the value of insight that the researchers can offer.

Road Map to Safe, Ethical Storytelling Spaces

We argue for an ethical roadmap that moves toward creating safe narrative spaces for PLWD as storytellers, participants, researchers, leaders and expert-knowers. Adjusting qualitative methodologies to accommodate all voices in storytelling spaces is not a loss of rigor, but a reflection of experiential reality, that is the work comes closer to the truth of living with disability. In so doing the wider community reaps the benefit of more stories and a greater understanding of the complexities of living with disability. Building the canon and decreasing data invisibility of the marginalized, allows for better resource allocation by social institutions. This creates a more epistemically just society.

We must begin from the operational platform of zero tolerance for epistemic injustice, ableism, and discrimination and outline here in Table 1.1, the key markers in a roadmap to creating safe narrative spaces. The principal considerations are:

- Acceptance of expert-knower status of PLWD.
- Active compliance with the protections, policies, and practices that underpin social justice and equity.
- Co-production, immersion, lived experience researchers, accessibility, methodological adjustments, allowances for the necessity of more time, budgeting for the inevitably increased costs, and equity in the ethics processes.
- Giving storytellers choices and control over the space/s, locations, timings and storytelling aides; embracement and openness to different ways of being, doing, and telling.

These are unpacked further and explicated individually in the following Table 1.1.

Table 1.1. Roadmap to safe, ethical storytelling spaces.

RESPECT EXPERT-KNOWERS	• The single most important principle underpinning roadmap is acceptance of PLWD as expert-knowers of their lives, impairments and needs. • PLWD are knowers of systems and institutions that fail to support, accommodate, and value them. • They are custodians of salutogenic knowledge of solutions—if asked in ways accessible to them.
COMPLY WITH PROTECTIONS	• Compliance with protections, policies and practices promoting inclusion, e.g., United Nations Convention on the Rights of Persons with Disabilities (UN CDRP) (2006, ratified by Australia 2008), Federal and state anti-discrimination legislation.
EMBRACE CO-PRODUCTION	• Recruit and remunerate PLWD as qualitative research team members, key informants, research assistants, researchers and leaders, as well as participants.
IMMERSION IN THE WORLDS OF PARTICIPANTS	• Crucial to ensure research and methods proposed are of benefit not harm, to the community. • Enables identification of prevailing barriers to participation; voicing of experiences and knowledge. • Allows consideration of intersectional influences. • Illuminates cultural norms and practices of particular groups and individuals.
VALUE LIVED EXPERIENCE RESEARCHERS	• Being "just like us" is a respected position and engenders trust in participants. • Create pathways and flexible workplaces with accommodations and adjustments, for PLWD to lead research, participate in research and find forums for telling their stories. • Ensure important cultural and accessibility requirements are planned for and built into the qualitative research space from its inception; not as an expensive, time-consuming add-on down the track.
SAFER, INCLUSIVE ETHICS PROCESSES	• Ethics applications to include completion of education modules on disability and accessibility for all applicants. • Accessibility and safety plans for all in the storytelling space to form part of the ethics application. • Participant information and consent forms provided in (or be readily made when needed) multiple formats. • Applications to contain explanation on how true informed consent is to be obtained and methods to obtain it.
ACCESSIBILITY	• Consideration of accessibility needs included at the beginning of research and continued throughout until the end of project. • Ask each participant and lived experience team member what is needed for inclusion. • Normalize as part of every space, every action, every document, every course, every project and every grant and ethics application. • Not prescriptive but rather adaptive and responsive to each individual and community.

ASK INDIVIDUALS	• Learn to ask each individual and group how they want to be identified (person-first, identity-first or other); • What their communication and access to information needs are; • What their physical access requirements for mobility and orientation are; • Any cultural practices and norms to understand; • Any other requirements for safety and trust in telling their stories and living their lives.
METHODOLOGY: ADJUSTMENTS & CHALLENGES	• Multiple methods may be needed and at different times in the same research when working with PLWD. • Adjustments of existing methods may be required to accommodate both participants and lived experience researchers. • Types of adjustments and accommodations for methodologies are wide and vast. • Dissemination of researcher experiences (the telling of the story of the story) is crucial to understanding more about methodological challenges, how they are met and what works; and what does not.
TIME	• Take time to dismantle barriers to accessibility, to prepare the research and storytelling spaces, to develop and produce accessible formats specific to the population, and to set up safe spaces. • Takes longer when kinetic communication methods are used i.e., sign or tactile language interpreters as rest breaks are needed for both storytellers and their interpreters. • Takes longer to source extra funding for provisioning safe, ethical narrative spaces.
BUDGETS	• Need to reflect cultural immersion and engagement of lived experience researchers, and key informants, accessibly provisioning, planning and setting safety plans and support, as well as extra time needs.
PARTICIPANT CHOICES & CONTROL	• Prior immersion enables researchers to plan for all that is required. • Participants to have choice and control of communication methods, environmental adjustments, and storytelling aids
COMMUNICATION	• Ability to select communication method that suits (note may need multiple methods and or different methods for different stages of the storytelling). • The interpreter of choice for those who need interpreters. • Ask participant storytellers to provide a list of their own preferred interpreters. • Project to engage and pay for interpreters and chosen communication formats.
PLACE	• Participant-storytellers free to choose location suited to them; what is most accessible and safe for them. • May be virtual, a national telephone relay service, paper-based questionnaires, or face-to-face.
ENVIRONMENT: ADJUSTMENTS	• When interviews take place in person, environment may need alteration to maximize accessibility, communication, and comfort.

	• May need a larger room as more people, devices and/or service animals in these physical narrative spaces. • Adjustments to space as needed, for example: seating, lighting, positioning of tables, positioning of a tactile table, water bottles, and space for a service animal.
STORYTELLING AIDS	• Aids to storytelling and story receiving may be needed. • Technical glitches can affect any storytelling session: aids often fail, run out of battery life, or simply not function as intended, for example, communication boards, hearing aids, cochlear implants, accessibility software, braille teletypers, or speech-to-text devices. • Approach with humor and quickly investigate alternative communication methods.
POSITIVE FRAMINGS	• Research must be beneficial and solutions-oriented. • Use lived experience team members to ensure salutogenic focus. • Ask the expert-knowers themselves how to make things better.
BEING OPEN TO DIFFERENT WAYS OF BEING DOING AND TELLING	• These ways may run counter to old-style qualitative methods. • Examples include: "yarning" by First Nations People in Australia, touch-centricity of many with Deafblindness; visual storytelling of sign language users; reduced English idioms and metaphors of PLWD marginalized from education; tense instability when recounting traumatic events/experiences; chaotic, fragmented or splintered narrative styles of those with post-traumatic stress disorder; dissonance where words have a different meaning e.g. the use of the word "good" to mean to the researcher that an experience is positive but actually to the storyteller signifies survival of the events.

The road map is not proscriptive, but rather a platform from which to begin considering how to collaborate and co-create safe and ethical narrative spaces for researchers and storytelling participants. Asking (and then providing) what everyone needs for inclusion and safety in qualitative inquiry, remains the epitome of ethical practice.

Conclusion

We have an ethical and legal obligation to engage with storytellers who live with disability in safe and inclusive ways. To fail to do so enables the flourishing of epistemic injustices, as Fricker contends (2007). People living with disability can experience trauma often in conjunction with a disabling experience, and also as part of the events of living a human life. But if we don't provide safe ethical storytelling spaces, we further traumatize by adding epistemic injustices.

A failure to honor diverse knowledge constitutes a failure to construct bodies of knowledge that are *indeed* knowledgeable. The goal then of our roadmap, is to bridge this gulf in such a way that knowledge is no longer lost nor discarded. An ethical storytelling space is one that does not commit epistemic injustices to its participants; one which constructs itself in ways that, to the best of its ability, mitigates the risk of silencing knowledge, and losing it in the gulf.

We cannot offer readers a list of comprehensive accessibility considerations to tick, such is the enormity of the heterogeneity of needs in the population. What works for some, may be a disabler for others, e.g., environmental lighting adjustments of bright light for some with night blindness may be a barrier to others with light sensitivity who need dimmed lighting. Formats, aids and physical room requirements vary vastly. Some PLWD take up no extra room as they prefer virtual spaces.

These accessibility, budget, safety, methodological and time considerations should be a normal part of all storytelling projects. Not only is disability common but it comes to all of us one way or another, at one time or another. We need to elicit stories about how our institutions really function so that we can move towards a more equitable, just society inclusive of all. If we are to build up the canon of literature on living with, understanding and explaining disability, if we are to avoid epistemic injustices and to hear everyone, not just some stories, we must collectively take these steps. We cannot, as researchers and writers, claim to offer insights and understandings into phenomena if we have not sought all the voices we can. In the post-COVID era, when so much of our research and storytelling has moved online, we know that not all are seen here, not all are heard in these virtual ways and so epistemic injustices continue. Some final words of warning, however, that to position ourselves as righting epistemic wrongs and liberating silenced voices is a power play. We are not liberators and our storytelling participants, and selves, are not "the liberated." Rather, we are all collaborators in knowledge creation and discovery.

Reference List

Avery, S. (2018) *Culture is inclusion: a narrative of aboriginal and Torres Strait Islander people with disability*. Sydney: First Peoples Disability Network Australia.

Australian Bureau of Statistics (2018) *Disability, ageing and carers, Australia: summary of findings*. ABS. Available at: https://www.abs.gov.au/statistics/health/disability/disability-ageing-and-carers-australia-summary-findings/latest-release (Accessed: 30 November 2023).

Biggeri, M. and Ciani, F. (2019) 'Emancipatory research as empowerment: an illustration from a research study of persons with disabilities in Palestine,' in Clark, D.A., Biggeri, M. and Frediani A.A. (eds.), *The Capability Approach, Empowerment and Participation*. Rethinking International Development series. London: Palgrave Macmillan, pp. 339-359. doi: https://doi.org/10.1057/978-1-137-35230-9_13

Fricker, M. (2007) *Epistemic injustice: power and the ethics of knowing*. Oxford: Oxford University Press. doi: https://doi.org/10.1093/acprof:oso/9780198237907.001.0001

United Nations (UN) (2006) *Convention on the rights of persons with disabilities (CRPD)*. Available at: https://www.un.org/development/desa/disabilities/convention-on-the-rights-of-persons-with-disabilities.html (Accessed: December 29, 2022).

Mellifont, D. et al. (forthcoming, 2023) 'Participation of people with disabilities in research – problematizing vulnerability,' in Watharow, A. (ed.) *Advances in Disability Research Ethics*. Sydney: Emerald Press.

Mellifont, D. et al. (2019) 'The ableism elephant in the academy: a study examining academia as informed by Australian scholars with lived experience,' *Disability & Society*, 34(7-8), pp. 1180-1199. doi: https://doi.org/10.1080/09687599.2019.1602510

Moodley, J. and Graham, L. (2015) 'The importance of intersectionality in disability and Gender Studies,' *Agenda*, 29(2), pp. 24-33. doi: https://doi.org/10.1080/10130950.2015.1041802

Oliver, M. (1996) *Understanding disability: from theory to practice*. Basingstoke: Palgrave Macmillan. doi: https://psycnet.apa.org/doi/10.1007/978-1-349-24269-6

Reindal, S.M. (2008) 'A social relational model of disability: a theoretical framework for special needs education?,' *European Journal of Special Needs Education*, 23(2), pp. 135-146. doi: https://doi.org/10.1080/08856250801947812

Shakespeare, T. (2013) *Disability rights and wrongs revisited*. 2nd edn. London: Routledge, Taylor & Francis Group. doi: https://doi.org/10.4324/9781315887456

Shakespeare, T. and Watson, N. (2001) 'The social model of disability: an outdated ideology?,' in Barnartt, S.N. and Altman, B.M. (eds.) *Exploring Theories and Expanding Methodologies: Where we are and where we need to go (Research in Social Science and Disability, Vol. 2)*. Bingley: Emerald Group Publishing Limited, pp. 9-28. doi: https://doi.org/10.1016/s1479-3547(01)80018-x

Scheman, N. (2011) *Shifting ground: knowledge and reality, transgression and trustworthiness. Studies in Feminist Philosophy*. New York: Oxford University Press.

Stone, E. and Priestley, M. (1996) 'Parasites, pawns and partners: disability research and the role of non-disabled researchers,' *The British Journal of Sociology*, 47(4), p. 699-716. doi: https://doi.org/10.2307/591081

Thomas, C. (2004) 'Rescuing a social relational understanding of disability,' *Scandinavian Journal of Disability Research*, 6(1), pp. 22-36. doi: https://doi.org/10.1080/15017410409512637

Watharow, A. and Wayland, S. (2022) 'Making qualitative research inclusive: Methodological insights in disability research,' *International Journal of Qualitative Methods*, 21. doi: https://doi.org/10.1177/16094069221095316

1.1.2
An Embodied Narrative Perspective on Transforming Trauma and Illness Experience

Sarah Pini

University of Southern Denmark, Denmark

Lillian Wilde

IU International University of Applied Sciences, England

Abstract

Trauma is notoriously difficult to communicate, as it often defies understanding. It unfolds over time and cannot be told through linear narratives. Nevertheless, we show that narratives can become a medium through which experiences of trauma may be shared, alleviating the sense of alienation common to post-traumatic experience.

Drawing from one of the authors' lived experiences of cancer and her illness narrative, we focus on the question of whether traumatic events can be narrated, known, and shared. In conversation with one another, and building on phenomenological literature on trauma (Husserl, 1973; Walther, 1923), illness (Carel, 2021, 2016), and working with an autoethnographic approach to cancer (Pini, 2022; Pini and Maguire-Rosier, 2021; Pini and Pini, 2019), we address the ways in which creative and expressive illness narratives—particularly the sharing of such experiences—can help patients heal or repair from trauma.

We identify the moment of the cancer diagnosis as a traumatic event, as it constitutes the expulsion of the individual into an *alienworld:* the world of the sick. We demonstrate how a philosophical account of unification (Walther, 1923) may help shed light on the complexities of traumatic experience and highlight the potential of embodied narratives to re-establish a sense of belonging through sharing trauma experiences. We present a case in which performance art serves not only as an act of creatively re-modelling the performer's illness narrative, but as a means to communicate this experience.

Sharing the experience of trauma and recovery contributes to a re-constitution of a sense of belonging.

We highlight that the (re-)constitution of feelings of belonging is a dyadic process between the traumatized individual and others. An illness narrative needs to be heard, seen, or otherwise witnessed in order to fulfill its full healing potential. In this way, we hope to contribute to a better understanding of how a narrative approach can be fruitfully applied in clinical practice.

***

Trauma is difficult to describe. There does not seem to be one definition that captures the multifaceted nature of the experiences usually traded under this term. Potentially traumatizing experiences are said to present the individual with "actual or threatened death, serious injury, or sexual violence" (American Psychiatric Association, DSM-5 Task Force, 2013, p. 271). Not only do these kinds of events range from natural catastrophes over interpersonal or sexual violence to terror and war—they are experienced *as* traumatic only by some of the people who are exposed to them. Post-Traumatic Stress Disorder (PTSD) is the most dominant framework used to classify the pathological experience in the aftermath of a traumatizing event (ibid., 2013). However, PTSD and other psychopathologies (such as anxiety, depression, and eating disorders) are not the only forms of experience common in the aftermath of trauma. Other possible reactions are more or less subtle, long-term alterations of lived experience, such as the feeling of alienation and not being understood, that color the individual's overall experience of being in the world. It is the latter in which we are particularly interested.

We thereby distance ourselves from the DSM's classifications. This is not meant as a critique of the framework; "PTSD" accurately describes the experience of many trauma survivors; it is just not the only way in which trauma may impact human experience. Moreover, according to the DSM-5, "non-immediate, non-catastrophic life-threatening illness, such as terminal cancer, no longer qualifies as trauma, regardless of how stressful or severe it is" (Pai, Suris and North, 2017). However, we are aware that these experiences can bring with them significant alterations of the most fundamental structures of experience.

We identify the moment of the cancer diagnosis as a traumatic event. Like other experiences that pose a severe threat to the life and bodily integrity of a person, it constitutes the expulsion of the individual into an alienworld: the world of the sick. Through trauma, the world may come to feel unfamiliar, strange, and devoid of meaningful social connections (Assing Hvidt, 2017; Ueland et al., 2021). This is not to say that all cancer patients feel the same, or that each traumatizing event brings with it the same alterations of lived experience. Human experience is highly heterogeneous.

In conversation with one another, and building on phenomenological literature on trauma (Husserl, 1973; Walther 1923, Wilde 2021), illness (Carel, 2021, 2016), and working with an autoethnographic approach to cancer (Pini, 2022; Pini and Maguire-Rosier, 2021; Pini and Pini, 2019), in this work, we address the ways in which creative and expressive illness narrative—particularly the sharing of such experiences—can help patients recover in the aftermath of a traumatizing event. Narratives can become a medium through which experiences of trauma may be shared, alleviating the sense of alienation common to post-traumatic experience.

Dancing the *Alienworld*: Illness Narrative in the Short Film *ABISSO*

Research on the existential challenges faced by cancer patients highlights that journeying with cancer entails an alienating experience since receiving a cancer diagnosis breaks with one's formerly familiar *homeworld* (Husserl, 1973), leading to a sense of homelessness that biomedical efforts are not well-equipped to address (Assing Hvidt, 2017; Ueland et al., 2021).

Things no longer seem to make sense the way they used to, and the affected individual can be left feeling estranged from their formerly familiar world and the people who shape it, "trapped in a separate dimension" (Pini, 2022, p. 29). This sense of alienation, of being different and somehow beyond understanding is an experience that frequently crops up in trauma narratives (Assing Hvidt, 2017; Stolorow 2019; Stern 2010). It is also an experience one of the authors is familiar with. Drawing from Pini's lived experience of cancer and her illness narrative (Pini, 2022; Pini and Pini, 2019), we focus on the question of whether and how traumatic events can be narrated, known, and shared.

In her early twenties, Pini (SP) was diagnosed with Hodgkin's lymphoma, a type of haematological cancer most frequently diagnosed in teens and young adults or among elderly people over seventy-five. Before receiving a cancer diagnosis, SP was pursuing a professional dance career, working as an apprentice within international dance companies and touring and performing across Europe with renowned choreographers and ensembles. Following her diagnosis, SP's dance career came to a sudden halt. She underwent oncological treatments which ended up stretching into a 10-year-long medical journey: a long residency in "the kingdom of the sick" (Sontag, 1977, p. 3).

During this time, SP developed and elaborated an autoethnographic embodied practice, a lived illness narrative (2019). In collaboration with her brother, a professional video maker, SP performed, recorded, and collected video dance improvisations performed and enacted either during, before or after her medical treatments and appointments. Elaborating her illness narrative in the form of improvised dance performances provided SP with a creative space to reshape her illness experience. In her words: "These performances became my coping strategy to simply find a hospitable locus after having been cast out from what once was a familiar habitat" (Pin and Pini, 2019, p. 7). SP later analyzed and developed this video material into a short dance film series. The first episode of this collection of video dance performances, the short film *ABISSO* (2018) aims to capture the feeling of being immersed in a different dimension, separate from the rest of the world, a dimension where it is impossible to breathe.[1]

ABISSO was filmed and performed underwater in Tenerife in 2014, recorded by Pini's brother Ruggero with a GoPro camera.

Figure 1.1. Picture still from *ABISSO*.

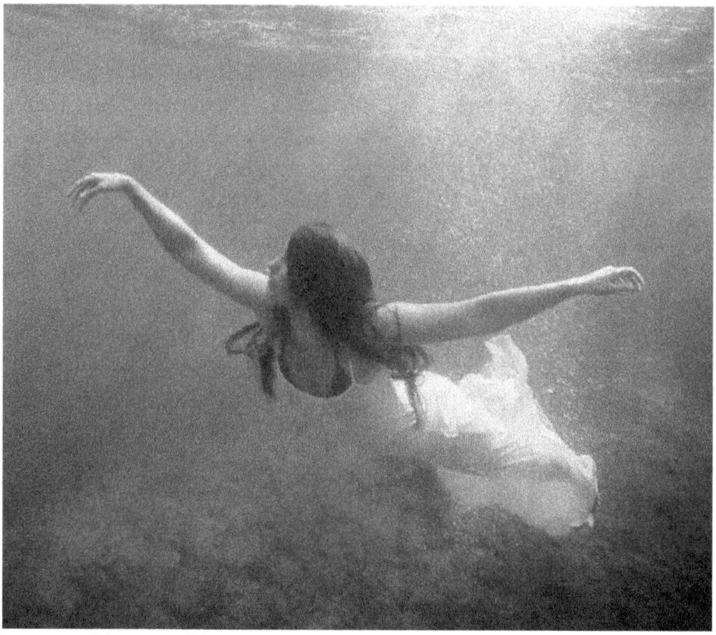

Production still from the filming of *ABISSO* by Sarah and Ruggero Pini. Photo credits by Ruggero Pini, 2014.

---

[1] The short film *ABISSO* (2018) can be watched at the following link https://vimeo.com/user17123701

ABISSO was premiered at the Australian Anthropological Society Annual Conference in Cairns in 2018. The same year the short film *ABISSO* won the Visual and Creative Ethnography Competition organized by the Australian Anthropological Society (AAS) and Australian Network of Student Anthropologists (ANSA). The film has been selected for international film festivals and recognized by, amongst other accolades, the 2019 CHASS Australia Prize for a Student in the Humanities, Arts and Social Sciences. For further information on the creative process underlying the development of the film *ABISSO*, hear Sarah Pini's interview on https://soundcloud.com/artemis-projects/dance-cinema-sarah-pini-abisso.

> After eight years of recurring cancer treatments, I was confronted with the necessity of receiving a bone marrow transplant. A profound fear was gripping my soul, along with the increasing awareness that the transplant might have been the last chance to cure my disease. I was feeling like I was stuck in a separate dimension, where I couldn't breathe. In December 2014, I decided to enact this feeling and filmed an underwater dance in Tenerife. This dance became a visual metaphor of my inner landscape at this phase of my medical journey. With my brother we later framed this performance into a short film named ABISSO. As a performative act, ABISSO marks the acknowledgment of my deepest fears and the courage to embrace my fate. (Pini and Pini, 2019, p. 8)

Home and Alien: A Dialog

SP: The film provides a visual kinesthetic metaphor of living with cancer. It also testifies to the struggle of making bearable, understandable, what illness unleashes: the fear of death, of the unknown.

Phenomenologist Havi Carel stresses the role played by the illness event as a disruptive force that pushes the perception of our body into the foreground of our conscious experience, disrupting the "normal" mode in which our body recedes into the background of awareness (Carel, 2016, 2008). According to Carel, illness is a violent and radical invitation to a "unique form of reflection" (2021, p. 212). Illness is something that usually happens unwillingly and unexpectedly, that abruptly challenges and transforms the experiences of one's own body and mind, and it can be considered a profound and radical form of reflection and philosophical inquiry.

The cancer diagnosis not only drastically shortened my dance career but had a profound impact on my sense of self. One of the first challenges I encountered during my illness journey was finding a way to reshape my identity and sense of self in relation to my illness experience. The cancer diagnosis and relative treatments became my passport to the kingdom of the sick. From that moment I felt like I was somehow trapped in a liminal space between life and death. Although the treatments made me very sick, and oftentimes that possibility of death became tangible, I was not dying, but I did not feel like I was alive either. I felt as if I was observing my life from behind a glass: my life was there, I could see it, but I could not reach it. Somehow, illness entails a long process of identity transformation, not only because of the physical transformations occurring to the body during oncological treatments, but also because of the felt reality of one's existence and the ways one relates to the world. I felt like I became a spectator of my own life, *alien* even to myself.

LW: The video allows the viewer, almost paradoxically, to share this sense of alienation. Watching *ABISSO*, I get a sense of what it might be like to be stuck in a different dimension, alone. I, too, feel unable to breathe.

Borrowing from Edmund Husserl's terminology, receiving a cancer diagnosis can be framed in terms of an expulsion into an *alienworld*: the world of the sick. He defines the alienworld in contrast to a *homeworld*, the shared, meaningful space of everyday experience, which is marked by a sense of familiarity and taken-for-granted-ness. Importantly, the homeworld is intrinsically intersubjective. That is, it is made meaningful in relation to others, constituted as that which is familiar to me and those like me and contrasted with the world of the alien, unfamiliar. The alien is not to be understood as something evil or threatening, it is simply that which is not-home, not part of *our* world (Husserl, 1973, p. 174f., Husserl, 2008, p. 157f.; Steinbock, 1995, p. 179).

How can a cancer diagnosis be said to constitute an expulsion from our homeworld? We are not the first to suggest this. Elisabeth Assing Hvidt argues that the moment of the cancer diagnosis presents a "heavy break with the homeworld" (2017, pp. 377, 380), and Ueland et al. (2021) state that: "Existential suffering after cancer treatment involves living on the edge of the old homeworld and the experience of a new alienworld" (p. 701). A cancer diagnosis threatens not only the integrity of our own body, but the entire taken for granted sense of safety that the homeworld offers. It is not only unfamiliar (we encounter many things that are strange, without being shaken to the core) but it affects the most fundamental assumptions we hold about our lives, of safety and health. As Steinbock puts it in his interpretation of Husserl: "through a transgressive liminal encounter there is a becoming alien of the home" (Steinbock, 1995, p. 210).

This results in a chasm between the cancer patient and the non-traumatized, healthy individual. The theme throughout both Assing Hvidt (2017) and Ueland et al. (2021)'s articles is that of not being understood. In fact, describing trauma, authors often resort to terms like "unimaginable," "unintelligible," and "unbelievable" (Herman, 1992; Brison, 2003; Kolk, 2015, p. 195). Trauma defies understanding. This is not a matter of a cognitive failure, of an inability to find the right words or to follow the reasoning of the trauma survivor or the cancer patient. Rather, narrating trauma is particularly difficult because of an absence of a pervasive background feeling of belonging to the same, meaningful, shared world, which is fundamental to feeling understood (Wilde, 2022). Framing the moment of the cancer diagnosis in terms of an expulsion from one's homeworld highlights the very fundamental, world-altering nature of the experience.

SP: The life I knew before the cancer diagnosis, the "world of dance," came to clash against Sontag's "kingdom of the sick." A diagnosis of cancer, much like other traumatizing experiences, is world-changing. With this change comes a sense that you no longer belong: you are alienated from your own life. In this sense, the expulsion from your homeworld results in a sense of disconnection from others. While both Assing Hvidt and Ueland acknowledge the intersubjective nature of the homeworld as Husserl defined it, they neglect the devastating impact the expulsion from one's homeworld has in these terms. A central aspect of the experience of expulsion from one's homeworld is that of alienation *from others.* I no longer felt like I was part of what was formerly *our* shared (home)world.

LW: Gerda Walther's work on unification further emphasizes the role others play in constituting this shared horizon of experience and thus highlights the way in which trauma may disrupt our sense of belonging to a shared homeworld (Walther 1923; Wilde 2022). *World-experience is intrinsically social.* The world is experienced as a shared place, becoming meaningful only in the encounter with others who are experienced as "humans, who also…," in Walther's words (1923), or "fellow humans" in Husserl's (1973, pp. 137, 141). The ellipsis in Walther's expression allows for a wide range of features, anything that might prompt a sense of unification or togetherness: e.g., sharing the same values, world views, or outlook on life. The one at stake in experiences of trauma can be framed in terms of a world-experience: the perception of what is possible shapes our world *as ours.* Edmund Husserl describes this as a horizon of possibilities that is constitutive of our homeworld (Husserl, 1973, p. 222; Zahavi, 2003, pp. 98f). In short, this means that we who share a common horizon of possibility have a shared way of relating to the world: some things are (perceived to be) possible in our world, while others are not. This shared experience is the basis for a pervasive feeling of togetherness.

It appears that receiving a cancer diagnosis changes the patient in a way that they no longer feel like a "human, who also…," someone who is at home in their once familiar homeworld. Instead, they become a resident in the alien "kingdom of the sick" (Sontag, 1977). The expulsion from the formerly familiar homeworld results in a sense of alienation and not feeling understood that goes beyond an inability to describe one's experience to a bystander.

How can an embodied narrative practice—like your film *ABISSO*—alleviate this sense of alienation through a (wordless) performance? How does it create a sense of understanding between the cancer patient and the healthy individual? It appears that this happens on an affective rather than a linguistic level. It is a form of communication across worlds that does not rely on words (which are notoriously world-bound).

Belonging to a Shared World: Sharing Trauma Through Narrative

SP: Illness narratives play a crucial role in the rehabilitation of people experiencing illness and trauma (Mattingly, 1994). The practice of documenting my illness through video dance performances provided me with a mean to express and modulate the extent of psychological, emotional, physical, and social pain tied to my condition. As I discussed elsewhere, "these performances acted as practices of resistance to counteract the dispossession of my body and to restore a form of agency, necessary to navigate what became a disrupted alien world." (Pini and Pini 2019, p. 7).

Dance and movement, and a reflexive embodied practice can help shape one's identity. Arthur W. Frank observed that "people telling illness stories do not simply describe their sick bodies; their bodies give their stories their particular shape and direction. People certainly talk about their bodies in illness stories; what is harder to hear in the story is the body creating the person" (Frank, 1995, p. 27). The healing potential of embodied art therapy in cancer is well known (Sibbett, 2008). In my case, the therapeutic value of sharing an embodied narrative consisted in the fact that I worked with my own body as a vehicle of sense-making and that process sustained the development of a meaningful narrative (Pini and Maguire-Rosier, 2021). Frank argued that:

> The stories that ill people tell come out of their bodies, the body sets in motion the need for new stories when its disease disrupts the old stories. The body, whether still diseased or recovered, is simultaneously cause, topic, and instrument of whatever new stories are told. These embodied stories have two sides, one personal and the other social. (Frank, 1995, p. 2)

LW: Trauma is notoriously difficult to communicate. We struggle to make sense of an experience that is not part of our familiar, safe homeworld. We struggle to put words to it, to tell a linear story with a clear causal structure because trauma often lacks a clear causal structure (Wilde, 2021). All of this makes it particularly difficult to share. An embodied narrative practice like *ABISSO* not only creates meaning but also allows to communicate it to the viewer. Which role did the gaze of the other, the availability of the performance to others, play in your creation of the video? Did it impact on your sense of "being immersed in a different dimension"? Did you think about the audience, the viewer, when creating your performances, and if so, in what way did it influence the narrative?

SP: In my experience, the lived trauma may become an aesthetic experience for the gaze of others. In the short film *ABISSO* for example, the feeling of alienation, of being trapped in an *alienworld* became an artistic artefact that can be seen and experienced by others. By creatively re-modelling my illness narrative I aimed to rewrite my medical and life history. Performing my illness, and the process of transforming it, shaping it into an artistic work that can be experienced and shared with other people allowed me to construct a different meaning for it. By enacting my illness narrative, I sought to shape my identity in other terms than the ones provided by the medical system. Through the sharing of my embodied illness narrative, I could be seen not only as an ill body, a disease, a cancer case, but as a person, as an individual, a performer, a doer. Eric Cassell pointed out how the experience of "suffering" in illness "occurs when an impending destruction of the person is perceived" (1982, p. 640). According to this view, suffering is understood as the fracturing of "personhood," that calls for "unification" of health, conceived as both a social and a personal event. In my experience, engaging with and developing such embodied illness narrative practice is what enabled a healing process.

Inviting audiences to take a dive into the fear and feeling of alienation that is living with a life-threatening illness helped me in regaining a feeling of belonging to the world, of becoming part of a new *homeworld.* When others can see it, can recognize it, the trauma tied to the illness experience is no longer mine, it is no longer mine alone to bear, but it is narrated, shared with others. An evocative quote from Fernando Pessoa recites that only "what we dream is what we really are, everything else, because of the simple fact that it exists, belongs to the world and to everyone else ... Life lobs us into the air like a stone, and we fly along, saying as we go: "You see, I'm moving." (Pessoa, 2017, p. 384).

LW: On Walther's account, communal experiences are made possible through a process of what she calls "unification." Through the recognition of the other as "humans, who also..." Walther 1923), someone's first-person perspective on the world comes to be intimately linked to the other's experiential relation to the world. The other's point of view now informs and alters one's own, and vice versa (Walther, 1923; Wilde, 2022). *We* now experience the world *together.* So, not only are there two (or more) people who have the same experience, "you and me"; the quality of the experience itself changes and is colored with a sense of experiencing things not individually but as a "we."

Narrative practice enables re-establishing this feeling of being together, of being part of the same homeworld. Although trauma may defy understanding and be described as unintelligible, unbelievable, and so on, it can still be shared in this way. Watching *ABISSO,* the viewer comes to experience something that they had not formerly recognized as part of their homeworld. It allows the viewer to experience the performer as another "human who, also..." despite their residence in a seemingly alien world.

By making your experience of alienation accessible to an audience through your performance, you allow the viewer to share the experience, to understand what it is like, and thereby create a bridge to a shared homeworld. In this way, the narration of your experience becomes a key to a newfound sense of connection and belonging. An illness narrative needs to be heard, seen, or otherwise witnessed by another human who is willing to accept this experience as a possibility in their world to re-create a sense of togetherness.

While there may not be a sense of "us" being trapped in a different dimension, the performance enables a form of communication about the unfamiliar and a connection with the alien. The viewer comes to gain an understanding of the experience of the other that was perhaps hidden amongst the medical equipment, obscured by the disease, and can re-connect with the identity of the performer as a person, a "human, who also...," as a first step towards unification. In the case of *ABISSO*, it does so without the use of words. Words are not necessary to witness the other as another person, another "human, who also..." that I, the viewer, can relate to.

Conclusion

We identified the moment of the cancer diagnosis as a traumatic event, as it constitutes the expulsion of the individual into an *alienworld*: the world of the sick. We presented a case in which dance and the performing body serves not only as an act of creatively re-modelling the performer's illness narrative, but as a mean to communicate this experience. Sharing the experience of trauma and recovery in this way contributes to a re-constitution of a sense of belonging to a shared, meaningful *homeworld*.

We demonstrate how philosophical accounts of the homeworld (Husserl, 1973) and of unification (Walther, 1923) may help shed light on the complexities of traumatic experience and highlight the potential of embodied narratives to re-establish a sense of belonging through sharing trauma experiences. The world is an intersubjective, shared space. We highlight that the (re-)constitution of feelings of belonging is a dyadic process between the traumatized individual and others. An illness narrative needs to be heard, seen, or otherwise witnessed in order to fulfill its full healing potential.

World-experience is intrinsically social. Narratives enable a connection which is fundamental to world experience. Embodied narratives can bridge the chasm between home- and alienworld without the use of words. They allow for a sharing of the experience in which the viewer comes to experience the performer as another "human, who also..." who is relatable in their experience. In this way, we hope to contribute to a better understanding of how a narrative approach can be fruitfully applied in clinical practice.

Reference List

ABISSO (2018) Directed by Sarah and Ruggero Pini [short film], Italy, Spain, 2:38 mins. Available at: https://vimeo.com/302645384 (Accessed: 31/01/2023).

American Psychiatric Association, DSM-5 Task Force (2013) *Diagnostic and statistical manual of mental disorders: DSM-5.* 5th edn. Arlington, VA: American Psychiatric Publishing, Inc.

Assing Hvidt E. (2017) 'The existential cancer journey: travelling through the intersubjective structure of homeworld/alienworld,' *Health,* 21(4), pp. 375-391. doi: https://doi.org/10.1177/1363459315617312

Brison, S. (2003) *Aftermath: violence and the remaking of a self.* New Jersey: Princeton University Press.

Carel, H. (2021) 'Pathology as a phenomenological tool,' *Continental Philosophy Review,* 54, pp. 201–217. doi: https://doi.org/10.1007/s11007-021-09538-9

Carel, H. (2016) *Phenomenology of illness.* Oxford: Oxford University Press.

Carel, H. (2008) *Illness: the cry of the flesh.* Stocksfield: Acumen Publishing Limited.

Cassell, E J. (1982) 'The nature of suffering and the goals of medicine,' *The New England Journal of Medicine,* 306(11), pp. 639-645. doi: https://doi.org/10.1056/NEJM198203183061104

Frank, A.W. [2013 (1995)] *The wounded storyteller: body, illness, and ethics.* 2nd edn. Chicago: The University of Chicago Press.

Herman, J. (1992) *Trauma and recovery.* New York: Basic Books.

Husserl, E. (1973) *Zur Phänomenologie der Intersubjektivität, Texte aus dem Nachlass Dritter Teil: 1929-1935,* hg. von Kern, I., HUA XV. Den Haag: Martinus Nijhoff.

Husserl, E. (2008) *Die Lebenswelt: Auslegungen Der Vorgegebenen Welt Und Ihrer Konstitution.* Edited by Rochus Sowa. HUA XXXIX. Dordrecht: Springer.

Mattingly, C. (1994) 'The concept of therapeutic "emplotment,"' *Social Science & Medicine,* 38(6), pp. 811-822. doi: http://dx.doi.org/10.1016/0277-9536(94)90153-8

Pai, A., Suris, A.M., and North, C.S. (2017) 'Posttraumatic stress disorder in the *DSM-5*: controversy, change, and conceptual considerations,' *Behavioral Sciences,* 7(1), 7. doi: https://doi.org/10.3390/bs7010007

Pessoa, F. (2017) *The Book of Disquiet: The Complete Edition.* New York: New Directions Books.

Pini, S. (2022) 'Autoethnography and "chimeric-thinking": a phenomenological reconsideration of illness and alterity,' *The Australian Journal of Anthropology,* 33(1), pp. 34-46. doi: https://doi.org/10.1111/taja.12420

Pini, S. and Maguire-Rosier, K. (2021) 'Performing illness: a dialogue about an invisibly disabled dancing body,' *Frontiers in Psychology,* 12(566520), pp. 1-6. doi: https://doi.org/10.3389/fpsyg.2021.566520

Pini, S. and Pini, R. (2019) 'Resisting the 'patient' body: a phenomenological account,' *Journal of Embodied Research* [Video Article] 2(1), 2 (20:05). doi: https://doi.org/http://doi.org/10.16995/jer.11

Sibbett, C.H. (2008) 'Liminal embodiment: embodied and sensory experience in cancer care and art therapy,' in Waller, D. and Sibbett, C.H. (eds.) *Art therapy and cancer care*. Seoul: HakJiSa Publisher/OUP, pp. 50-81.

Sontag, S. (1977) *Illness as metaphor*. New York: Penguin Books.

Steinbock, A.J. (1995) *Home and beyond. Generative phenomenology after Husserl*. Evanston: Northwestern University Press.

Stern, J. (2010) *Denial: a memoir of terror*. New York: Harper Collins.

Stolorow, R. (2019) 'A phenomenological-contextual, existential, and ethical perspective on emotional trauma,' in Stanghellini, G. et al. (eds.), *The Oxford Handbook of Phenomenological Psychopathology*, Oxford: Oxford University Press, pp. 895-906.

Ueland, V. et al. (2021) Homeworld/Alienworld: a qualitative study about existential experiences after cancer treatment, *Scandinavian Journal of Caring Sciences*, 35(3), pp. 701-709. doi: https://doi.org/10.1111/scs.12902

van der Kolk, B.A. (2015) *The body keeps the score*. New York: Penguin.

Walther, G. (1923) 'Zur Ontologie der sozialen Gemeinschaften,' in Husserl, E. (ed.) *Jahrbuch für Philosophie und phänomenologische Forschung VI*. Halle: Niemeyer, pp. 1-158.

Wilde, L. (2021) 'Trauma: phenomenological causality and implication,' *Phenomenology and the Cognitive Sciences*, 21, pp. 689-705. doi: https://doi.org/10.1007/s11097-020-09725-8

Wilde, L. (2022) 'Background feelings of belonging and psychological trauma,' *Psychopathology*, 55(3), pp. 190-200. doi: https://doi.org/10.1159/000518327

Zahavi, D. (2003) *Husserl's Phenomenology*. Stanford: Stanford University Press.

1.1.3

Grieving in the Everyday: Metastatic Cancer, Life Writing and the Grief of the Dying

Astrid Joutseno

University of Turku, Finland

Abstract

This chapter draws attention to the grief of those living with terminal cancer. Often the grief of the dying remains unaddressed in the clinical setting and in culture at large. With the concept of the grief of the dying, I consider its likeness to everyday trauma, and suggest non-subsumptive ways of looking for the narratives of such grief. I offer a case study of my experience as a researcher-artist living with metastatic breast cancer, followed by a discussion on how grief figures in the life narratives of the terminally ill. I present four aspects of the grief of the dying: unending uncertainty, the oscillation between immersion and avoidance, fragmented narrative styles and the mourning of one's own death. I suggest that life writing is a useful site for expressing the grief of the dying and for examining it in critical medical humanities.[1]

***

In her essay "On Being Ill," Virginia Woolf noted how literature and culture lacked descriptive language for the experience of illness. According to Woolf, the position of the ill is starkly separate from the healthy. She saw illness as a critical perspective that the healthy lack: "We become deserters ... We float with the sticks on the stream; helter-skelter with the dead leaves on the lawn, ... perhaps for the first time for years to look round, to look up – to look, for example, at the sky." (2009). Since Woolf, much has been written about the

[1] This chapter is part of Finnish Research Council project: Counter-Narratives of Cancer: Shaping Narrative Agency (2023-2027), 354789.

difficulty of conveying illness in narrative form. Still, during the late twentieth and early twenty-first centuries, the experience of illness became a popular theme in memoirs and other forms of life writing (Jurecic, 2012; Nesby and Johansen, 2019). In a sense, illness has been hiding in plain sight in narrative expression. I suggest that the same is true for grief.

This chapter examines the grief of those dying from cancer. Kathryn Schulz has noted that against common misconception, sadness isn't the key emotion linked to grief (2022, p. 64). Instead, as Brené Brown has stipulated, grief is made of loss, longing and feeling lost (2021, pp. 110-11). In this chapter, I define grief not as a procession of uncomfortable feelings with an end goal, but a life-altering temporally ambiguous state. Grief that is hidden or hiding is *disenfranchised* (Doka and Davidson, 2016). It is not recognized or acknowledged and therefore, systems of care and/or entire cultures lack awareness of it. Grief is always related to loss, but not all loss means death. Neil Thompson describes: "… tendency to equate loss with bereavement and thereby artificially restrict grief to situations involving death serves to distract attention from the often major role of grief in our lives in relation to losses that have no connection with death." (2020, p. 21). Losses pile up when life with incurable illness is prolonged. Compounding losses can lead to the experience of everyday trauma, which while becoming repeated and commonplace, does still cause harm (Bordere, 2017). This is why awareness of grief is paramount in considering trauma and narrative ethics. Robert Eaglestone has characterized "traumatic texts" as disrupted, often referential to history and intra-textual containing portions about writing and remembering, as well as ending without closure (2018). Contrary to expectations, trauma-related narratives reveal that "the trauma is constantly there" (ibid., p. 63), permeating narratives of grief. The everydayness of trauma and grief is present in the life writing section of this chapter.

The development of life-extending medicines for metastatic cancer has led to new trajectories of long-term living (in the case of breast cancer in Finland, see Jääskeläinen, 2022). Living with MC (metastatic cancer) is defined by various and individual embodied challenges, one of those is grief. Quite often research that proposes to study grief as an experience of the ill slides into discussing bereavement. Tackling grief from the perspective of the dying seems to be missing, although Kübler-Ross' seminal study from 1973 examined the grieving of the terminally ill (2014). In writing about death from cancer, Stephen P. Hersh does what often happens: quickly slides from end-of-life symptoms to the grief of those who are left behind (2016, pp. 100-03). Understandably, the dying process has to be considered from the perspective of the bereaved, but what about the grief of the dying? How does prolonged illness impact the narrative expressions of grief? Do they answer to the stark stereotypes of the gravely ill cancer patients or narrate inexpressible traumatization? What is it like to permanently reside in the impermanence of the horror cabinet of death's vestibule? This chapter is the beginning of an exploration of the grief of the dying. First I present an autoethnographic study of *the grief of the dying* (Jones, Adams and Ellis, 2013; Lykke, 2014; Ettorre, 2017). Then I outline characteristics and concepts, suggesting that life writing provides a resource for studying non-subsumptive narratives of grief, illness and dying (Meretoja, 2018a). I write from a crip studies (Chen et al., 2023) and critical medical humanities stance, underlining the epistemological significance of the ones with the illness experience, who are not just informants or bodies in trouble, but fundamentally humans engaged in living (Whitehead et al., 2016, pp. 35-38). Upon embarking on a situated story (Haraway, 2016), I note that my experience unfolds in Finland where I receive cancer care through the public healthcare system.

Grieving in the Everyday

On the 5th of January 2023, I received news: my treatment was working again! Metastasis in my cerebellum were shrinking. After a six-month breather, I had resumed treatment in fall 2022 once activity appeared on the MRI scans. It was three years from the start of treating brain metastasis of my breast cancer and nearly 9 years since my initial diagnosis at 32. In September 2021 a novel targeted chemo became available in Finland, and I have received it ever since. The medicine saved me from immediate death that fall, as all other treatments had failed.

On this January morning, while my oncologist delivered the good news, I thought: *Now I can fly to Catalonia as planned in two weeks.* Only later did I remember that tomorrow I would have to endure another chemo infusion and survive the aftermath. I was excited yet anxious. Counterintuitively, I felt no relief, but a sense of rightness. Things were as they should be.

The next day, I received my treatment at the local cancer ward and then stayed home for a week, taking my medicine on a schedule to fight nausea and exhaustion. I had learned to deal with symptoms a little better in the last months: a palliative doctor was trying therapeutic exercises with me to break the mental association linked to severe nausea. I was learning to take care of myself rather than abandoning and ignoring my body in sadness and rage. I was learning to weather the week a little better. Still, or maybe because of this, a few days after my treatment I became deeply sad over the tufts of hair falling from my head. Despite me wearing an ice hat during treatment, my hair has consistently gotten thinner and bald patches have begun to appear. Over the years I've experienced hair loss four times, but there is no getting used to it. The feeling of my balding scalp under my fingers extenuates my sense of unfamiliarity and loss. It reminds me that almost nothing is in my control. That I am dying.

Laying on the double bed at home, I feel twinges of nausea. I don't want to eat or go for my usual walk. I feel sad. As I write this, I can feel the nausea mildly clenching my diaphragm, turning my throat into a slippery rejection pipeline. It is a memory my body keeps. As I am feeling lousy, I avoid talking to my partner. Instead, I just lie in bed fighting tears. I stay there a long while away from activities that usually occupy the ill days. I feel despair. I remain close to the idea of death. I think about talking to my partner at night. I plan what I will say, but never do. Somewhere in this mush I remember my vacation plans. I will travel with a childhood friend who is an artist. It is our first overseas holiday after Covid-19. I haven't left Finland for three years—an eternity for the terminally ill. This is an adventure I never thought I would participate in. During the past years, I have lost most of my cancer sisters—also living with MBC—and regarding my own mortality, the last years have been a sequence of pessimistic predictions and increasing uncertainty. *I know that I am not supposed to be here.*

By the evening I have spent hours looking at the map of Spain. Instead of grief, I want to talk about restaurants. Then, every day I walk a little, I talk a little longer, finally finding the energy to put the washing machine on, and to wash my hair. A week and a half later I cook for the first time. Then I take my 10-year-old to a café after school. We eat cake and talk about our upcoming birthdays.

Two weeks later I fly to Barcelona. I feel my lungs restrict as the air pressure changes. For a few hours, we wander around Barcelona admiring the architecture before taking the train to Girona in the afternoon. The train station is a maze we almost do not survive. It takes me a day to stop feeling like I have a lung infection. I often feel like that when I am exhausted. In our room on the hillside of Girona overlooking the old town, I lie in child's pose and worry that I will ruin our holiday. Then my exhaustion disappears. We walk every day, eat beautiful meals and look around. I am joyously alive. When my muscles ache in my legs, I walk more and patch my toes with plasters where they blister. On the train to Figueres to a Dalí Museum we talk about my imminent but postponed death and the death of my friend's father. He died of cancer nearly 15 years ago. We agree that Dalí's playful absurdity reminds us to embrace life, to create instead of dwelling. I take in the beauty, the sunlight, the mountains and the signs of disarray and decay around us.

On the last day of our vacation, we stay in Barcelona and visit the Museum of Contemporary Art (MACBA). We see a Maria Teresa Hincapié exhibition, "If This Were a Beginning of Infinity" (2023). The Colombian artist died in 2008 of breast cancer and left behind an archive of performance art. Hincapié began as a feminist artist commenting on gender and sexuality, particularly women's role in the patriarchy. Her focus was on the everyday. In time, her works grew toward addressing the planetary suffering from capitalism and environmental disconnection. I move slowly through the large spaces where screens and photographs of different sizes have been arranged. Hincapié's works are presented retrospectively and in 2d-form, altering them from their original three-dimensional performance-art format. The body of the artist is missing. Still, I feel soothed in residing in her archive. I am consoled by the acts of preservation that her son and others have taken. This is a space where I can celebrate Hincapié's life, mourn her death, while also grieving my own vulnerability. The exhibition leaflet showcases a quote: "I am not interested in dead art. I believe that life is art, and my body is my living art. It is my body that has to move, that is looking, that is tired, that is exhausted. This is what I propose" (ibid., 2023). The words send a jolt of energy down my spine. I am taking in something new and abundant. I feel energized as we return to the city bustling around us in the velvet light of the early evening.

Arriving home, my liver markers are nearly normal. I am ready for another round of chemo that promises extended time. Before then, I host a birthday party for my 11-year-old. I am lucky to be baking and arranging green napkins, balloons and golden candles. Each birthday is a benchmark: *we made it together*. I make big gestures to mark time. Mixed in the elation is anxiety: *is this the last birthday with her mother alive?*

After chemo, I lie in bed for the rest of the day. My child comes and goes bringing nuggets about school and toys. I ask her to stay in the other rooms. I am too unwell to listen. In the evening she cuddles up to me and I hold her. As our bodies relax, she shares with me a quote from the mother of her favorite Star Wars actress: "a cuddle always helps." We agree.

The Grief of the Dying

Next, I discuss four aspects of the grief of the dying: unending uncertainty, oscillation between acknowledgment and avoidance, the fragmentation of narrative, and the mourning of one's own death. The grief of the dying is shaped by continuous uncertainty. This is evidenced in the narratives of terminal illness. This instability has been discussed as a source of "chronic trauma" and can be a therapeutic issue, but grief cannot be simply equated with trauma (Mitchell, 2020, p. 153). Grief needs to be considered alongside it, appearing in partnership with everyday losses caused by MC. According to Linda Nesby and May-Lil Johansen the widely popular memoir *When Breath Becomes Air* (2016) by Paul Kalanithi, emphasizes "the importance of the individual ... acknowledging that truth is not necessarily only a biomedical fact but also a vague or subjective phenomenological experience of what it feels like to be ill." (2019, p. 196). For Nesby and Johansen, Kalanithi's prose—a neurosurgeon who died of lung cancer at the age of 37—is an example of illness writing that more broadly acknowledges the limits of what can be known. This is the scope of the uncertainty. I add that perhaps the entire definition of knowledge is dislodged in the vicinity of death. If knowledge is associated with power, then grief acknowledges what is beyond knowing and therefore, also control. As such, grief should be a central interest in medical humanities.

Metastatic cancer unfurls as a sequence of medical interventions and side-effects—they puncture the everyday and the orientation to past and future narratives. The everyday occurrence of losses has been recognized in the research of non-death losses (Doka and Davidson, 2016; Harris, 2020a; Thompson, 2020). Harris suggests that the dual process model of loss in bereavement can be applied to understanding how non-death losses are dealt with by oscillation between immersion in the experience and avoidance or "getting on with life" (Harris, 2020a, p. 10). I propose this model useful in describing the waning and waxing of grief with MC. Importantly, it describes the experience of grief and grieving as intermingling with everyday life (ibid., p. 11). In the life writing segment, I described how in receiving the good news about my health, I turned to an immediate outcome, a vacation while avoiding addressing the contradictory feelings that arose. The segment then exemplifies oscillation as bursts of grief appear everywhere—even on holiday. The illness and its conditioning refuse narrative linearity. In making sense of this, I suggest a non-subsumptive narrative model, which has implications both on how we interpret and create narratives (Meretoja, 2018a, pp. 105-09; 2018b). This narrative hermeneutic approach relinquishes ideals of control, completeness and assimilation to what is already known. Non-subsumptive narrative understanding approaches storytelling as dialogic (Meretoja, 2018b, p. 265), radically relational (2018a, 106); and as explorative counter-narratives to hegemonic narrative practices (ibid., p. 107). From this interpretation, a single situated narrative is not by default representative of a whole, but life writing becomes part of the specificity of the narrative and its interpretation. Yet, this particularity does not diminish the narrative because it does not have to fit into pregiven modes. Referring to Hannah Arendt among others, Hanna Meretoja proposes that this is an ethical approach to narratives because it does not presuppose their value, but facilitates the reading of unique identity/story in a state of becoming (2018a, pp. 108-109). Previously, I have presented this potency of life writing with Eve Sedgwick's concept of reparative writing, emphasizing the potential for new insights and new kinds of agency in writing about grief (Sedgwick, 2003; Joutseno 2021). Meretoja stipulates that "understanding, mediated by language, neither necessarily perpetuates dominant sense-making practices, nor is inevitably oppressive ... it can also open new possibilities, experiences and realities" (ibid., p. 104). In my view, grief narratives often do just that and benefit from being interpreted with this model.

In life writing, the grief of the dying is evidenced in narrative fragments; it is in bits and pieces often referring to the everyday. In my archive of art and research, grief flares up at seemingly unrelated instances (Swan, 2019, 2021; Joutseno, 2020). For example, in my PhD, I examined two memoirs and blogs by mothers dying from MC (Riggs, 2017; Yip-Williams, 2019; Joutseno, 2021). I propose that to study the grief of the dying, we must closely read memoirs, fiction and other forms, but also consider grief's presence in archives such as Hincapié's artistic archive. If we are to look for the grief of the dying in non-subsumptive narratives, we cannot assume to find neatly ordered linear storytelling. Grief narratives demand acute awareness of the unexpected or new, as well as skilled interpretation of the way in which grief is cocooned not just in narrative but within experience: recall my description at the Hincapié exhibition, where I experienced a spaciousness for grief as energizing. The non-linear, self-reflexive and multi-dimensional narrative may also discuss the mechanics of narration and its impact on experience. Meretoja stipulates that non-subsumptive narratives "lay bare their own constructedness, processuality and the movement of telling rather than the told" (Meretoja, 2018a, p. 108). In his discussion on the impact of trauma on narrative, Robert Eaglestone suggests that ethical storytelling is intertwined, "jagged" and its foundation is "the rubble of history …" (2018, pp. 64-65). Here lies the ethical potential of narratives in relation to the grief of the dying.

Finally, the grief of the dying is tied to a process of disappearing from life. It includes the mourning of one's own death. It is existence on the precipice of the unknown. Even in the ebbs and flows between "ordinary life" and *illness time* (Joutseno, 2020) MC intrudes into dreams and commitments – every facet of relationships, how a past is assessed and future (not) imagined. In celebrating my daughter's birthday, I immediately sensed the edges of melancholia, the anticipation of my absence. As a terminally ill mother, I expect to die while my child is young. This is an example of a changed assumptive world (Harris, 2020a, p. 10). The assumptive world shattered by illness is an inner schema based on our earliest life experiences. It guides us in making sense of our role in the past, present and future (ibid., pp. 8-9). Compounded losses require the readjustment of the narrative of the self; the "reweaving" of this new temporary position (Meretoja, 2018b; Harris, 2020a, p. 13). I propose that this rewiring does not mean the expulsion of grief nor the acceptance of illness or nearing death—these are too difficult things to completely process. Instead, narratives of the grief of the dying describe the process of reconfiguration; a way of *living with*, permitting the ever-occurring ruptures, changes and losses. Grief cannot be cured or finished. In my view, this is not anticipatory grief (Doka, 2020). Dying is not a process of anticipation but living through tangible and intangible losses (Harris, 2020b, p. 240) while embodying disintegration. The intangible losses that lack physical resemblance entangle with the tangible: for example, the hair loss I describe becomes metaphoric expressing the intangible losses that are difficult to address. *It is never just hair.* Many MC losses remain unexpressed. Yet, the grief of the dying hides and is made sense of in the body (Brinkmann, 2019). The body is that which is dying. It might be impossible to differentiate between nausea as a side effect of treatment and as an expression of grief because grief is entangled and experienced as embodiment. In the life writing section of this chapter, I suggested that once I began to address the presence of my grief, I became more able to receive help for my physical symptoms (Joutseno, 2021, pp. 4-5). What I do not wish to suggest is that the symptoms would now be under control. They are not. Time or grieving do not make death any more acceptable. Acceptance should not be required. Grief of the dying is not processual but existential. It is a philosopher's predicament in a world that has little time for philosophy.

Conclusion

Metastatic cancer can be accompanied by long-term grieving, much like everyday trauma. I suggest that in critical narrative medicine (Whitehead et al., 2016) fiction and life writing can be analyzed for better attunement to the grief of those who live with incurable illness; realized via an understanding of what happens to narrative. Combining narrative studies, life writing and insights from hospice and palliative care can aid in the project of critical narrative medicine, which allows for rigorous multi-disciplinarity and is focused on dismantling the dichotomy between medicine, humanities and arts in favor of the non-subsumptive and particular. Hanna Meretoja has suggested that it is in *the narrative imaginary* that our unconscious norm-assimilating and the possibility of subversion—imagining differently—exist (2018b, pp. 18-21). In a wider social context, locating the grief of the dying in our narrative imaginary may allow connections where disconnection often takes hold. This means that narratives of grief, illness and dying may contribute to the transformation of understanding and the alleviation of loneliness. Acknowledging the existence of the grief of the dying helps those living with incurable illness and those closest to them. Further research will yield a well-rounded picture of the linkages between everyday trauma, compounding losses and the grief of the dying.

I have begun to suggest that the grief of the dying is varied, challenging, yet potentially enriching. Its archive needs to be named. I suggest that illness experience is a potential position of knowledge; its expression and exploration are fruitful. Yet, the grief of the dying is not to be mined for knowledge. In their delicate rebellion, non-productive affective existence, such grief narratives may occur as generous gifts in the shared process of coming to understanding. My illness narrative is offered as an example of the multitude of positions and possibilities of reflection and expression. In the absence of a definitive characterization of the grief of the dying, I propose that the variability of grief matters.

Reference List

Bordere, T.C. (2017) 'Disenfranchisement and ambiguity in the face of loss: the suffocated grief of sexual assault survivors,' *Family relations*, 66(1), pp. 29-45. doi: https://doi.org/10.1111/FARE.12231

Brinkmann, S. (2019) 'The Body in Grief,' in *Mortality*, 24(3), pp. 209-303. doi: https://doi.org/10.1080/13576275.2017.1413545

Brown, Brené (2021) *Atlas of the heart: mapping meaningful connection and the language of human experience*. New York: Penguin Books.

Chen, M.Y. et al. (eds.) (2023) *Crip genealogies*. Durham: Duke University Press.Doka, K.J. (2020) 'Disenfranchised grief and non-death losses,' in Harris, D.L. (ed.) *Non-death lossand grief: context and clinical implications*. New York: Routledge, pp. 25-35.

Doka, K.J. and Davidson, J. (eds.) (2016) *Living with grief: when illness is prolonged*. 2nd edn. New York: Routledge.

Eaglestone, R. (2018) 'Forms of ordering: trauma, narrative and ethics,' in Meretoja, H. and Davis, C. (eds.) *Storytelling and ethics: literature, visual arts and the power of narrative*. New York: Routledge, pp. 55-67.

Ettorre, E. (2017) *Autoethnography as feminist method: sensitising the feminist "I."* London and New York: Routledge.

Haraway, D.J. (2016) *Manifestly Haraway*. Preface by Cary Wolfe. Minneapolis: University of Minnesota press.

Harris, D.L. (2020a) 'Non-death loss and grief: laying the foundation,' in Harris, D.L. (ed.) *Non-death loss and grief: context and clinical implications*. New York: Routledge, pp. 7-23.

Harris, D.L. (2020b) 'Tangible and intangible losses,' in Harris, D.L. (ed.) *Non-death loss and grief: context and clinical implications*. New York: Routledge, pp. 237-242.

Hersh, S.P. (2016) 'Death from the cancers,' in Doka, K.J. and Davidson, J. (eds.) *Living with grief: when illness is prolonged*. 2nd edn. New York: Routledge, pp. 99-104.

Hincapié, M.T. (2023) *Maria Teresa Hincapié: if this were a beginning of infinity*. Co-production of Corporación Museo de Arte Moderno de Medellín (MAMM) and Museu d'Art Contemporani de Barcelona (MACBA). Available at: https://www.macba.cat/en/exhibitions-activities/exhibitions/maria-teresa-hincapie-if-this-were-a-beginning-of-infinity (Accessed: 2 March, 2023)

Hubara, K. and Swan, A. (2019) 'Post-Äiti.' Helsinki: Hubara & Swan.

Jääskeläinen, A. (2022) 'New prognostic factors and long-term prognosis of different breast cancersubtypes.' Acta Universitatis Ouluensis. D, Medica, 1672. Oulu: University of Oulu. Available at: http://jultika.oulu.fi/files/isbn9789526232997.pdf (Downloaded: 22 February 2022).

Jones, S.H., Adams, T.E. and Ellis, C. (eds.) (2013) *Handbook of autoetnography*. Walnut Creek: Left Coast Press.

Joutseno, A. (2020) 'Becoming D/Other: life as a transmuting device,' *a/b: Auto/biography Studies*, 35(1), pp. 81-96. doi: https://doi.org/10.1080/08989575.2020.1720180

Joutseno, A. (2021) 'Blogging to let go: life writing, maternal cancer and illness,' *On_Culture: The Open Journal for the Study of Culture*, 11, pp. 1-22. doi: https://doi.org/10.22029/oc.2021.1212

Jurecic, A. (2012) *Illness as Narrative*. Pittsburgh: University of Pittsburgh Press. https://doi.org/10.2307/j.ctt5hjr8p

Kalanithi, P. (2016) *When Breath Becomes Air*. London: The Bodley Head.

Kübler-Ross, E. (2014) *On Death and Dying*. London: Routledge.

Lykke, N. (ed.) (2014) *Writing academic texts differently: intersectional feminist methodology and the playful art of writing*. New York: Routledge. doi: https://doi.org/10.4324/9781315818566

Meretoja, H. (2018a) 'From appropriation to dialogic exploration,' in Meretoja, H. and Davis, C. (eds.) *Storytelling and ethics: literature, visual arts and the power of narrative*. New York: Routledge, pp. 101-121. Available at: https://library.oapen.org/handle/20.500.12657/47709 (Accessed: 13 March 2023)

Meretoja, H. (2018b) *The ethics of storytelling: narrative hermeneutics, history, and the possible*. New York: Oxford University Press.

Mitchell, M.B. (2020) 'Non-Finite and cumulative loss in foster care,' in Harris, D. L. (ed.) *Non-death loss and grief: context and clinical implications*. New York: Routledge, pp. 147-156.

Nesby, L. and Johansen, M.-L. (2019) 'Why do we read illness stories? Paul Kalanithi's When breath becomes air (2016) read in the light of Rita Felski,' *Tidsskrift for Forskning i Sygdom og Samfund*. Det Kgl bibliotek, Danmark, 16(31), pp. 187-202. doi: https://doi.org/10.7146/tfss.v16i31.116964

Riggs, N. (2017) *The bright hour: a memoir of living and dying*. New York: Simon & Shuster.

Schulz, K. (2022) *Lost & found: a memoir*. London: Picador.

Sedgwick, E.K. (2003) *Touching feeling: affect, pedagogy, performativity*. Durham: Duke University Press.

Swan, A. (2019) *Viimeinen kirjani: kirjoituksia elämästä*. [My Last Book: Writings About Life]. Helsinki: Nemo.

Swan, A. (2021) 'D/other.' Helsinki: Soliti.

Thompson, N. (2020) 'The social context of loss and grief,' in Harris, D.L. (ed.) *Non-death loss and grief: context and clinical implications*. New York: Routledge, pp. 17-23.

Whitehead, A. et al. (2016) *The Edinburgh Companion to the Critical Medical Humanities*. Edinburgh: Edinburgh University Press (Edinburgh companions to literature).

Woolf, V. (2009) 'On Being Ill,' in Bradshaw, D. (ed.) *Selected essays*. Oxford: Oxford University Press, pp. 101-110.

Yip-Williams, J. (2019) *The unwinding of the miracle: a memoir of life, death and everything that comes after*. New York: Randomhouse Books.

Part 2:
Narrative Methods and Ethics in Trauma Care

2.1. Health Care-Centered

2.1.1

Supervising the Traumatized Practitioner Using a Narrative-Based Approach

John Launer

University College London, England

Abstract

In the United Kingdom, an approach to narrative medicine has developed with roots in systemic and narrative family therapy, emphasizing the use of narrative skills and ideas in interactions with patients and other professionals. This approach has been described as "narrative-based practice" and is associated with a training method known as 'Conversations Inviting Change' (CIC). It is taught largely through the medium of peer supervision, on the principle that practitioners who bring narratives about cases or encounters that have caused them concern can be coached in narrative skills while supervising each other in small groups. They can then apply these skills across the whole range of their work including patient care, training, teamwork and management.

This chapter describes the application of this approach in multi-professional supervision groups attended by practitioners sharing narratives of encounters in their work they have experienced as traumatizing—for example arising from abuse by patients (who may themselves have been traumatized), entrenched conflict in the workplace or an unsustainable workload with inadequate collegial and emotional support. As well as describing the general principles of applying narrative skills to help colleagues, the chapter includes two case examples.

***

A few years before Rita Charon published the ground-breaking book on narrative medicine (Charon, 2006), two British professors of family medicine, Trisha Greenhalgh and Brian Hurwitz edited a volume of essays with the title Narrative-Based Medicine*: Dialogue and Discourse in Clinical Practice* (Greenhalgh and Hurwitz, 1998). Like Charon's book, its aims were to act as a counterpoise to evidence-based medicine and to restore humanity to the practice of medicine. It included contributions from interdisciplinary scholars, healthcare professionals, patients and carers from around the world demonstrating how much could be learned from exploring narratives of health and illness experiences.

In its eclecticism and orientation towards clinical practice, *Narrative-Based Medicine* can be seen as establishing a different tradition to that of the Columbia school of narrative medicine, yet in their origins and aims, these two foundational texts on narratives and medicine were not so very different. They shared the same historical and theoretical roots (Jones and Tansey, 2015). Their editors and authors shared the convictions that narratives are central to medicine, and that competence in engaging with them, however acquired, is a pre-requisite for ethical practice. Given the diversity and cross-fertilization that has occurred in the field since those early years, one could argue that any distinction between narrative-based medicine and narrative medicine is probably now redundant (Launer and Wohlmann, 2023).

One contribution to the volume edited by Greenhalgh and Hurwitz was a chapter I wrote on narrative and mental health (Launer, 1998). I drew on my experience as both a family physician and family therapist, engaged in exploring what the two professional fields could learn from each other. As a family physician, I was familiar with the worlds of positivistic science, evidence and guidelines. As a systemic family therapist, I was trained to pay attention to the complex, polyphonic and often contradictory narratives brought by different family members or participants in other human systems such as work teams. In the context of *Narrative-Based Medicine* I examined how medical practitioners might navigate the uncomfortable no-man's land between conventional medical science and a search for meaning through witnessing stories and inquiring into them.

This question and the search for answers were part of a wider project. Together with my colleagues at the Tavistock Clinic in London, I ran a training for primary care workers based on principles from systemic and narrative therapy (Launer and Lindsey, 1997). Its name was "Conversations Inviting Change." Its aim was to teach family physicians and their teams how to practice in a way that was both safe and sensitive, in a world where the authority of the health professions could no longer be taken for granted, and where they needed to share power with patients who had divergent views of the world. This divergence might be on account of gender, generation, social class, culture, religious and political beliefs, or many other factors (Burnham, 1992).

Over the subsequent 25 years, training in CIC has developed into a range of activities that have been delivered widely around the UK and Europe, as well as internationally including the United States and Japan. These activities range from one day introductory workshops to multi-professional courses and supervision groups lasting a year or more (Launer, 2020). We describe what we teach as "narrative-based practice," or more simply "narrative practice" (Launer, 2018). In what follows, I describe its application in supervision, and then focus specifically on its use in supporting professionals who feel traumatized.

Narrative-based supervision

When we first created trainings in narrative practice, we employed many of the familiar methods of postgraduate training in interactional skills. These included role play, case discussions, and reviewing video recordings. We soon discovered that course participants wanted two things above all. Firstly, they wanted to see live examples of narrative practice in action. Secondly, they found that the most useful way of acquiring narrative skills was to apply these directly in conversations with each other about their cases. In addition, we found that many of the clinicians who enrolled in our courses declared themselves to be "on the edge." They felt overwhelmed by the scale and nature of their workload. Some had chosen to undertake our training knowing that it took place in a mental health institution and expected it, while not being explicitly a form of therapy, to have a therapeutic effect.

We settled on the design that we now use throughout our trainings. We give an opening presentation on the theoretical origins of narrative practice and its relation to narrative medicine. We provide a live demonstration of narrative practice in a conversation between a trainer and a course member about a predicament that person is facing. Following this, we divide people into small supervision groups to practice the techniques themselves (Launer, 2013). During this group work, participants are effectively both learning narrative practice and also receiving direct support with issues that are troubling them, in the form of therapeutic conversations rather than psychotherapy. In the cases presented later in this chapter, there is an example of one case narrative told in the context of a demonstration and another recounted within a supervision group.

For the purposes of a demonstration, we ask if someone is willing to recount a story of a difficulty in the workplace, and to be interviewed about this by a trainer while the rest of the group observes the conversation. We emphasize the importance of confidentiality, and of emotional safety: the person who volunteers to tell their story has the right to withdraw at any point, and the trainer will make sure to "take the temperature" of the conversation throughout. We usually find that three or four people in any course group volunteer a brief "headline" of their workplace issue, and we choose one that appears to offer the most promise for a demonstration.

The trainer then interviews the volunteer in a "fishbowl," applying the elements of narrative practice. These include questioning styles originally derived from the practice of family therapy, such as so-called "circular questioning" (Cecchin, 1987; Selvini et al., 1980; Tomm, 1988) and as used in narrative therapy (White, 2007). Although there is some resemblance to coaching and counseling, our emphasis is on linguistic attentiveness, with encouragement to pay precise attention to such aspects of language as metaphor or cues that carry emotional weight. In this regard, the method can be considered analogous to the close reading of literary texts. We also stress the importance of following the narrator's flow with questions arising through natural curiosity rather than being determined by a predetermined goal. We draw on the principles of narrative ethics by trying to make sure that each choice of question, comment, or use of silence by the interviewer guided by a sense of what matters to the narrator and is likely to lead to narrative development (Launer, 2017).

In discussions following the demonstration interview, group members who have observed it generally comment on two features. One is the ability of the trainer to avoid "nudging" the conversation in any predetermined direction, through withholding any advice, guidance or even reformulation, but instead following only the narrative flow of the storyteller. The other observation is how the story appears to shift onto new ground under its own momentum. This may be because it has been energized by the quality of the interviewer's questions and focused curiosity. It may also result from the reflective capacity of the narrator, who can discover new perspectives through the very act of narration, in a process that is similar to reflective writing.

The majority of time during any course is taken up with practice in small supervision groups of four or five people. In these, we invite one person (termed the supervisee or narrator) to recount a clinical case or workplace encounter that has caused them ongoing concern. Another member of the group acts as a peer supervisor, interviewing them about the narrative. Meanwhile, the other members of the small group act as observers, while a trainer accredited in teaching narrative practice acts as a coach or facilitator. The coach may pause or "freeze frame" the conversation and invite the observers to comment on the conversational process or ask them to function as a "reflecting team" (Andersen, 1987), for example by proposing hypotheses about the narrative or suggesting further questions the interviewer might pose.

We allow around 30 minutes for each piece of supervision and ask members of the small group to change roles for the next round. Group members are free to bring any professional problem concerning either patients or colleagues and others they encounter in the workplace, although we specify that these must have live dilemmas, involve real people and situations and be narrated spontaneously as one would to any trusted colleague ("real play" and not "role play").

The commonest feedback we receive from narrators is that it is an extraordinarily helpful experience (and sometimes an unprecedented one) for them to receive such intense attention for a dilemma or predicament, without any attempt to tell them what to do. This is often accompanied by surprise at how far they have been able to think through their problem—and find their way towards a resolution. Feedback from those who carry out supervision often relates to how difficult they find it to hold back their automatic interviewing behaviors, such as trying to nudge the narrator towards their own preferred ideas or solutions. Conversely, they often report how surprised they are to discover the energy for narrative change brought about by curiosity alone.

Almost everyone who has undertaken training reports over time that they have gained an enhanced ability to apply narrative skills with patients and colleagues, empowering others and lessening their own sense of burden from the responsibilities they carry (Bullock et al., 2011). In the words of one course participant: *"I have been liberated from the role of Dr Fixit."* Regular attendance on a course or at a workshop also means that participants can report on work issues as these evolve over time and as they develop ways of dealing with them.

Over the many hundreds of workshops and trainings we have run, participants have shared a huge variety of narratives concerning patients they have found it difficult to help or who have caused them emotional distress. Some narratives have related to conflict with particular workmates or to people finding themselves isolated and in opposition to management or certain factions within the workplace. In the context of this book, I will give two examples that relate to practitioners who felt themselves to have been traumatized and were reporting or displaying features of a trauma response. The cases illustrate some of the forms in which traumatization of health professionals occurs, and how narrative-based supervision can help.

While not as dramatic or life-threatening as many other examples of traumatization described elsewhere in this book, they illustrate how health practitioners, through acute or chronic exposure to adverse professional experiences, can undergo processes akin to those who encounter these in their personal lives. Both cases are anonymized and each draws on details from several different pieces of supervision.

Case 1

Ben is a young doctor who qualified in the United Kingdom around two years ago. He attended a course in "Conversations Inviting Change" arranged by his local department for medical education, designed to support doctors in their early years of practice. During the first session of the course, he volunteered to speak about his work, with the other course participants as observers. The trainer explained the ground rules for their conversation, including Ben's right to terminate this at any time.

Ben began by telling the trainer that his first year after qualification had been fine. His seniors had given him a lot of support and teaching and he had looked forward to moving on in his career. However, his application for the next job he wanted had been unsuccessful. He had been assigned instead to work on a unit for elderly mentally infirm patients, mostly with dementia. From the first day, he was shocked to find that a large part of his role consisted of identifying patients who could be discharged, in order to free up beds to admit other patients for assessment.

Ben told the supervisor that he had to have conversations with patients' families on a daily basis that he found extremely distressing. He had to explain that their relatives would be discharged home or to nursing homes, while the families protested that the facilities available to support the patients were inadequate. He described how his consultant avoided these conversations himself and offered little supervision. Ben explained he was finding the situation intolerable. His sleep was poor, he had lost weight and his family had told him he was "a shadow of his former self." He was contemplating resignation from his job but was frightened of the adverse effect this might have on his career prospects.

The trainer supervising him explored the background to his current predicament, evoking positive memories of the previous year when he had felt *"it was grand to be a doctor"* and his disappointment when the application for his preferred job was rejected. In response to questions about Ben's consultant, he said the man was unlikely to respond well to requests for sympathy because of service pressures. The trainer then asked if he was able to describe one of the conversations he had had with a family in his current job. As he did so, Ben started to cry. "The family were devastated," he said. "They were lovely people. I felt like a member of the Gestapo. This wasn't why I trained as a doctor."

The supervisor asked if it was all right to continue and to do so with observers present. Ben said he would like to: in spite of his tears, he was finding the conversation helpful because he urgently needed to find a way forward. The trainer asked him what form "a way forward" might take. They spent several minutes exploring this.

Ben then recalled something he had known before but forgotten to mention: his predecessor in the same job had resigned because she had found it intolerable too. She had gone to receive formal therapeutic help. Afterwards she had a "bumpy ride" in terms of her career but had eventually won a place on a training program for general practice, which is what Ben himself hoped to do in due course. "I do have options, and maybe I need to take some risks. If she did it, I could too." Before bringing the supervision to a close, the supervisor asked him who in his support system might be most helpful in considering this matter further. Ben remarked: "I think what the doctor before me did was actually very sensible. I want to check with her how she got professional help."

Case 2

Isabella is a physiotherapist who works in a private clinic in Italy. She attended a series of multi-professional supervision workshops there to learn narrative practice, but remained fairly silent for the first three sessions. At the fourth session, she asked her supervision group if she could tell them about a case she had seen a couple of months previously, but had not felt able to speak about. It concerned a truck driver, who suffered a neck injury following a collision in the course of his work. He had already consulted a lawyer specializing in accident compensation, who told him how to claim the maximum sum in damages, and a private doctor, who advised him what treatment a physiotherapist should give him. He arrived to see Isabella with precise written instructions for extensive treatment that the doctor had written out, and a form for her to sign that he could forward to his insurance company to claim the large sum needed to fund the treatment.

Isabella told her supervision group that she had examined the patient and reached the conclusion he had a fairly minor injury, which was likely to resolve quickly. When she explained this, he became abusive and questioned her authority to disagree with his doctor, whom he named as an eminent orthopedic surgeon. When Isabella explained to the patient that he was free to seek another opinion, he stood up and shouted and swore at her. She feared he was going to hit her before he stormed out of the room. He subsequently sent a complaint to the manager of the clinic. Isabella felt undermined and shaken by the experience and was visibly agitated when telling her story. She said: "Since this happened, I've been completely drained of confidence. My sense of security has gone. I face every patient I see with dread, even ones I really used to trust."

The person supervising Isabella in the small group was a palliative care physician called Max. He explored several different dimensions of Isabella's story. The truck driver had been a large, muscular man and she felt very intimidated by his presence. She had had previous experiences involving doctors giving patients inappropriate advice, and of patients pursuing legal claims that were disproportionate to their injuries, but the combination of factors in this case had overwhelmed her. She was concerned she should have handled the situation better. The clinic manager (a man she described as "overbearing" himself) had written what she felt was a mollifying response to the client. She suspected the manager was mainly concerned about the loss of fees that extensive treatment would have brought in.

Max checked out with her several times if it was all right to proceed. In the course of the supervision, the group took a couple of pauses. During these, the trainer invited the three observers—a nurse, a psychiatrist and a family physician—to offer their reflections on the conversation, in the hearing of Isabella and Max. In accordance with our ground rules, the observers held back from offering advice, but simply shared their thoughts in response to the emerging narrative. In the first pause, they raised questions about gender, the difference in prestige between different occupations, and the tension between profit and professionalism. They also raised the possibility that the patient might himself been traumatized by his accident, psychologically if not physically, and had behaved as he did because of this. In the second pause, they reflected on the challenges of addressing bullying by clients, especially where there was a lack of support from employers.

After each pause, Max invited Isabella to offer her responses on what she had heard and to continue talking in any way she wished. Following the first pause, she explained that she felt she had judged herself too harshly: her professional decision had been the right one since the man had been very pressurizing and had left her no space for doing anything except acceding to his demands. After the second pause, she said she felt very supported. She had also reached a resolution (not previously suggested by any of the group). She now felt the manager's attitude was entirely unacceptable in not taking a robust attitude to protecting staff, especially women. She wanted to speak about the experience with other woman colleagues in the clinic and approach the manager as a group to ask for some quite specific actions. These would include the introduction of an explicit "zero tolerance" policy and the installation of panic buttons in recognition of the risks faced by staff.

Conclusion

Supervision is no panacea for professional trauma. It cannot address the genuinely intolerable conditions in which many health professionals find themselves working. It is not therapy, nor should it be. However, it can explore avenues that might otherwise have seemed unavailable. Narrative-based supervision does not aim intentionally for emotional catharsis. Indeed, we emphasize in our teaching that the uninvited exploration of painful feelings can be experienced as deeply intrusive and itself traumatic. At the same time, opening up someone's story through narrative inquiry, done sensitively, can give people access to emotions and thoughts that they may not have expected. If we invite stories to evolve in directions they had not previously gone, both the teller and listener may be surprised by where they end up. We take seriously our responsibility not to cross the boundary into areas that legitimately belong to personal therapy. At the same time, we also make it clear that, if we are asked or if we consider it professionally advisable, we are able to direct people towards formal psychological help.

Almost all health professionals start out with idealism like Ben in Case 1. They may be ill-prepared for a working life where they may find themselves as functionaries within a system that is bureaucratic and under-resourced. The discrepancy between the care they hoped to give and what they had the resources to offer in their working lives was causing them a form of distress that has aptly been described as "moral injury" (Dean et al., 2020). They may work under the tremendous pressure of unrealistic expectations, both from others and themselves. This may be compounded by difficult domestic circumstances or personal illness (Bovo and Launer, 2022). This can lead to early burnout, being forced into choices that may put their chosen career at risk, and even more tragic outcomes including suicide (Gerada, 2018; Gunja et al., 2022).

Professionals can also be traumatized in other ways, including through abuse as Isabella was in Case 2, or even assault. They may also be caught up in networks of power that can leave them feeling the victims of sexism, racism and other toxic prejudices, as well as in conflicts involving hierarchies, money and organizational politics. This can make them vulnerable not only to isolated incidents of trauma but to chronic exposure. Isabella had remained almost silent for the first few sessions of her supervision group, as if it was too hard for her to speak about what she had experienced as unspeakable. Once she trusted the supervision process enough to do so, she not only found her own voice, but a resolution to speak with others.

Clinicians need to be able to provide patients with trauma-informed care, but supervisors and teachers need to create the conditions for trauma-informed training in interactional skills as well. If patients need time and space to tell their narratives, and for these to be heard and sensitively explored, so do health professionals. In many countries and in many professions, people working in health care receive inadequate supervision for the traumatizing experiences they may have regularly in their working lives. The most important mission of narrative medicine may be to increase narrative competence among practitioners for the benefit of patients, but a pre-requisite for this may be to expose them to conversations where they can be the recipients of this as well. There may be no more crucial task for teachers and practitioners of narrative medicine.

Reference List

Andersen, T. (1987) 'The reflecting team: dialogue and meta-dialogue in clinical work,' *Family Process*, 26(4), pp. 415-428. doi: http://dx.doi.org/10.1111/j.1545-5300.1987.00415.x

Bovo, M.V. and Launer, J. (2022) "Tell me about that colleague': long COVID, narrative medicine, and a remarkable conversation,' *British Journal of General Practice*, 72(719), pp. 278-279. doi: https://doi.org/10.3399/bjgp22X719669

Bullock, A., Monrouxe, L. and Atwell, C. (2011) 'Evaluation of the London Deanery training course: supervision skills for clinical teachers,' *Cardiff School of Social Sciences Working Paper Series*. Working Paper 141. Cardiff: University of Cardiff School of Social Sciences. Available at: https://orca.cardiff.ac.uk/id/eprint/26441/ (Accessed: 11 March 2023).

Burnham, J. (1992) 'Approach-method-technique: making distinctions and creating connections,' *Human Systems*, 3(1), pp. 3-26.

Cecchin, G. (1987) 'Hypothesising, circularity, and neutrality revisited: an invitation to curiosity,' *Family Process*, 26(4), pp. 405-413. PMID: 3319683. doi: https://doi.org/10.1111/j.1545-5300.1987.00405.x

Charon, R. (2006) *Narrative medicine: honoring the stories of illness*. New York: Oxford University Press.

Dean, W., Talbot, S.G. and Caplan, A. (2020) 'Clarifying the language of clinician distress,' *JAMA: Journal of the American Medical Association*, 323(10), pp. 923-924. doi: http://dx.doi.org/10.1001/jama.2019.21576

Gerada, C. (2018) 'Doctors and suicide,' *British Journal of General Practice*, 68(669), pp. 168-169. doi: https://doi.org/10.3399/bjgp18X695345

Greenhalgh, T. and Hurwitz, B. (eds.) (1998) *Narrative based medicine: discourse and dialogue in clinical practice*. London: BMJ Books.

Gunja, M.Z. et al. (2022) *Stressed out and burned out: The global primary care crisis. Findings from the 2022 international health policy survey of primary care physicians* (Commonwealth Fund, November 2022). doi: https://doi.org/10.26099/j2ag-mx88

Jones, E.M. and Tansey, E. M. (eds.) (2015) *The development of narrative practices in medicine c.1960–c.2000*. Wellcome witnesses to contemporary medicine, vol. 52. London: Queen Mary, University of London. Available at: http://www.histmodbiomed.org/witsem/vol52.html

Launer, J. (1998) 'Narrative in mental health in primary care,' in Greenhalgh, T. and Hurwitz, B. (eds.) *Narrative based medicine: dialogue and discourse in clinical practice*. London: BMJ Books, chap. 10.

Launer, J. (2013) 'Training in narrative-based supervision: conversations inviting change,' in Sommers, L.S. and Launer, J. (eds.) *Clinical uncertainty in primary care: The challenge of collaborative engagement*. London: Springer, pp. 163-176.

Launer, J. (2017) 'Narrative ethics in primary care,' in Spicer, J. and Papanikitas, A. (eds.) *Handbook of primary care ethics*. Abingdon: CRC Press, pp. 259-265. doi: https://doi.org/10.1201/9781315155487

Launer, J. (2018) *Narrative-based practice in health and social care: conversations inviting change*. Abingdon: Routledge.

Launer, J. (2020) *Conversations inviting change. Effective dialogue for health and social care.* Available at: https://www.conversationsinvitingchange.com/ (Accessed: 24 January 2023).

Launer, J. and Lindsey, C. (1997) 'Training for systemic general practice: a new approach from the Tavistock Clinic,' *British Journal of General Practice,* 47(420), pp. 543-456. PMID: 9281876, PMCID: PMC1313059.

Launer, J and Wohlmann, A. (2023) 'Narrative medicine, narrative practice and the creation of meaning,' *Lancet,* 401(10371), pp. 98-99. doi: https://doi.org/10.1016/s0140-6736(23)00017-x

Selvini, M.P. et al. (1980) 'Hypothesising-circularity-neutrality: three guidelines for the conductor of the session,' *Family Process,* 19(1), pp. 3-12. PMID: 7364036. doi: https://doi.org/10.1111/j.1545-5300.1980.00003.x

Tomm, K. (1988) 'Interventive Interviewing: Part III. Intending to ask lineal, circular, strategic or reflexive questions?,' *Family Process,* 27(1), pp. 1-15. doi: https://doi.org/10.1111/j.1545-5300.1980.00003.x

White, M. (2007) *Maps of narrative practice.* New York: W. W. Norton & Company.

2.1.2
The Dangers of Collecting Small Trauma

Colleen McMillan

University of Waterloo, Canada

Aaron Smith

Yorkville University, Canada

Abstract

Working with individuals who have experienced trauma requires a deeply personal and intimate relationship to create a place of safety and healing. This process requires the provider to be unconditionally present, empathic, and suspend their own emotions and reactions while vicariously listening to traumas, often on a daily basis.

As practicing clinicians and academics, we are aware of how collecting stories of trauma over one's career impacts one's sense of self and capabilities. Regularly hearing "small traumas" from patients disrupts the line between "them" as the patient and "us" as the helper. At some point the issue of ethics enters, when the provider is forced to reflect upon the accumulation of small trauma stories, and to what degree this line has become blurred and unrecognizable. While most literature focuses on large trauma events, this chapter explores the impact of "small trauma" occurrences, a nuanced kind of relational ruptures, hurts, anger, losses, grief, and abandonment, among other emotional injuries, that regularly and routinely enter our caseload. The occurrence of small traumas may suggest to the provider they are not "big enough" to pause and process and so this kind of trauma lies under one's radar undetected.

In this chapter, we explore the phenomena of collecting small traumas: what are they? What shape do they take? And what is their impact on provider efficacy? A review of the literature combined with personal stories from a therapist, physician, psychiatrist, and a nurse highlight this little understood issue that obliquely finds its way into the psyche and practice of front-line providers.

We end the chapter with new insights for those who devote their practice to the healing of others and in the process collect small incidental traumas that not only impact their professional practice, but also impact the stories of their own lives.

***

Many of us in health care or other helping professions regularly collect small emotional injuries as part of our professional self. Our day is devoted to emotionally attending to the pain of others, listening to stories of suffering, and offering solace in the name of healing. This routine is then repeated the next day and the next day and before one realizes, one has sojourned through a career composed as a compilation of small traumas. Despite this collection however, small traumas are seldom, if ever, acknowledged let alone discussed among peers or colleagues. The silence surrounding such daily occurrences, or small traumas, suggest that such innocuous injuries are considered the "garden variety" of trauma when compared to events such as natural disasters, pandemics, plane crashes, or mass shootings. The sheer magnitude of human suffering marking such tragedies overshadows the daily relational ruptures a practitioner might hear about sadness, heartache, grief, or loneliness. Stories containing such emotions seem too ordinary to share, and the banality of small traumas goes unnoticed.

A review of the literature identifies the occurrence of trauma on a spectrum ranging from secondary traumatic stress (STS) to the more significant vicarious trauma (VT) which can alter basic cognitive beliefs within a helper. While STS can result in burnout, depersonalization, and reduced feelings of personal accomplishment (Craig and Sprang, 2010), the incidence of VT among professional helpers is receiving more attention due to the pandemic (Leo et al., 2021). VT can have lasting impact on basic cognitive schemas, such as safety, trust, esteem, intimacy, and control (Pearlman and Saakvitne, 1995). The mention of small traumas is absent in the literature, and we wonder if the absence reflects the need for this chapter. The scale of these daily traumas flies below the radar archived into memory without being first identified, recorded, or processed.

In critically reflecting on our own experiences, we began to question how we have changed as a result of small traumas in our practice lives. Discussion with colleagues working in the helping professions revealed that while some have experienced STS or VT, almost all acknowledged similar small, emotional ruptures experienced on a daily basis. Often obscured under the global phrase, "having a bad day," deeper deconstruction identified small incidences of loss, anger, judgment, and disappointment resulting from listening and responding to stories from those we are employed to serve. Such injuries go undetected, absorbed into one's psyche or cognitive map of how one perceives themselves and their world.

Literature Review

As mentioned previously, there exist numerous concepts related to the occurrence of trauma as experienced by helpers. We intentionally step outside of the definition of trauma found in the *DSM* 5 and instead embrace the description coined by Scaer (2005), a neurologist whose work suggests accumulative daily traumas hold greater capability to be debilitating in one's personal and professional life. Similarly, the wider term "trauma-related stress conditions" is found in discussions related to helpers and trauma and includes compassion fatigue and professional burnout (Newell and MacNeil, 2010). Though disagreement remains regarding whether these stress conditions are necessarily related to trauma (van Mol et al., 2015), generally most agree they are risks inherent for those working in the helping professions (Ondrejková and Halamová, 2022). As such, and as each is related to the current discussion of small traumas, a brief overview is warranted.

Burnout has been described as "a state of physical, emotional, psychological, and spiritual exhaustion resulting from chronic exposure to (or practice with) populations that are vulnerable or suffering" (Newell and MacNeil, 2010, p. 58). Compassion fatigue (CF) has been described as "the cost of caring for others or their emotional pain, resulting from the desire to relieve the suffering of others" (Ruiz-Fernández et al., 2020, p. 4322). Similar to compassion fatigue, secondary traumatic stress (STS) is defined as "the emotional duress experienced by persons having close contact with a trauma survivor" (Jenkins and Baird, 2002, p. 424). Conversely, vicarious traumatization is described as "transformation in the inner experience of the therapist that comes about as a result of empathic engagement with clients' trauma material" (Pearlman and Saakvitne, 1995, p. 31). Finally, Post-Traumatic Stress Disorder (PTSD) is best understood as an individual's response to an event or events that "pose significant threat (physical, emotional, or psychological) to the safety of the victim or loved ones/friends and are overwhelming and shocking" (APA, 2016, p. ES-3).

There are also various types of trauma: attachment trauma, autonomy or identity trauma, interdependence trauma, achievement or self-actualization trauma, and, perhaps the most commonly discussed, survival trauma (Kira, 2001). Further, all traumas—which Kira describes as "events that are outside the range of the individual's usual experience, that constitutes, for him [sic], exceptional mental and physical stressors" (ibid., p. 73)—can occur at any and every stage in the life cycle, and can result from single events, repeated events, or, as is proposed in this chapter, can be accumulative in nature. Given the variation in both form and type of trauma, as well as when and how it is encountered, it is little surprise that trauma is a highly subjective experience. Or, as Kira notes, "what is traumatic for an individual, may not be as traumatic for another" (ibid.).

Despite the subjective nature of trauma, there is consensus regarding symptomology indicating some sort of "stress reaction" to trauma. These can include burnout, depersonalization, reduced feelings of accomplishment, and changes to one's cognitive frameworks. As noted by Jason Newell and Gordon MacNeil, reactions to trauma—regardless of type or form, as well as when and how it is encountered—often also include "a full range of PTSD symptoms" such as "intrusive thoughts, traumatic memories or nightmares associated with client trauma, insomnia, chronic irritability or angry outbursts, fatigue, difficulty concentrating, avoidance of clients and client situations, and hypervigilant or startle reactions toward stimuli or reminders of client trauma" (2010, p. 60).

Similar to how trauma is experienced subjectively, so too is the concept itself defined differently according to various researchers and authors. For example, the APA defines trauma as:

> Exposure to traumatic events can occur in one (or more) ways: 1) direct experiencing; 2) witnessing, in person; 3) learning that the traumatic event(s) occurred to a family member, or someone else in close relationship; 4) experiencing repeated or extreme exposure to aversive details of the traumatic event(s) ... typically involving major threat to the physical, emotional, or psychological safety and well-being of the individual victim(s) and loved ones and friends. (2016, p. 6)

Conversely, Francine Shapiro defines trauma as "any event that has had a lasting negative effect upon self and psyche" (2017, p. 39). Such a definition, as noted by Valery Krupnik, "blurs the distinction between trauma and adversity, placing them on a continuum from 'small trauma' to 'big trauma'" (2019, p. 256). It is in this blurry place that we find stories of helping professionals who, on a daily and often moment-by-moment basis, collect small traumas.

Small Trauma Stories – How do They Happen?

Regardless of discipline, training in the helping professions stresses the importance of presence, active listening, and empathy (Kahrima et al., 2016). All three are considered core concepts necessary for the development of a therapeutic relationship, providing the motivation for therapeutic change (King, 2011). Maria Moudatsou and colleagues found that helping professionals with high levels of empathy "operate more efficiently as to the fulfillment of their role in eliciting therapeutic change" (2020, p. 3). This change is more likely to occur when the end user feels understood by the health care professional, as users feel secure and trust the professional's abilities and advice. If this dynamic is present, the distance between the helper and the helped shortens and both parties come closer. While enjoying mutual benefits as a result of this dynamic (Kliszcz et al., 2006), it also blurs the line between "us" as the helper and "them" as the service user. While this type of empathic response is valued by the helping professions, and can strengthen the therapeutic alliance, it also results in the helper unconsciously absorbing emotions that accumulate over time. Unlike feelings, emotions are chemical reactions occurring in the amygdala and prefrontal cortex of the brain in response to stimuli, also referred to as triggers (Bechara, Damasio and Damasio, 2000). The amygdala becomes activated in response to being exposed to hearing or seeing upsetting things, such as stories containing pain, anger, loss, or that may feel threatening. In short, the heightened ability to feel what our clients or patients are experiencing as a therapeutic tool becomes an emotional liability in protecting ourselves from collecting small traumas.

What do these small traumas look like? Informal conversations with a family physician, nurse, social worker, and psychiatrist, in addition to our own practices of a combined 50 years, suggest several defining traits. The first trait is that small traumas generally go undetected; partially because they are subconscious reactions but also because we are *trained*, as helping professionals, to not prioritize ourselves. Instead, we are taught to mute if not mask our reaction in deference to preserving the therapeutic alliance, the cornerstone for healing of others (Farber, 2006). The psychiatrist we spoke to explained it by saying:

> I see some very damaged people who are in unimaginable emotional pain. For many, I am the only support they have in their lives. I can't imagine what harm it would do if I showed the slightest emotion to the stories they share with me every week. I am their secure base in attachment terms, so I have to be objective and absorb some of that pain so they can continue with life.

The second trait is the presence of a persistent, low-level distraction during a session when stories contain emotions that hold the potential to harm the listener. While distraction is a shared trait with the phenomena of burnout, particularly within the helping professions (Gabassi, 2002), we differentiate by suggesting that small traumas are unique due to the frequency by which they occur and go undetected. Distraction may be a response by the amygdala sensing harm to the self, triggering the coping mechanism of flight or fight. The social worker explained:

> I never really thought about why I am distracted in so many sessions. I do grief counselling so I assumed it's just part of the job to feel flat at the

> end of the day. During some stories, particularly those involving suicide, I find myself daydreaming about totally unrelated things ... it's not that I don't care ... (pause) ...

The last trait is seen in our ability to dismiss and absorb. Indicative of responses to trauma, over time we normalize uncomfortable emotions as a way to manage our professional lives, but also as a response to the systems that employ us. The family physician we asked about small traumas stated:

> I see five to six patients every hour during a typical eight-hour day. I simply do not have time to pause and think about the content I hear so I just move on. Sure, many times I hear horrible situations; but what can I do about it? Such stories are part of the human condition and it's my job as a physician to be available and just do the best I can. Is this trauma? Is it how workplaces are structured? I don't know.

Similarly, a nurse working in tertiary care during the pandemic shared her experience of small trauma, saying:

> To be honest I never thought of what I hear as small stories of trauma. I always thought that the role of a nurse is to hear these stories and just listen. But you know I do carry these stories with me; back home, to the gym, to bed, watching TV. I haven't figured out a way to deal with them. I don't see anything changing in how I do my work.

These last two comments raise the question of how organizations perpetuate the occurrence and maintenance of small traumas. Are small traumas individually situated or rather a response to how organizations and institutions are structured?

Small Trauma and the Structure of Systems

Given its subjective nature as well as the lack of a consensus definition (Krupnik, 2019), it is difficult if not impossible to definitively label certain experiences as trauma. In the words of Mark Seery and colleagues, "it is important to note that adversities that fail to meet typical definitions of 'trauma' nonetheless contribute to predicting psychiatric disorder onset" (2010, p. 1027). In other words, whether one is exposed to "big" trauma or "small" trauma, whether this happens one time or repeatedly, and whether one chooses to do so or does so involuntarily, such exposure is likely to have significant impacts on one's story and deleterious impacts on one's wellbeing.

To describe the experience of being exposed to, and thereby (un)intentionally collecting, small trauma, O'Rourke and Dufour's description of working in palliative care is helpful: though small traumas "may not seem to bother us in our day-to-day living, they can cause physical symptoms including insomnia, aches and pains, headaches or stomach ailments," and a whole host of other symptoms consistent with trauma (2012, p. 19). One does not always notice when they are exposed to small traumas nor realize the accumulative impact.

According to an informal poll conducted by the authors, on average mental health social workers see approximately five to six clients per day. For example, one author of this chapter recently experienced a clinic morning that consisted of the following cases during a four-hour timeslot:

- 9:00 am – 85-year-old women diagnosed with Parkinson's Disease seeking medically assisted death.
- 10:00 am – 25-year-old woman coping in a physically violent relationship.
- 11:00 am – 32-year-old woman grieving over the loss of her brother who died on the weekend from an opioid overdose.
- 12:00 pm – 12-year-old girl self-injuring as a way to manage past sexual assault.

This type of schedule and case content is not uncommon for many social workers. Though exceptions exist, there is a tendency among many healthcare systems to prioritize efficiency of service (Gavurova et al., 2021; McArdle, 2008). As such, it is unsurprising that, whereas a therapist might see five to six patients in an eight-hour day, many physicians, on average, will spend approximately 10-15 minutes per patient (Das et al., 2021; Elmore et al., 2016), thereby seeing upwards of four-six plus patients per hour and 30 or more patients each day. That many of these patients communicate small, distilled stories of trauma makes it all but certain that these physicians will unintentionally, and perhaps unknowingly, collect multiple stories of trauma throughout any given workday.

In his book, *The Wounded Storyteller*, sociologist Arthur Frank suggests that when stories are told in the context of healthcare and other helping professions, they are done so "in conditions of fatigue, uncertainty, sometimes pain, and always fear" (1995, p. 54). Many of these stories, argues Frank, are uncomfortable not only for patients to tell, but also for physicians to hear. When such stories are encountered, "the modernist bulwark of remedy, progress, and professionalism cracks to reveal vulnerability, futility, and impotence" (ibid., p. 97). Stories of fatigue, uncertainty, pain, and fear – in other words, stories of (small) trauma—thus impact not merely the professional role of the helper, but their personal story as well.

The notion that cultural narratives impact an individual's experience is not new. Michael White and David Epston, for example, suggest that we "consider the stories that provide the broader sociopolitical context of the person's experience" (1990, p. 18). For example, one such story that informs the experience and even sense of self for many helpers is the notion that helpers should not ask for help. Evidence of this is seen in a recent ACEP (2020) survey that found that 45% of emergency room physicians are not comfortable seeking mental health treatment even when they realize it is needed. As such, if one of these physicians who has collected small traumas, both realizes they have done so and recognizes it is harming their wellbeing, the system in which they exist not only limits how they can and do respond, but also impacts their life story more broadly.

Are Systems to Blame for Small Trauma?

The idea that principles within organizations may set individuals up to experience small traumas is not a new one but has received more attention since the COVID-19 pandemic. Often cited for this result are reasons of profit or political gain (Liaropoulos and Goranitis, 2015). When a system such as healthcare sustains chronic strain that exceeds its resources, it fractures and is unable to support those who work there or seek medical or psychological services. The unrelenting demands on mental and medical staff during the prolonged pandemic highlighted systems which also experienced daily traumas, manifested by burgeoning wait rooms, endless waitlists, and weary or sick providers who themselves carried internal small traumas.

Institutional trauma is a concept that recognizes the "ubiquity of trauma in our every day lives" (Tosh and Thompson, 2021). We extend Jem Tosh and Lucy Thompson's definition to suggest that systems, as an entity, also experience trauma which is overlooked. In this context, the idea of small traumas, the focus of this chapter, became even more invisible as such stories appeared too frivolous to share, particularly within a workplace that too was suffering.

While the typical individual and community response has been to blame the system, shifting blame to a larger lens opens a space to explore what can be different for the future. Scholars are highlighting the role of resiliency in organizations and institutions by adopting a trauma informed approach or TIA (Poole, 2020; Poole and Greaves, 2012). Shifting to view a system not as the problem but the outcome of intersecting societal, cultural, political, and financial discourses avoids simplifying a complex issue. Resisting the urge to totalize an institution is the reason so many people experience small traumas, some feminist theorists propose disentangling contributing discourses to find pockets of opportunities for change. In rejecting the binary of "people versus the organization," framing the issue as relational, meaning that small trauma is shared, and both impacts and is impacted by both individuals and institutions, promotes a culture of collaboration rather than blame (Fotaki, 2021).

Writing of new Stories Into Practice – New Insights in Moving Forward

A trauma informed approach is a universal strategy for addressing the range of traumas that occur as a collective response that aligns practices and policies to support resilience and healing across an organization, institution, or service delivery system. Such an approach makes room for small traumas to be known and acknowledged toward what Michael White (2004) refers to as recreating an alternative storyline or different outcome. Transferring White's theory to the topic of small traumas offers a re-envisioning of how we learn, work, and live. Alan Carr explains White's theory this way:

> The narrative approach rests on the assumption that stories are not representations of reflections of identities, lives and problems. Rather narratives constitute identities, lives and problems. According to this position, the process of therapeutic re-authoring personal narratives changes lives, problems and identities because personal narratives are constitutive of identity. (2020, p. 17)

Simply put, the therapeutic relationship holds the power to *listen differently* to each story we hear with a client/patient. When we listen for threads of resiliency within a story, we hold the power to support the individual to think about the strengths they already hold but are buried. White's other concept of a "reflexive practitioner" is also helpful here. Translating a problem saturated patient story into conversing about hope shifts the burden neither to the provider nor the user, but rather externalizes the issue outside of the therapeutic relationship. Both parties think differently, yet equally important, and both feel differently at the end of the exchange. White's theory applies to organizations as well; by avoiding totalizing organizations as "all bad," they become places where opportunities for change can occur.

Conclusion

There is a dearth of discussion regarding small traumas located in the literature, discussed in professional circles, and routinely dismissed by even those who experience them. Couched with stories shared by patients and helpers, small traumas are painful human emotions that routinely occur within the therapeutic relationship and are absorbed into the story of the helper. The presence of high provider empathy and full booking schedules combine to build a slow swelling of small traumas impacting provider mental health. Taking a holistic view that both individuals and systems share this phenomenon, we suggest first externalizing the issue and seeing it for what it is. Doing so, while also acknowledging its occurrence, and working within systems to bring about change, reducing small trauma is not only possible, but critical for the wellbeing of helping professionals, their stories, and the workplaces that employ them.

Reference List

American College of Emergency Physicians (ACEP) (2020) *Mental health among emergency physicians.* Available at: https://www.emergencyphysicians.org/globalassets/emphysicians/all-pdfs/acep20_mental-health-poll-analysis.pdf (Accessed: 30 January 2023).

American Psychological Association (APA) (2016) *Clinical practice guideline for treatment of posttraumatic stress disorder (PTSD) in adults.* Available at: https://www.apa.org/ptsd-guideline/ptsd.pdf (Accessed: 30 January 2023).

Bechara, A., Damasio, H. and Damasio, A. (2000) 'Emotion, decision making and the orbitofrontal cortex,' *Cerebral Cortex,* 10(3), pp. 295-307. doi: https://doi.org/10.1093/cercor/10.3.295

Carr, A. (2000) 'Chapter 2: Michael White's narrative therapy,' in Carr, A. (ed.) *Clinical psychology in Ireland volume 4: family therapy theory, practice and research.* Wales: Edwin Mellen Press, pp. 15-38.

Craig, C.D., and Sprang, G. (2010) 'Compassion satisfaction, compassion fatigue, and burnout in a national sample of trauma treatment therapists,' *Anxiety, Stress, & Coping,* 23(3), 319-339. doi: https://doi.org/10.1080/10615800903085818

Das, M.C. et al. (2021) 'Appointment length with patients in medical consultations in Bangladesh: a hospital-based cross-sectional study,' *Healthcare,* 9(9). PMID: 34574938 PMCID: PMC8466760. doi: https://doi.org/10.3390/healthcare9091164

Elmore, N. et al. (2016) 'Investigating the relationship between consultation length and patient experience,' *British Journal of General Practice,* 66(653), pp. e896-e903. doi: http://doi.org/10.3399/bjgp16X687733

Farber, B.A. (2006) *Self-disclosure in psychotherapy.* New York: Guilford Press.

Fotaki, M. (2021) 'Feminist research changing organizations and societies: taking stock and looking to the future,' *European Journal of Work and Organizational Psychology,* 30(3), pp. 390-399. doi: https://doi.org/10.1080/1359432X.2020.1765862

Frank, A.W. (1995) *The wounded storyteller: body, illness, and ethics.* Chicago: University of Chicago Press.

Gabassi, P.G. et al. (2002) 'Burnout syndrome in the helping professions,' *Psychological Reports,* 90(1), pp. 309-314. doi: http://doi.org/10.2466/pr0.2002.90.1.309

Gavurova, B., Kocisova, K. and Sopko, J. (2021) 'Health system efficiency in OECD countries: dynamic network DEA approach,' *Health Economics Review,* 11(40). doi: https://doi.org/10.1186/s13561-021-00337-9

Jenkins, S.R. and Baird, S. (2002) 'Secondary traumatic stress and vicarious trauma: a validation study,' *Journal of Traumatic Stress,* 15(5), pp. 423–432. doi: http://doi.org/10.1023/A:1020193526843

Kahrima, I. et al. (2016) 'The effect of empathy training on the empathic skills of nurses,' *Iran Red Crescent Medical Journal*, 18(6). doi: http://doi.org/10.5812/ircmj.24847

King, S. (2011) 'The structure of empathy in social work practice,' Journal of Human Behavior in the Social Environment, 21(6), pp. 679-695. doi: http://doi.org/10.1080/10911359.2011.583516

Kira, I.A. (2001) Taxonomy of trauma and trauma assessment. *Traumatology*, 7(2), pp. 73-86.

Kliszcz, J. et al. (2006) 'Empathy in health care providers – validation study of the Polish version of the Jefferson Scale of Empathy,' Advanced Medical Science, 51, pp. 219-222. Available at: https://pubmed.ncbi.nlm.nih.gov/17357313/ (Accessed: 30 January 2023).

Krupnik, V. (2019) 'Trauma or adversity?,' *Traumatology*, 25(4), pp. 256-261. doi: https://doi.org/10.1037/trm0000169

Leo, C.G. et al. (2021) 'Burnout among healthcare workers in the COVID 19 era: a review of the existing literature,' *Frontiers in Public Health*, 9. doi: https://doi.org/10.3389/fpubh.2021.750529

Liaropoulos, L. and Goranitis, I. (2015) 'Health care financing and the sustainability of health systems,' *International Journal for Equity in Health*, 14. doi: https://doi.org/10.1186/s12939-015-0208-5

McArdle, P. (2008) *Relational health care: a practical theology of personhood.* Germany: VDM Verlag.

Moudatsou, M. et al. (2020) 'The role of empathy in health and social care professionals' *Healthcare*, 8(1). doi: http://doi.org/10.3390/healthcare8010026

Newell, J.M. and MacNeil, G.A. (2010) 'Professional burnout, vicarious trauma, secondary traumatic stress, and compassion fatigue: a review of theoretical terms, risk factors, and preventive methods for clinicians and researchers,' *Best Practices in Mental Health*, 6(2), pp. 57–68. Available at: https://psycnet.apa.org/record/2010-23187-006 (Accessed: 30 January 2023).

Ondrejková, N. and Halamová, J. (2022) 'Prevalence of compassion fatigue among helping professions and relationship to compassion for others, self-compassion and self-criticism,' *Health and Social Care in the Community*, 30(5), pp. 1680-1694. doi: http://doi.org/10.1111/hsc.13741

O'Rourke, M. and Dufour, E. (2012). *Embracing the end of life; Help for those who accompany the dying.* Toronto: Novalis Publishing.

Pearlman, L.A. and Saakvitne, K.W. (1995) *Trauma and the therapist: countertransference and vicarious traumatization in psychotherapy with incest survivors.* New York: W. W. Norton.

Poole, N. (2020) *Trauma-informed teams and organizational culture.* 6 October. Available at: https://www.youtube.com/watch?v=B21j-8-vJdM (Accessed: 15 January 2023).

Poole, N. and Greaves, L. (eds.) (2012) *Becoming trauma informed.* CAMH: Centre for Addiction and Mental Health.

Ruiz-Fernández, M.D. et al. (2020) 'Compassion fatigue, burnout, compassion satisfaction and perceived stress in healthcare professionals during the COVID-19 health crisis in Spain,' *Journal of Clinical Nursing*, 29(21-22), pp. 4321-4330. doi: http://doi.org/10.1111/jocn.15469

Scaer, R. (2005). The trauma spectrum: Hidden wounds and human resiliency. W.W. Norton & Co.

Seery, M.D., Holman, E.A. and Silver, R.C. (2010) 'Whatever does not kill us: cumulative lifetime adversity, vulnerability, and resilience,' *Journal of Personality and Social Psychology*, 99(6), pp. 1025-1041. doi: https://doi.org/10.1037/a0021344

Shapiro, F. (2017) *Eye movement desensitization and reprocessing (EMDR) therapy: basic principles, protocols, and procedures.* 3rd edn. New York: Guilford Press.

Thompson, L. and Tosh, J. (2021) 'Understanding institutional trauma,' *Psygentra*, 28 July. Available at: https://www.psygentra.com/post/understanding-institutional-trauma (Accessed 30 January 2023).

van Mol, M.M.C. et al. (2015) 'The prevalence of compassion fatigue and burnout among healthcare professionals in intensive care units: a systematic review,' *PLoS ONE*, 10(8). doi: https://doi.org/10.1371/journal.pone.0136955

White, M (2004) 'Working with people who are suffering the consequences of multiple trauma: a narrative perspective,' *The International Journal of Narrative Therapy and Community Work*, 1, pp. 44-75. Available at: https://dulwichcentre.com.au/wp-content/uploads/2020/01/Working_with_people_who_are_suffering_the_consequences_of_multiple_trauma_Michael_White-2.pdf (Accessed: 30 January 2023).

White, M. and Epston, D. (1990) *Narrative means to therapeutic ends.* New York: W.W. Norton.

2.1.3

Making Narrative Medicine Practices Trauma Informed

Elizabeth Lanphier

University of Cincinnati College of Medicine, US

Abstract

This chapter focuses on narrative medicine practices of close reading and reflective writing and the "narrative medicine workshop" developed and taught by Rita Charon and colleagues, and why trauma informed practice is an integral supplement for the narrative medicine workshop. Like Charon's account of narrative medicine, this chapter unfolds in three movements. The first describes core narrative medicine methods, narrative medicine's alignment with social justice, and concerns regarding its susceptibility to unintended injustice. The second introduces principles and practices of trauma informed care arguing for its natural affinity with narrative medicine methodology and practice. The third movement proposes trauma informed care is an extension of the goals of narrative medicine practice, arguing for a relationship of "supplementarily" between narrative medicine and trauma informed care.

***

In what follows I deploy "narrative medicine" to describe the practices of close reading and reflective writing, and the "narrative medicine workshop," developed and taught by Rita Charon and colleagues in the Program in Narrative Medicine at Columbia University and elucidated in their *Principles and Practices of Narrative Medicine* (Charon et al., 2016). I argue for an ethical imperative that this narrow, *technical* account of narrative medicine become trauma informed to respond to the pervasiveness of trauma and to meet this specific account of narrative medicine's self-described orientation to social justice.

This argument unfolds in three movements, paralleling Charon's three "movements" of narrative medicine. The first orients to the core methods of narrative medicine *training and practice* designed to develop and refine narrative medicine's movements of "attention, representation, and affiliation" specifically through narrative medicine workshops. It also considers putative social justice goals of these narrative medicine practices, and touches on social justice critiques of narrative medicine in the literature.

The second movement describes trauma informed care and its affinity with narrative medicine. Trauma informed care is not an explicit competency or approach within traditional narrative medicine methodology and practice though could become one. The third movement illustrates a relationship of supplementarity between trauma informed care and narrative medicine, arguing for explicitly integrating trauma informed principles into narrative medicine training and practice.

Narrative Medicine: Definitions and Ambitions

The diversity of chapters in this volume makes plain the many meanings and uses of "narrative medicine." However, I deploy a narrow definition of narrative medicine throughout this chapter, what I have elsewhere described as a *technical* definition (Lanphier, 2021a; Lanphier, 2021b). For my purposes, "narrative medicine" means the practices of close reading and reflective writing first developed by Charon and colleagues at Columbia University, which are learned and refined through the "narrative medicine workshop," both of which the editors discuss in the introduction to this collection. I adhere closely to Charon's account of "attention, representation, and affiliation," as the tripartite process and goal of a technical meaning of narrative medicine, in the service of which close reading, reflective writing, and the narrative medicine workshop are tools.

Working from within this technical definition permits clarity about the scope of my arguments and precision regarding the critiques to which this technical account of narrative medicine is, and is not, susceptible. It also hones the activities which I argue a trauma informed supplement ameliorates. Furthermore, I deploy this technical definition not at the exclusion of others, but instead to recognize the heterogeneity of "narrative medicine" and narrative *in* medicine (Lanphier, 2021a) and acknowledge that other accounts and meanings are outside the scope of this chapter.

Close Reading and Reflective Writing

Charon initially described narrative medicine as a tool to refine a clinician's skill by developing "narrative competencies," which Charon suggests occurs through literary practices of close reading and reflective writing (2006). According to Charon, close reading skills like learning to "identify frame, form, time, plot, and desire" can help clinicians to consider "the enduring narrative features of medicine and of illness—temporality, singularity, causality/contingency, intersubjectivity, and ethicality" (ibid., p. 126). Moreover, lessons learned through close reading form "habits of readerly reflection" that "are highly valuable for the clinician who listens to the patient, reads a note in a medical chart, or rereads what she has written" (ibid.). While some critique narrative medicine for being instrumentally in the service of clinician skill-building (Neilson, 2022), clinician competency may have been the start, but is far from the exclusive scope, of what I am calling a *technical* account of narrative medicine.

As narrative medicine has developed into a field of study (see introduction to this volume), its skills, tools, and teachings reach beyond the practicing clinician. They are broadly applicable to those who encounter medicine and illness (typically all of us, at some point). Those trained in the technical narrative medicine methodology that is my focus are from humanist, artistic, and clinical backgrounds. They run narrative medicine workshops for patients and caregivers, but also organizations and groups oriented around non-medical topics. As I will discuss below, the Columbia program ran a narrative medicine workshop addressing anti-racism, and not limited to anti-racism in clinical environments. At the start of the Covid-19 pandemic, they also launched virtual narrative medicine workshops open to all-comers, connected only through their shared experience of living through a global pandemic.

Thus, anyone can train in narrative competencies and pursue the three "movements" of narrative medicine. Close reading practices support attention and representation in the work of noticing that goes on when reading closely and representing the narrator's concerns, interests, motives, and meanings. Representation further occurs in the practice of reflective writing when one's words may be explicitly or implicitly in conversation with the closely read text.

The Narrative Medicine Workshop

The work of close reading and reflective writing, especially when done in community, as in the narrative medicine workshop, "spiral toward affiliation," to borrow from the active process of affiliation that Charon describes when "attention and representation culminate in action" that builds "community," (ibid., pp. 149-150) but also occurs *in* community. The typical narrative medicine workshop is a physical and temporal space in which (generally) two trained narrative medicine facilitators lead a group through close reading and reflective writing. Facilitators select a text that the group typically reads aloud several times. Then participants notice, paying attention to the text ("frame, form, time, plot, and desire") and attempting at representation: What is the text *doing* and *meaning*?

The workshop then shifts to reflective writing. Facilitators introduce a prompt, derived from, or inspired by, the closely-read text. Participants (sometimes facilitators, too) write, briefly. Finally, everyone in the workshop is invited to read their writing, and the group directs attention and representation to these new texts. This process builds community within the workshop itself, spiraling toward affiliation with and between texts and group. The workshop is a tool for teaching skills to support attention, representation, and affiliation beyond the workshop. It is also an iteration of attention, representation, and affiliation, actively doing the work of these three movements and the community building that they are designed to foster.

Social Justice Goals and Critiques

In an article describing "an intensive three-day workshop" addressing anti-racism "using the methods and principles of narrative medicine" Charon and colleagues (2021, p. 160) describe these practices as creating space—presumably both literally and figuratively—a point I return to when considering becoming trauma informed. Here, I want to reflect on how Charon and colleagues articulate an aim of narrative medicine "to create spaces – or 'clearings,' … where persons gather to discuss and confront serious elements of their work and of the culture to which it belongs" (ibid., p. 162). In this study the aim of creating clearings to discuss serious elements of work and culture is specifically in the service of "anti-racism and anti-bias work" (ibid., p. 161), an explicitly social justice-oriented objective.

Other programs have also pursued narrative medicine workshops to teach diversity, equity, and inclusion topics, using the principles and practices of narrative medicine to enhance self-reflection in anti-racism and social justice curriculum (Holdren et al., 2022). Narrative medicine's movements of attention, representation, and affiliation, align with practices of attending to and centering voices of individuals or groups experiencing injustice or oppression, representing stories and experiences as they are understood by the individual or group, and affiliating as a form of solidaristic community building. The "clearing" created by narrative medicine can create and hold space for typically marginalized voices, whether from clinical encounters, like patient and caretaker voices, and experiences, such as emotional or personal ones, that may be absent from medical *or* social and political contexts. This reflects potential political commitments to inclusive social practices, and also potential ethical methodologies that center experience or attend to emotion.

At the same time, reasonable concerns exist within the literature that narrative medicine can implicitly, and sometimes explicitly, uphold and even reinforce injustice. According to such arguments, the "narrative" demands of narrative medicine risk perpetuating epistemic injustice when they fail to accommodate those unable to "narrate" their experiences due to physical or intellectual disability (Leichter, 2019). Paul Ricoeur, in connecting narrative practices to self-formation, posits narrative capacity as a uniquely human ability, contrary to animals or non-living entities (Ricoeur, 1991). Yet this view may diminish—even dehumanize—the experiences of individuals who cannot or do not self-narrate in the ways Ricoeur postulates, or not in ways clearly legible to others who Ricoeur views as part of an active process of receiving and completing a story. Illegibility to others may be due to emotional or psychic states, physical abilities of expression, language differences, age (being preverbal, or being in cognitive decline), etc.

So, while narrative accounts of self and experience exist throughout the philosophical literature (Taylor, 1989), they also face critique for their inability to accommodate diverse experiences that may depart from narrowly understood narrative capacities. Moreover, while the "clearing" of narrative medicine *can* create space to empower those historically or systematically marginalized, it is not to say that they *necessarily* achieve inclusion simply by virtue of using narrative methods. Katie Saulnier (2020) observes that some tellers are subject to "narrative neglect"—their accounts receive unequal attention or consideration. In Saulnier's examples, a teller's gender impacts perceived credibility. As Saulnier's concept of "narrative neglect" demonstrates, narrative methods are not intrinsically anti-oppressive and inclusive. Uncritical reliance on narrative concepts and approaches can in fact reify oppression and marginalization and undermine individual or group standing. Yet Saulnier suggests a critical approach to narrative can overcome these injustices, offering tools for ameliorating oppression and marginalization.

I agree that narrative reliance risks these harms, but narrative engagement can also afford avenues for their rectification. Elsewhere I have addressed why a *technical* definition of narrative medicine can resist certain epistemic injustice critiques (Lanphier, 2021a, Lanphier 2021b). Crucially, attention, representation, and affiliation as core practices and aims of narrative medicine do not impose a specific concept of what is or is not "narrative." If anything, they make demands on a listener to train attention on another, no matter how that individual communicates, and to do the work of representation and affiliation. Arguably, refining attention, representation, and affiliation can and should occur *especially* when narrative modes are least legible and therefore require rapt attention and more careful representation and affiliation.

Narrative medicine's social justice commitments are thus also reflected in how it conceptualizes narrative experience and form. Charon acknowledges that "visual arts, performance arts, music" and "philosophical thought" are also "full partners" in narrative, and that "some of the most important events" in clinical practice "happen without words" (Charon, 2015, p. 1). In the context of the narrative medicine workshop, the selection of "texts" for close reading presents another opportunity for inclusion, but also risks reinforcing practices of marginalization or exclusion, by virtue of which texts, topics, experiences, and authors or creators are represented—or absent.

There is an open and worthwhile question regarding whether expanding what is properly understood as narrative (McKechnie, 2014; Lupton, 2017) is superior to engaging in a more radical practice of upending the primacy of narrative reliance to address social justice concerns and meet social justice aims. However, I suggest in the remainder of this chapter that there are alternatives to a radical upending (though by no means am arguing against it), through the tools of trauma informed care.

Trauma Informed Care

Here I briefly outline the assumptions and principles of trauma informed care as developed by the Substance Abuse and Mental Health Administration (SAMHSA, 2014) and note its uptake in clinical and non-clinical settings. Contrasting trauma informed care with "cultural competency" suggests one, though not the only, reason why narrative medicine ought to be explicitly trauma informed.

Principles and Practices of Trauma Informed Care

Trauma informed care is a set of principles and practices based on an understanding about the impact of trauma on individuals and society. Developed by SAMHSA, it provides approaches for addressing the residual impact of trauma even in settings not focused on *treating* trauma. While trauma informed care is becoming more common in clinical practices, not all trauma informed services are necessarily related to clinical (medical, psychological) *care*. Trauma informed *approaches* are also incorporated into domains ranging from education to policing to movement and bodywork practices. Such domains may not engage in activities typically circumscribed by "care," although being trauma informed in them may be a way to show or practice care.

The foundation of trauma informed care is the understanding that trauma is pervasive in at least two ways: trauma is widespread, and trauma's impact on individuals and communities runs deep. Studies suggest that most adults will have experienced at least one traumatic event by middle-age. The trauma informed literature typically defines "trauma" broadly to include not only objectively experienced events corresponding to a psychological definition of trauma in the DSM. For trauma informed care, trauma also includes subjectively felt singular or recurring experiences of violence or abuse, natural or human-made disaster, collective or individual oppression, if and when these events or experiences disrupt someone's coping mechanisms or inhibit their ability to form coping mechanisms (Lanphier and Anani, 2021).

Trauma informed care meets these understandings about the widespread experience and impact of trauma with commitments to learning signs and symptoms of trauma and responding in ways that minimize retraumatization. Trauma informed practices include promoting physical and emotional safety, enhancing transparency, practicing inclusion, working to level hierarchy, empowering voices and choices, fostering peer support, and remaining mindful of bias, stereotype, cultural difference, and historical or ongoing exclusion and marginalization. While the practices can be social or political, as well as interpersonal, trauma informed care also responds to an ethical imperative to attend to trauma (Lanphier, 2023).

Trauma informed care fundamentally shifts from encountering an individual or behavior experienced as discomforting away from asking "what is wrong with them?" toward curiosity about "what happened to them?" or "what is going on for them?" It recognizes that the answers may be personal, individual, collective, cultural, structural, contemporary, or historical. In this way, trauma informed care shares affinities with other narrative practices, including feminist" methodologies that center narrative and experience (ibid.).

Trauma Informed Care over Cultural Competency

The vision of narrative medicine, and particular the narrative medicine workshop, articulated by Charon and colleagues shares goals and practices with trauma informed care and principles. Trauma informed care's invitation to narrative resonates with the "openness to the world of others – and of ourselves" (Charon et al., 2021, p. 162) that narrative medicine can yield. Charon and colleagues argue that this openness can address issues of inclusion, exclusion, bias, cultural awareness and makes narrative medicine workshops superior to what they characterize as "non-narrative" endeavors such as "sensitivity" or "implicit bias training" (ibid.) for fostering anti-racism.

Uchenna E. Anani and I have suggested that narrative practices provide a supplement to intersectional frameworks attending to the unique ways in which multiple identity markers interface and compound for individuals and in situations, shaping their experiences, particularly experiences of oppression (Lanphier and Anani, 2019). We have built upon this idea to suggest that teaching and implementing trauma informed practices better addresses the goals and objectives of activities like "cultural competency training" in healthcare (Anani, Lanphier and Feltman, 2021). Like Charon and colleagues, we see limitations, and potentially harms, in non-narrative approaches to teaching concepts like "cultural sensitivity" or "anti-racism." Here I am suggesting that it is the narrative method *in combination with* trauma informed method that can better meet social justice aims such as anti-racism and anti-oppression, and avoid unintended harm, than narrative medicine can alone.

In their essay reporting on a narrative medicine workshop approach to anti-racism, Charon and colleagues describe the "narrative medicine clearing" created in a workshop in ways that resonate with trauma informed principles. Through the "pedagogic methods and actions of the facilitator" the clearing supports "safety and non-hierarchical participation" (2021, p. 162). This aligns with principles of safety and leveling hierarchy. Participants "work as a group" in the close reading exercises, promoting "an engagement that builds mutual discovery, attunement, and self-reflective awareness" (ibid.). Such objectives align with inclusion, collaboration, and, to some extent, peer support (if done in environments where participants understand themselves as peers). The writing to a prompt that follows the close reading is met with an "invitation to all participants to read aloud what they have created" (ibid.), a form of empowering participants' voices, while permitting their choice whether to share.

While trauma informed care and narrative medicine (on my *technical* definition) share overlapping principles and objectives, the exact practices—the "pedagogic methods and actions of the facilitator"—to enact these principles within the narrative medicine workshop require further exploration. Certainly, narrative methods *can* achieve these intended aims, and Charon and colleagues (2021) report an apparently successful instance of implementing narrative medicine for anti-racism. Yet narrative methods alone, while potentially an opportunity to develop openness and curiosity that *could* mitigate bias, should not be presumed, necessarily, to do so. At least not without greater elucidation of the precise pedagogical methods involved.

Recall that there are active critiques within the existing scholarship that narrative methods can, at times, risk perpetuating bias, hierarchy, exclusion, or oppression, especially when "narrative" is narrowly construed. Taking these critiques seriously is to neither overpromise what narrative can do, nor dismiss possibilities to do better. One reason I motivate this chapter with a *technical* definition of narrative medicine is that the focus on the *process* of attention, representation, and affiliation, does not rely on any specific account of what constitutes "narrative," nor expectations for how or if one communicates a narrative. It can accommodate an inclusive view of narrative and expressive form. Yet it also requires supplementation to fill in how, exactly, the narrative medicine processes of close reading and reflective writing, and the literal and figurative space of the workshop, designed to teach and foster attention, representation, and affiliation, can actively work against social injustices, and be a tool for social justice. Trauma informed principles can enter as supplement.

Making Narrative Medicine Trauma Informed

The supplement I propose between narrative medicine and trauma informed practice borrows from a reading practice. According to Jacques Derrida's (1967) logic of supplementarity, the "supplement" is that which makes up for something lacking in the nature of the thing supplemented. Yet it is also derived from the very nature of the supplemented thing. This logic of supplementarity affords a way to read and synthesize philosophical texts that may appear in tension with each other but need not be in contradiction.

Narrative medicine can appear as an alternative or response to, even a rejection of, other methods in medicine and practice. Cheryl Misak (2008, 2010) points to the apparent disjunction, for example, between "narrative medicine" and "evidence based" medicine, but argues they are not in fact in a binary relationship. Misak points out that collecting and evaluating "evidence" relies on at least some "narrative" practices regarding how data are collected, framed, and interpreted. Hypothesis and analysis are not free-floating a priori facts but are generated through (narrative) thinking and shaped by (narrative) language. Similarly, narrative medicine and trauma informed practice are not in a disjunctive or binary relationship. A decision to engage one methodology is not a choice to reject the other.

Supplementarity puts narrative medicine and trauma informed care in a relationship to each other that is more than simply additive. My claim is not that narrative medicine can benefit from being trauma informed. It is instead to suggest that for narrative medicine to meet its aims, particularly related to social justice, it *must* be trauma informed. But this relationship also works in the other direction, given the reliance on narrative in trauma informed practice. Trauma informed narrative medicine practice gives shape and structure to the "pedagogic methods and actions of the facilitator" guiding narrative medicine workshops, establishing clear principles to inform practices, and minimizing potential risks of unintended perpetuation of injustice, harm, exclusion, or retraumatizing that may be present without this supplement, as critics of narrative medicine worry about.

Without being explicitly trauma informed, a well-run narrative medicine workshop may happen to instantiate certain trauma informed principles. It may also theoretically aim to promote safety and trust, transparency and peer support, collaboration and empowerment, and flattening hierarchy. However, explicitly integrating trauma informed care into narrative medicine as supplement moves theoretical commitments into practice and supports consistent and intentional, rather than ad hoc or coincidental, integration of trauma informed principles. It creates an imperative to shape the literal and figurative spaces of narrative medicine—from setting up and facilitating interactions in the space to support physical and emotional safety, to selecting inclusive texts and empowering voice in reading and writing, while being sensitive to bias and exclusion—by following trauma informed principles.

Trauma informed care also aligns with narrative medicine's movements. It *attends* to someone's story and experience, *represents* that story through recognizing signs and symptoms of trauma, and *affiliates* through efforts to minimize retraumatization. Trauma informed principles share values with narrative medicine regarding inclusion, voice, and justice. The principles also add explicit attunement to present and historical oppression, bias, stereotype, structures, and culture, affording a supplement for narrative medicine to support its social justice aims and mitigate risk of unintentionally undermining those goals.

A core component of trauma informed care is that it is a universal precaution. I have focused on an example of a narrative medicine workshop for anti-racism as an example of its social justice commitments, uses, and potential shortcomings, to argue for a trauma informed supplement. But it is not only when focusing on anti-oppression that narrative medicine must be trauma informed, nor only when narrative medicine is responding to trauma sourced in social oppression. Trauma informed practice should be implemented as a universal precaution in any narrative medicine setting, regardless of target population or topic of the workshop. Again, trauma is pervasive, and trauma informed care is meant not to treat trauma (similarly to how narrative medicine is not designed to be therapeutic) but to respond to its prevalence and impact.

Finally, trauma informed care is ideally integrated throughout an organization or institution. As organizations and institutions succeed at integrating trauma informed care in holistic ways, its supplementarity with narrative medicine provides a model, and potential argument, for the similar integration of narrative medicine as universal precaution. Yet a trauma informed supplement to narrative medicine does not afford a simple how-to manual for running effective, trauma informed, socially-justice-minded, narrative medicine workshops. The diversity of needs, groups, sources of trauma, and trauma responses resist any singular approach to what is trauma informed for all persons at all times in all places. There remains active work to be done regarding how, exactly, to transform trauma informed principles and general practices into specific actions. Narrative medicine, its theory and practice, can support such refinement in addition to benefitting from it.

Conclusion

Narrative medicine has grown exponentially since its inception. Yet it also remains a young field continuing to develop and evolve. As it does, particularly in its commitments (and deployment as a response) to social justice—being trauma informed aligns with and furthers these aims. Systematically integrating trauma informed principles into narrative medicine practice in a relationship of supplementarity recognizes the necessity of narrative, broadly construed, in trauma informed practice. This integration also brings narrative medicine in alignment with trauma informed care through a set of adaptable yet actionable principles and practices.

Reference List

Anani, U., Lanphier, E. and Feltman, D. (2021) 'Trading cultural competency for trauma informed care,' *The American Journal of Bioethics*, 21(9), pp.13-16. doi: https://doi.org/10.1080/15265161.2021.1952348

Charon, R. (2006) *Narrative medicine: honoring the stories of illness.* New York: Oxford University Press.

Charon, R. (2015) 'Embodied narrative: living out our lives,' *The Journal of the Humanities in Rehabilitation*, 14, pp. 1-4. Available at: https://www.jhrehab.org/2015/02/01/embodied-narrative-living-out-our-lives/ (Accessed: 12 March 2023).

Charon, R. et al. (2016) *The principles and practice of narrative medicine.* New York: Oxford University Press. doi: https://doi.org/10.1093/med/9780199360192.001.0001

Charon, R. et al. (2021) 'Racial justice in medicine: narrative practices toward equity,' *Narrative*, 29(2), pp.160-177. doi: https://doi.org/10.1353/nar.2021.0008

Derrida, J. [1998 (1967)] *Of grammatology.* Translated from the French by Gayatri Chakravorty Spivak. Baltimore and London: Johns Hopkins University Press.

Holdren, S. et al. (2022) 'A novel narrative medicine approach to DEI training for medical school faculty,' *Teaching and learning in medicine*, pp. 1-10. PMID: 35608161. doi:https://doi.org/10.1080/10401334.2022.2067165

Lanphier, E. and Anani, U.E. (2019) 'Narrative ethics and intersectionality,' *The American Journal of Bioethics*, 19(2), pp. 29-31. doi: https://doi.org/10.1080/15265161.2018.1557282

Lanphier, E. and Anani, U.E. (2021) 'Trauma informed ethics consultation,' *The American Journal of Bioethics*, 22(5), pp. 45-57. PMID: 33684027. doi: https://doi.org/10.1080/15265161.2021.1887963

Lanphier, E. (2021a) 'Narrative and medicine: premises, practices, pragmatism,' *Perspectives in Biology and Medicine*, 64(2), pp. 211-234. PMID: 33994393. doi: https://doi.org/10.1353/pbm.2021.0013

Lanphier, E. (2021b) 'Breaking down communication: narrative medicine and its distinctions,' *Social Philosophy Today*, 37, pp. 197-205. doi: https://doi.org/10.5840/socphiltoday202181181

Lanphier, E. (2023). 'Trauma-Informed Ethics,' In: Sellers, M., Kirste, S. (eds) *Encyclopedia of the Philosophy of Law and Social Philosophy.* Springer, Dordrecht. doi: https://doi.org/10.1007/978-94-007-6730-0_1031-1

Leichter, D.J. (2019) 'Communication breakdown: probing the limits of narrative medicine and its discontents,' *Social Philosophy Today,* 35, pp. 59-73. doi: https://doi.org/10.5840/socphiltoday201981263

Lupton, E. (2017) *Design is storytelling.* New York: Cooper Hewitt.

McKechnie, C.C. (2014) 'Anxieties of communication: the limits of narrative in the medical Humanities,' *Medical humanities,* 40(2), pp. 119-124. PMID: 248 69471. doi: https://doi.org/10.1136/medhum-2013-010466

Misak, C. (2008) 'Experience, narrative, and ethical deliberation,' *Ethics,* 118(4), pp. 614-632. doi: https://doi.org/10.1086/589529

Misak, C. (2010) 'Narrative evidence and evidence-based medicine,' *Journal of Evaluation in Clinical Practice,* 16(2), pp. 392-397. PMID: 20367872. doi: https://doi.org/10.1111/j.1365-2753.2010.01407.x

Neilson, S. (2022) 'A logical development: biomedicine's fingerprints are on the instrument of close reading in Charonian Narrative Medicine,' *Medical Humanities,* 48(3), pp.: e1-e4. doi: http://dx.doi.org/10.1136/medhum-2021-012301

Ricoeur, P. (1991) 'Life in quest of narrative,' in Wood, D. (ed.) *On Paul Ricoeur.* New York: Routledge, pp. 34-47.

Substance Abuse and Mental Health Services Administration [SAMHSA] (2014) 'SAMHSA's concept of trauma and guidance for a trauma-informed approach,' HHS Publication No. (SMA) 14-4884. Rockville, MD.

Saulnier, K.M. (2020) 'Telling, hearing, and believing: a critical analysis of narrative bioethics,' *Journal of Bioethical Inquiry,* 17(2), pp. 297-308. PMID: 32180110. doi: https://doi.org/10.1007/s11673-020-09973-y

Taylor, C. (1989) *Sources of the self: the making of modern identity,* Cambridge, MA: Harvard University Press.

2.1.4
Care Amidst Chaos: Narrative Medicine and the Holocaust

Mark Celinscak

University of Nebraska Omaha, US

Abstract

The Allied medical personnel who entered Nazi camps at the end of the Second World War in Europe were confronted with profound medical and ethical dilemmas. At the outset, medical personnel were not ready to handle the large numbers of survivors in urgent need of attention and treatment. Consequently, difficult decisions about patient care had to be made.

Doctors and nurses were often faced with tens of thousands of undiagnosed patients who had been worn down by years of abuse, neglect, and starvation. Medical personnel had to deal with unfamiliar languages, cultural differences, inadequate supplies, limited and untrained staff, as well as rare illnesses. During the first several days after the liberation of the Bergen-Belsen concentration camp, for example, not everyone was given adequate care. In that case, thousands of inmates died, and this weighed heavily on the British medical relief teams. Due to staffing shortages, German military personnel were later employed, much to the consternation of the survivors. In short, the work of British medical personnel was vital, complex, and contentious. While thousands of former inmates died, many more thousands were saved.

This chapter explores the narratives offered by British medical personnel who worked at the Bergen-Belsen concentration camp during the spring and summer of 1945. How did they deal with their enormous responsibilities? What medical, moral, and ethical dilemmas were confronted? How did medical personnel describe the situation they encountered at Bergen-Belsen? These questions and more will be examined.

This chapter will argue that the responsibilities delegated to and generally accepted by doctors, nurses, and other staff often went beyond their typical duties. Medical personnel took on tasks outside their regular roles, including sanitation work, evacuation of the sick and the distribution of food and water. With added weight, heavy decisions concerning life and death were made regarding the sick. Above all, those who would survive with only basic care were prioritized over those in greater need and who were less likely to survive over the next few hours or days. Lastly, the language used to portray the scenes encountered by medical personnel illustrates the degradation of the human condition. Allied military personnel thus employed language, such as animal metaphors, to compare an environment they understood to contrast a world that defied their imagination.

***

Narrative medicine has been defined as an act "practiced with the narrative competence to recognize, absorb, interpret, and be moved by the stories of illness" (Charon, 2006, p. vii). When British medical personnel entered the Bergen-Belsen concentration camp in April 1945, they were met with a situation for which they were not prepared or trained. While doctors and nurses often stressed that the situation put them at a loss for words, many were compelled to document what they witnessed. As Rita Charon notes, "sickness calls forth stories" (ibid., p. 203). For both survivors and medical personnel there was a desire to narrate their experiences offset with the difficulty of finding appropriate words and metaphors for what they wanted to tell. The enormity of the task of locating those words and phrases that captured the emotions they felt and the decisions they were required to make was overwhelming.

Charon advises that we must be alert to the "divides between the sick and the well" (ibid., p. xi). Upon entering the camp, medical personnel entered another realm, one that has been called the "kingdom of night" (Celinscak, 2022). David Biro argues that pain creates an "ontological divide" between those in pain and those who observe it, noting that "From the perspective of the sufferer, there is nothing more real ... But for the observer, it is the exact opposite. The pain is so remote, it becomes unreal" (2010, p. 33). Accordingly, metaphors are frequently employed to create a tangible connection to those in pain. Comparisons were made with familiar images to help make sense of the surreal or unimaginable.

Metaphors symbolically transfer characteristics of one object or thing to that of another. Accordingly, this transfer can offer a new way of understanding complex subjects. A metaphor can alter perceptions and offer a reflection on values and meanings. Moreover, what is reproduced in language is a construct and not necessarily reality. Therefore, our experiences are structured by conceptual systems, which are basically metaphorical. James Geary has argued that "The logic of metaphor is the logic of our lives. Metaphor impinges on everything, allowing us—poets and non-poets alike—to experience and think about the world in fluid, unusual ways. Metaphor is the bridge we fling between the utterly strange and the utterly familiar … between I and the other" (Geary, 2011, pp. 224-25). In short, British medical personnel tried to locate suitable metaphors and images for what they wished to represent in their narratives.

Medical narratives can be assessed in relation to how care was ultimately delivered and received. In *The Principles and Practice of Narrative Medicine*, it is suggested that "attention, representation, and affiliation [are] the three movements of narrative medicine that emerged from our commitment to skilled listening, the power of representation to perceive the other, and the value of the partnerships that result from narrative contact" (Charon et al., 2016, p. 3). "Attention" relates to what the listener can offer to the storyteller; in other words, what the doctor extends to a patient by listening. "Representation" relates to how the narrator frames and shares the story. Lastly, "affiliation" is the relationship between storyteller and listener, doctor and patient, writer and reader; the community that engages with the narrative and the experience of care.

Those who narrate their experience will select and contemplate different aspects of it, making associations to form patterns of meaning. Therefore, narratives offer both empirical data and parts representing a meaning or a moral. As Sissela Bok explains, narratives comprise "empirical and moral claims that individuals stake out about their lives and, in the process, about the lives of others they have known" (2000, p. 308). Medical personnel who offered narratives about their experience at Bergen-Belsen, did so from a distinct point of view and for a particular reason. And while they often struggled to adequately detail and explain what they saw, their responses are critical and with meaning, often containing a moral or ethical component.

Craig Irvine and Rita Charon argue that "Narrative ethics as we understand it in narrative medicine reminds writers and readers that narratives of any kind by necessity privilege certain perspectives and positions, that marginalized voices are often silenced, and that commitments to equality require 'equal access' to the author/teller position" (2016, p. 113). Multiple narratives of a historical event can be used to narrow the gap on historical truth and counterbalance privileged positions.

Thomas Murray suggests four possible concepts for narrative ethics, which include moral education, methodology, discourse, and justification (2013, p. 6). He argues that narratives help us understand ourselves and the world around us, which plays an important role in making moral judgments and helping us to live more humane lives. Accordingly, how did British medical personnel understand what they discovered in the camps? How did they justify the choices that were made about patient care? What follows below is an exploration and assessment of the narratives offered by British medical personnel. But first, the liberation of the Bergen-Belsen concentration camp must be placed in historical context.

The Liberation of Bergen-Belsen

The liberation of Nazi concentration camps in Europe is frequently neglected in the history of the Holocaust. One reason for this disregard is that scholars often prefer clear endpoints for their subject matter. For many, the history of the Holocaust culminates with the death marches, or Germany's unconditional surrender in Europe, and yet, liberation and the immediate period following it, including life in the displaced persons camps, are crucial to our understanding of the Holocaust and its long-term impact.

In April 1945 the British Army liberated the Bergen-Belsen concentration camp. Canadian military personnel joined in the relief efforts (Celinscak, 2015). The British became involved at the camp because the Germans turned it over to them. Recognizing that the war was all but lost on 12 April 1945 a representative from the 1st German Parachute Army crossed British lines and declared that inmates in a nearby concentration camp were ill. An agreement was signed the next morning. However, due to fighting in the surrounding area, the Allies were delayed from entering the area by forty-eight hours, thus the camp was formally entered on 15 April 1945. In the ensuing days, weeks and months, British and Canadian forces arrived at Bergen-Belsen to assist, witness and document the scene.

Much like other Nazi camps, Bergen-Belsen developed over time. While it was initially constructed to house laborers, in 1940, it began to take in prisoners-of-war. By 1943, parts of the complex were converted into a concentration camp. As a concentration camp, Bergen-Belsen imprisoned approximately 120,000 men, women, and children during its existence. In April 1945, at the time of its surrender, there were around 60,000 prisoners still in the camp and many were terribly ill. Of the prisoners still alive in Bergen-Belsen when the Allies arrived, the majority, more than sixty percent, were Jews. The prisoners comprised a range of nationalities, although the majority were Polish and Russian; women made up more than half of the inmates.

In Bergen-Belsen, the death rate was extremely high. When it was surrendered, thousands of emaciated corpses were strewn around the campgrounds because the crematorium was overloaded by the total number of dead. Between January and March 1945, it is estimated that 35,000 people were killed. The death rate continued to accelerate, and in the month of March 1945 alone, 18,000 people died in the camp (Zander, 2006, p. 345). In total, 50,000 people perished in Bergen-Belsen prior to Allied personnel arriving at the camp. Disease and starvation were the primary causes of death.

Clearly, military personnel were unprepared for what they were to find at the camp. When it was initially surrendered, the war, of course, continued to rage on. Consequently, that meant supplies were limited, personnel were largely unavailable, and many resources were occupied elsewhere. Those who remained to work at the camp were left with monumental tasks much outside of their realm of expertise and past experiences.

The victims of Bergen-Belsen continued to die even after the camp was submitted to the Allies. Between 19 and 30 April 1945 another 9,000 people died. The following month 4,500 inmates succumbed to illness, while in June another 400 more would perish. In total, approximately 14,000 people died in the camp after its transfer. In other words, nearly a quarter of the total number of prisoners still alive when the British first arrived at the camp ultimately met their demise. These statistics outline that Allied control of Bergen-Belsen did not put an end to misery and to loss of life. Undoubtedly, the suffering weighed deeply on all involved, and while the situation slowly improved, the conditions in the camp remained grim even weeks after its surrender. How did medical personnel respond to the crisis during liberation?

Care Amidst Chaos

When the British arrived at the camp on 15 April 1945 it was readily apparent that assessments of this dire situation were needed. As they prepared to take control of the camp, it also became clear that British medical personnel were ill-prepared to handle the large number of survivors who needed critical care. As the war in Europe continued for another three weeks, medical teams at Bergen-Belsen were initially lacking personnel, supplies, equipment, facilities, and medications.

Plans were soon established to bury the dead in mass graves and to evacuate the living to the nearby Panzer Training School. Despite these early efforts, progress was slow. Removing those in need of immediate care became more complicated as the dead, dying and healthier survivors intermingled in the barracks. Consequently, difficult decisions regarding the prioritization of the inmates were needed. As senior medical officer, Brigadier Glyn Hughes, Deputy Director of Medical Services of the British Second Army, developed plans to deal with the sick and starving survivors. Regarding his experience in Bergen-Belsen, Hughes commented, "I have been a doctor for thirty years and have seen all the horrors of war, but I have never seen anything to touch it" (Phillips, 1949, p. 35). One of his first major decisions concerned how to deal with the tens of thousands of survivors in need of medical care. Regarding which survivors would receive priority treatment, the brigadier was pragmatic. According to Hughes:

> Under the conditions which existed it was obvious that thorough diagnosis and laborate treatment of individual patients ... would take up so much time that only a small fraction of them could be dealt with and that to the exclusion of the elementary care of the remainder. The principle adopted was that the greatest number of lives would be saved by placing those who had a reasonable chance of survival under conditions in which their own tendency to recover could be aided by simple nursing and suitable feeding, and in which further infection could be prevented. (n.d., p. 10)

The significant number of survivors in need of serious medical attention prompted British medical teams to adopt the practice of triage. Due to a lack of staff, time, and resources, only those who would survive with the most basic care received it. Those in greatest need were generally withheld treatment, a difficult and controversial decision. Survivors were placed into one of three categories: the first two comprised those who would likely survive and those who would likely die, regardless of the care they received; the third consisted of those for whom immediate care could mean the difference between life and death.

Consequently, patients had to be removed from the overcrowded, unsanitary barracks. Stretcher bearers were brought into the quarters and separated those who were deemed fit for care. Prior to their entry, a medical officer (MO) placed an identifying marker on the patient. According to Lieutenant-Colonel Mervin Willett Gonin, the officer commanding the 11th Light Field Ambulance:

> The MO went into each hut and marked on the forehead of each patient a cross to indicate to the bearers that this patient would be moved. The MO made no attempt to fix a diagnosis – all he did was decide whether the patient had any chance of living if he or she were moved or what the chance of survival might be if the patient were left in the camp for another week. It was a heart-rending job and amounted to telling hundreds of poor wretches that they were being left to die. But, as I have said, the individual did not count. (Flanagan and Bloxham, 2005, pp. 26-27)

Those in need of greatest care were passed over. In his narrative, Gonin attempts to justify this decision by rationalizing that the "individual did not count." The focus was to be on the "greater good," no matter how difficult or painful the choice. Nevertheless, the act of removing only some of the survivors led to chaos for the British. Those not selected, but who still had the strength, pleaded, hollered, demanded, and begged the relief workers in hopes of receiving some medical attention. Paul Weindling has argued that the relief efforts at Belsen lacked an "ethical concern" for the victims (2006, 417). The needs of those suffering the most were often set aside.

Myrtle Beardwell of the British Red Cross observed some of these stark judgments. In those first several days after liberation, medical teams quickly adapted strategies to remove some survivors while leaving behind others. According to Beardwell, the situation became so difficult that "they had to have decoy stretchers at one door of the hut whilst the doctor went in at the other and quickly grabbed a sick person" (1945, p. 39). Like Gonin, Beardwell called it an "impossible proposition" (ibid.). Her narrative, racked with guilt, justifies the decision as an attempt to save the greatest number of inmates. As these painful scenes continued, Allied medical personnel searched for different options to care for the thousands of survivors in urgent need of attention. Employing a ratio of one nurse for every ten patients, historian Joanne Reilly argues that Bergen-Belsen would have required 5,000 nurses at the time of the camp's surrender—an impossible number to secure (1998, p. 35). A team of ninety-six medical students from London, who already had basic medical training, were sent to assist at the camp, arriving in early May 1945. However, while their assistance was significant, it was nowhere near enough.

As Weindling has detailed, in May 1945 a group of German nurses from Hamburg were brought into the camp to assist the Royal Army Medical Corps (2006, p. 408). Their arrival was met with anger and protests from the survivors, as many were aware of the medical crimes and experiments in Nazi camps. Indeed, the psychological impact on the survivors was severe. According to Hadassah (Bimko) Rosensaft, a former internee of Bergen-Belsen who provided care to the inmates both before and after liberation, "We were obliged to take in German military doctors and nurses. They were in Wehrmacht uniforms, not SS, but the psychological effect was bad enough on me – imagine what it was like on the severely ill" (2005, p. 58). Later, German civilians and even former prisoners of war were brought into the camp to assist with medical care.

At Belsen Hospital, German staff were also retained. Canadian Lyle Creelman was chief nurse of the British zone of occupied Germany with the United Nations Relief and Rehabilitation Administration (UNRRA). Creelman was responsible for the supervision of nurses throughout the British zone, including those at Belsen hospital. She notes that Belsen hospital had a higher ratio of patients to nurses than any other hospital in Germany. According to Creelman, "the care given the patients [by German medical personnel] was of good quality ... [And yet] there was much criticism from many sources of the continued use of German personnel but ... it was not possible to obtain a sufficient number of qualified DP personnel in spite of the many statements made claiming that 'hundreds of qualified nurses were available'" (1947, p. 556). Like Brigadier Hughes, a pragmatic view was taken by someone in charge of a difficult situation. As British Red Cross nurse Beatrice Mary (Molly) Silva Jones explains, the decision to use German staff was a "detrimental move, but a practical necessity.... It was the job that mattered every time, not the person, [nor] the position ..." (1945, n.p.). For the survivors, their feelings on the matter were largely disregarded.

In addition to the number of patients and lack of staff, differences in language and culture also played a factor. Katherine J. Elvidge, a nursing sister with the Queen Alexandra's Imperial Military Nursing Service (QAIMNS), discussed this issue in her narrative. "The chief [difficulty] is that of languages," she recalled, "The majority of the patients have some Jewish origin, but are from all countries under the sun ... and only about four of them have a smattering of English" (1945, n.p.). Moreover, while the patients were from countries across Europe, as has been discussed above, the medical personnel brought in also had different backgrounds. Elvidge notes that she was assigned both Polish and Russian nurses who worked alongside Hungarian soldiers, who did the cleaning (ibid.). She also dealt with German nurses who worked in the evenings. Among the Poles, Russians, Hungarians, and Germans with whom she worked, only one nurse spoke some English. In other instances, the limits of language became dangerous, especially administering medication. As medical student Thomas Gibson recognized: "To explain to a Pole who speaks a little French how to give a course of sulphonamide to a Russian with erysipelas who only speaks Russian is no easy matter, and we had no means of ensuring the course was correctly given" (2005, p. 19). Therefore, the challenge of communicating to both staff and patients, made working conditions extremely challenging for British medical personnel.

Describing the Chaos

In the narratives offered by medical personnel assigned to work at the Bergen-Belsen concentration camp, the employment of harsh, distant language was all too common. Indeed, many of the words and metaphors offered by allied medical personnel demonstrate the employment of what can be referred to as zoomorphic language. Simply put, zoomorphism is the comparing or attributing of animal characteristics to people or to their behavior. It is the opposite of anthropomorphism, which is the assigning of human characteristics to animals. Examining the uses of such language can reveal the complexity of a situation whereby doctors and nurses wanted to help the sick and dying but were also greatly disturbed and disgusted by the appearance and behavior of those very same individuals.

Captain J. Grant of the 21 Light Field Ambulance was stunned by the behavior of the survivors. "If you want to strip off in public, no one will mind," he recalls, "Most people do it, for self-respect and decency are gone in the majority of cases. You do this, and then pick off the larger lice. They are reverting to animals" (Flanagan and Bloxham, 2005, p. 17). Lieutenant-Colonel James

Alexander Deans Johnston of the 32 Casualty Clearing Station admitted to the difficulty of describing the horrendous conditions inside the camp. He called the survivors a "dense mass of emaciated apathetic scarecrows together in wooden huts" (ibid., p. 9). The language that was easily classifiable, but often unsuitable to the victims of Nazi atrocities.

Many medical personnel had tremendous difficulty relating to, as fellow human beings, the survivors of Bergen-Belsen. The language offered to describe the inmates could often betray the lifesaving work they were providing. Indeed, human reactions to the unthinkable or the unimaginable are frequently primitive and visceral. Those working in the camp could be appalled and even disgusted by the gaunt, half-naked inmates in ragged prison uniforms. Moreover, barriers such as language, as well as religious and cultural differences made it difficult for many personnel to interact and even comprehend the inmates they were assisting.

Turning to biology, medical student Alan MacAuslan evoked the theory of recapitulation in his writings. Propagated by German biologist Ernst Haeckel in the nineteenth century, the much-criticized theory suggests that during its course of embryonic development, an organism passes through a sequence of stages representing our fully grown ancestors (i.e. ontogeny recapitulates phylogeny). While most biologists abandoned this concept in the early twentieth century, the theory points to a primitive or animal-like behavior at one end of the spectrum, and a higher-level, sophisticated civilization at the other. While the theory of recapitulation was meant to be taken in a factual sense, it has also found use as a metaphor. According to MacAuslan, while physical illnesses shocked, psychiatric conditions alarmed the British medical students. Referring to a specific group of internees, he wrote:

> What were we taught "ontology recapitulates phylogeny"? The development of the individual mirrors the development of the species. The human foetus goes through all the historical stages from single cell to tadpole, via fish with gills to mammal, climbing in the womb from primordial slime to human being. These bemused people seemed to have reversed the process, slipping down below herd consciousness, abandoning family and personal ties, to become more primitive than reptiles, more primitive than gastropods. They were exiled from civilisation, stunned into bare existence ... Perhaps this is what starvation does to you, would do to us. (n.d., p. 7)

Associating the behavior of inmates as something animal-like, overly instinctual, or as something irrational, immoral, or uncivilized, was all too common in the narratives offered by those who worked in the camp.

Conclusion

For the British medical personnel who entered the Bergen-Belsen concentration camp during the spring and summer of 1945, the experience was unthinkably challenging, and one that led to medical and moral dilemmas. Initially lacking staff, supplies, equipment, facilities, and medications, personnel frequently had to improvise and adopt roles they never had to perform. While the physical deterioration of inmates shocked them, it was often the moral and social collapse that disturbed many of the doctors and nurses. Struggling with issues of language limitations and isolation, medical staff treated rare and complex illnesses under trying circumstances. At times, medical care seemed to offer little optimism. Care amidst chaos was the experience they shared, and the medical narratives demonstrate the complexity of providing aid during what was a previously unimaginable situation.

Reference List

Beardwell, M. (1945) *Aftermath.* Ilfracombe: A. H. Stockwell.

Biro, D. (2010) *Listening to pain: finding words, compassion, and relief.* New York: W.W. Norton & Company.

Bok, S. (2000) 'Autobiography as moral battleground,' in Schacter, D. and Scarry, E. (eds.) *Memory, brain and belief.* Cambridge: Cambridge University Press, pp. 307-24.

Celinscak, M. (2015) *Distance from the Belsen Heap: allied forces and the liberation of a Nazi concentration camp.* Toronto: University of Toronto Press.

Celinscak, M. (2022) *Kingdom of night: witnesses to the Holocaust.* Toronto: University of Toronto Press.

Charon, R. (2006) *Narrative medicine: honoring the stories of illness.* New York: Oxford University Press.

Charon, R. et al. (eds.) (2016) *The principles and practice of narrative medicine.* New York: Oxford University Press. doi: https://doi.org/10.1093/med/978019 9360192.001.0001

Creelman, L. (1947) 'With the UNRRA in Germany,' *The Canadian Nurse,* 43(7), pp. 532, 552-556.

Elvidge, K.J. (1945) 'Letter dated 26 May 1945,' IWM, Department of Documents, 1029, private papers of Mrs. K.J. Elvidge, 89/10/1.

Flanagan, B. and Bloxham, D. (eds.) (2005) *Remembering Belsen: eyewitnesses record the liberation.* London: Vallentine Mitchell.

Gibson, T. (2005) 'Belsen 1945,' *BLC: Barts and the London Chroniclek,* 7(1), p. 19.

Gonin, M.W. (no date) 'Private papers of Lieutenant Colonel M.W. Gonin DSO.' Imperial War Museum, Department of Documents, 3713.

Geary, J. (2011) *I is an Other: the secret life of metaphor and how it shapes the way we see the world.* New York: Harper Collins.

Hughes, G. (no date) 'Report on medical aspects of Belsen,' Contemporary Medical Archives Collection, Wellcome Library, RAMC 1218/2/13.

Irvine, C. and Charon, R. (2016) 'Deliver us from certainty: training for narrative ethics,' in Charon, R. et al. (eds.) *The principles and practice of Narrative Medicine.* New York: Oxford University Press. doi: https://doi.org/10.1093/med/9780199360192.003.0006

Jones, S.M. (1945) 'From a Diary Written in Belsen,' IWM Department of Documents, 9550, from the private papers of Miss J. McFarlane (99/86/1).

MacAuslan, A. (no date) 'Private Papers,' IWM Department of Documents, 3042 (95/2/1).

Murray, T. (2013) 'What do we mean by 'narrative ethics'' in Nelson, H. (ed.) *Stories and their limits: narrative approaches to bioethics.* London: Routledge.

Phillips, R. (1949) *Trial of Josef Kramer and forty-four others: the Belsen Trial.* London: W. Hodge.

Reilly, J. (1998) *Belsen: the liberation of a concentration camp.* London: Routledge.

Rosensaft, H. (2005) *Yesterday: my story.* New York: Yad Vashem and the Holocaust Survivors' Memoirs Project.

Weindling, P. (2006) ''Belsenitis': liberating Belsen, its hospitals, UNRRA, and selection for re-emigration, 1945-1948,' *Science in Context,* 19(3), pp. 401-418. PMID: 17214437. doi: https://doi.org/10.1017/s0269889706000998

Zander, U. (2006) 'To rescue or be rescued: the liberation of Bergen-Belsen and the white buses in british and swedish historical cultures,' in Karlsson, K. and Zander, U. (eds.) *The Holocaust on post-war battlefields: genocide as historical culture.* Malmö: Sekel.

2.2 Patient-Centered

2.2.1

Repair and Re-enchantment: Reading and Writing Cancer

Oddgeir Synnes

VID Specialized University, Norway

Hilde Bondevik

University of Oslo, Norway

Abstract

Receiving a cancer diagnosis can be considered a traumatic life experience. The trauma of cancer concerns not just a *biological* disruption but also a *biographical* one (Hubbard and Forbat, 2012). Living with cancer, thus, might involve a loss of narrative and voice (Frank, 2014). According to Susan Gubar, author, professor of literature and cancer survivor, the reading and writing of literature can be an effective complementary therapy when living with cancer; writing can alleviate the loneliness of the disease, provide tools to understand how to live with cancer, and function "as a creative defense against present and future losses" (2016, p. 21). Furthermore, American poet Gregory Orr (2002) sees the ordering power of poetry as a crucial way of meeting the disordering experience of trauma.

In this chapter, we explore if and how reading and writing might be of help when living with cancer by looking at recent experiences from three creative writing courses we have given at Oslo University Hospital, Radiumhospitalet. The texts and experiences from the courses will be put in dialogwith theoretical perspectives related to narrative medicine, poetic language and meaning-making (Charon et al., 2017). In particular, we will draw on Paul Ricoeur's poetic and existential hermeneutics (2008) and post-critique's growing interest in the literary practices of lay persons to examine in what way reading and writing in the setting of a cancer hospital can open towards repair, of finding a voice, re-enchantment and affiliation to the world and others (Jurecic, 2012, Sedgwick, 2003; Felski, 2008).

***

There is a growing interest in the use of creative writing in healthcare settings. Creative writing is an umbrella term for various forms of writing practices that emphasizes the literary aspects of writing, such as the use of literary tools and genres like storytelling, fiction and poetry, both in groups and on an individual basis (see Costa and Abreu, 2018; Gillam, 2018 for a presentation of creative writing in healthcare settings). The available literature underscores that creative writing in general might promote wellbeing. More specifically research has shown that creative writing might provide a safe space for mastery and growth (Romm, Synnes and Bondevik, 2022), it can help see ones's life in a new light and in terms of potentiality and hope; and it might give validation of voice and offering a creative and supportive community (Gorelick, 2005; Synnes, Romm and Bondevik, 2021). Furthermore, creative writing can involve therapeutic aspects of externalizing emotions and finding a language that can (re-)describe difficult and traumatic events (Bundesen et al., 2020; Orr, 2002). As Birgit Bundesen and colleagues (2020) write, trauma is an event that has not yet been integrated or interpreted, but something that might be evoked and processed by writing within a safe framework.

Theoretical Perspectives

We frame creative writing in health care in light of larger debates on the uses of literature as found in Paul Ricoeur's existential hermeneutics (2008) and in the evolving fields of narrative medicine (Charon et al., 2017) and post-critique (Felski, 2008). This positioning opens for an understanding of the application of literature and writing, not merely as a form of method or individual therapy, but as a criticism of modern medicine's shortcomings of addressing loss of meaning and the loneliness of suffering. The above-mentioned positions thus see literature, not as something that is to be solely dealt with in the academic world of literary studies but is deeply connected to our way of being in the world. In Ricoeur's existential hermeneutics, he is concerned with how human existence is conditioned by the voluntary and involuntary. As human beings, we are part of nature, subject to diseases, trauma, and events outside our control. At the same time, our existence is not merely given but achieved, through interpretation and engagement with the available symbolic and linguistic resources in the culture. For Ricoeur, literature and poetic language thus play a particularly crucial part in how we come to understand ourselves in the world, not through the description of an objective reality but as potentiality: "Is it not the function of poetry to establish another world – that corresponds to other possibilities of existence, to possibilities that would be most deeply our own?" (2008, pp. 270-271). Literature, thus, plays a constitutive role in Ricoeur's existential hermeneutics. For Ricoeur, the reading of literature is not so much concerned with the author's intention or hidden meaning of a text; rather, we read to understand ourselves "in front of the text" (1981).

Ricoeur's argument for literature as existential self-understanding has been taken up in the literary field of what has been termed post-critique (Felski, 2008). As the name alludes to, post-critique attempts to go beyond literary studies' dominating practice of reading as criticism, of demasking the text as bearer of ideology etc. (Ricoeur's "hermeneutics of suspicion"). Instead, post-critique attempts to read in front of the text, engaging with literature, not as criticism, but as a way of understanding oneself in the world. According to Rita Felski, this is a way of reading that rarely has been the attention of literary studies but is how "ordinary" people often engage with literature. On a similar note, Eve Sedgwick has criticized cultural studies' shortcomings when it comes to assessing art-making practices of lay people. Instead of attending to these practices in the default setting of "paranoid reading" we need to acknowledge, e.g., the art-making practices of sick people with a "reparative reading" (Sedgwick, 2003) by tuning into and acknowledging how people engage with the objects of culture to find meaning and purpose.

Felski argues for four modes of textual engagement that offer an existential way of reading: *recognition*, *enchantment*, *knowledge*, and *shock*. We argue that several of these modes are helpful in understanding how reading and writing might alleviate the trauma of cancer. A cautionary note should be made on the fact that Felski's interest is in reading, not writing; still, we find her modes fruitful to understand aspects of the creative writing groups. We thus use these modes as *sensitizing concepts* (Blumer, 1954), not to be illustrated by the empirical material but rather to help us consider what affordances reading and writing might open towards. Furthermore, in the emerging field of narrative medicine, Rita Charon and her colleagues argue for creative writing and close reading as the "signature method" of narrative medicine in clinical education (Charon, Herman and Devlin, 2016; Charon et al., 2017). According to Charon close reading and creative writing involve *attention*, *representation*, and *affiliation*, underscoring how our attentive openness and curiosity are required for nuanced representations that might open for intersubjectivity and affiliation between caregiver and patients.

The Writing Groups

The participants in the three writing groups were recruited through a center for patient treatment at Oslo University Hospital, Radiumhospitalet, which published information on its website and on the Cancer Society's pages. Around 10 people signed up for each course, mostly women but also some men. All participants have or have had a cancer diagnosis, but they were in different treatment phases with different prognoses. The participants thus had common experiences related to receiving a cancer diagnosis and further treatment, but in terms of age and background, it was a heterogeneous group. No one knew each other from before. All the interviews in the first two courses were conducted digitally and then transcribed. In the last group, a questionnaire was distributed to participants.

As course managers, we strived to establish a safe and trust-based framework around the meetings. After all, the participants wrote about personal experiences and thoughts—often painful and difficult—and shared these with persons they had never met before. Sessions consisted of two hours in which the participants wrote based on tasks given by us. They also wrote at home to various writing prompts.

Each meeting was structured around specific themes that were introduced by us and exemplified through poetic texts written by established authors. The participants were then given a specific task and the writing session began. These sessions were short, rarely more than ten minutes. After the writing session, the participants read their own texts aloud, and all of us commented on and discussed them. The remarks were always constructive—we emphasized what we found interesting and what worked well, highlighting literary aspects of the texts such as details, rhythm, innovative metaphors, perspective, etc. It was never allowed to be critical towards the texts. We continued with more writing after a break and discussed the texts the participants had written at home.

The themes we introduced were, among others, how to use the imagination, how to use our senses, how to emphasize details and use metaphors, how to express abstract feelings, and how to create suspense. Examples of prompts given were: That day; A childhood memory; Trust; What we are looking for; What would you not change in your life? The tasks were open, but specific, and, with one exception, not related to cancer. The participants chose whether they wanted to write about cancer and share their own experiences of the disease and treatment or focus on other aspects. An important notion for us was that we always took the text and the writing self—the narrative self—as the point of departure, not the individual person and their experiences or medical histories. At the end of each course, the participants wrote a metatext about their thoughts and experiences from the group. Two groups met for eight sessions, the other for six.

Even though the feedback was overwhelmingly positive we would like to add that one of the participants did not feel she was ready to be exposed to writing about cancer and meeting the other cancer patients, and another mentioned that she would have liked more critical comments on her writings.

Reading and Writing in the Trauma of Cancer

Based on observations, interviews, and written texts from the participants we argue that reading and writing can be helpful through four dimensions: *(1) attention and recognition, (2) (re-)enchantment, (3) repair and (4) affiliation.*

(1) Reading and writing as attention and recognition

According to Felski, a central aspect of reading literature is how literary language opens toward forms of recognition. This is connected to the dialogic nature of selfhood where literature plays an important mediating role in self-formation, perhaps especially crucial in situations when one lacks acknowledgment or experiences feelings of estrangement: "I feel myself acknowledged; I am rescued from the fear of invisibility, from the terror of not being seen." For Felski, such experiences of recognition are not confined to "private or solitary reading; they resonate with special force when individuals come together to form a collective audience ... Aesthetic experience crystallizes an awareness of forming part of a broader community" (2008, p. 33).

Many of the experiences of the participants resonate with Felski's argument. The writing group opened for a verbalization of the cancer experience that was hard to voice in other parts of their lives, as one participant explained: "[cancer] is something that people would rather not have to deal with. And it's just so great to be part of a group who can bear to deal with it."

Another participant expressed her surprise and dismay that cancer was a word that was never used by the medical doctors or nurses at the treatment at the cancer hospital. She found this absurd and needed to write a text that explicitly could scream the word CANCER! out loud in capital letters. The writing group provided an arena for this where her reading led to a conversation where participants could share and discuss similar experiences. In the interview, this participant explained how her writing and the reception in the group opened another way of acknowledging cancer experiences:

> I've probably found my voice, I think, with a bit of gallows humour ... where I'm good ... it has opened a way to get out the gore that you don't share with people. I think that very often when you get out stuff in a group you get solace. But I'm not looking for solace, because it's not solace-able. And I think it's been wonderful to just get it out, whether it's gallows humour, anger or sadness or just sort of venting it to someone without someone giving me a hug or telling me that it's going to be all right ... so it has just been ... less false.

(2) Reading and writing as (re-)enchantment

The practice of writing and sharing, for many participants, is intimately connected with a re-enchantment of an often-disenchanted world.

> I think it has been incredibly interesting with the different ways [we] have attacked the tasks, because it makes you start to think about details. You start thinking about childhood memories. You start to think that almost anything can be rewritten, and it has been quite absurdly funny. I don't want to stop!

Furthermore, the enchantment is something that several of the participants relate to both one's own writing as well as the reception of the other participants' texts. As a young man in his late 20s explained:

> It's been great fun; I have been enthusiastically inspired by it … it caught my attention so much that I have not thought about anything else while the course has been running … it is moving in a very positive way. And then it is also very exciting to listen to all the others' contributions and versions, and I have learned a lot from that … It's a bit like when you've baked a fantastic cake and must deliver it after dinner, and everyone is looking forward to it. That's how I've felt. Hehe.

Several of the participants expressed similar experiences of euphoria and enthusiasm where the immersions in the group and the writing were deemed a form of enchanted self-forgetting and wonder. As one man expressed: "in terms of getting out of a cancer setting, it has been a very nice distraction. And not just a distraction, it has allowed me to focus on something very joyful, something very inspiring."

For some, the writing also involved a re-enchantment of the taken-for-granted everyday world. An example of the latter can be found in one text where a female participant writes about how she wakes up early due to the aftereffects of the treatment, but where this change of rhythm allows for a time of possibility where she can use that spare time to send off her children and husband with expressions of love: "how many times do I get to say I love you?" But as this woman also ponders: this opportunity in her everyday life is intimately linked to a literary language that makes the experience visible, explicit, and sharable.

(3) Reading and writing as repair

For several of the participants, the writing and its importance went beyond a recognition and enchantment and involved therapeutic aspects in how writing explicitly dealt with the trauma of cancer as a form of working through. As one man explained:

> I was given a space to look in the right direction in relation to my situation, which I think is one of the greatest strengths you can offer to a group of people with cancer ... The way you relate to it is almost the most decisive factor in how one feels. How you see the situation ... You may not have much power over the situation itself, but how you see it, you have all the power over that.

Similar expressions of writing as a way of interpreting and reconfiguring their situation were made by many participants. Others expressed that writing could be a way of documenting one's illness experience that otherwise was lost in a haze and how it could also help remember and process impressions during treatment.

A crucial part of writing as repair was how it facilitated verbalizing, at least partially, the trauma of the disease. For some, writing represented an opening for talking about cancer and their lives in the group that they rarely did with friends and family members. For others, their writing was a way of finding a language that could enable for conversations between the writer and family members around the most traumatic situations. "Liv," a woman in her 60s explained:

> ... the most important thing of all [I've learned] is to try ... and write, just put down the pen and write ... maybe not so much cancer experiences, but the fact that I'm going to die. Processing that thought ... and just writing it on a paper ... it does something to you when you dare to write it. It means that you might dare to say it to others. Because I hadn't even talked to the family about it before the writing course. But when I started writing it, it became real for me, and then I could also talk about it at home, which has been very good, above all for the children.

In her book *Unclaimed Experience: Trauma, Narrative, and History* Cathy Caruth sees trauma as "an unspeakable event," an experience that is not fully assimilated; it is a crisis without "simple knowledge" (1996, p. 5). According to Caruth, trauma thus asks questions that "can never be asked in a straightforward way, but must, indeed, also be spoken in a language that is always, somehow, literary: a language that defies, even as it claims our understanding" (ibid.).

Considering this in light of the quote from "Liv" might hint at the ability of literary language to verbalize aspects of trauma or represent openings out of trauma. Through her writing, "Liv" found another language that was productive, as it altered her ability to realize and talk about her condition and her future. According to Felski, the reading of literature can involve a "phenomenology of self-scrutiny" (2008). Looking at the quote of "Liv" as well as several of her poems we see how her writing also can involve, perhaps both a phenomenological and hermeneutical self-scrutiny, e.g., as seen in the following poem that reveals how poetic language and metaphor can give a *form* that opens for the contrasts between living with cancer and living with incurable cancer:

> Cancer sounds like the sound of the wind
> blowing through the trees
> when you are standing in an enchanted forest.
>
> Incurable cancer sounds like the silence
> in the conversation that never quite begins,
> the awkward silence that comes
> when you say you're going to die.

(4) Affiliation

A salient experience throughout the writing groups was the importance of the group that served as a creative community of exchanges of texts and discussions both on their cancer conditions as well as other aspects of life. For Charon and colleagues (2016), a crucial aspect of narrative medicine is how the sharing of reading and writing in groups in health care involves *affiliation*. The various texts' form-giving of experiences opened for an intersubjectivity and exchange between the participants that many deemed the most important aspect of the group practice. As a woman in her 40s explained:

> I felt a strong community with the others. And the reason for that is that we wrote and read to each other. It became such an extremely quick way to know the group. One thing is that we practiced expressing ourselves, another thing is that we practiced sharing with someone in a safe space with little performance anxiety. Being part of a group that has similar experiences was very strong and important. It was very special. ... this thing about cancer is quite taboo ... it's something people would rather not have to deal with. And it's so nice to be in a group where everyone is forced to deal with it.

Many participants highlighted the community of the group and how this was facilitated by the sharing and exchange of writing, making people feel they "knew each other, without actually knowing each other," as one said. Another aspect, as the quote above mentions, is how the group facilitated an openness to verbalize cancer experiences through writing and telling, underscoring the need for what William Randall (2016) terms *narrative care* and *narrative environments* in health care. And furthermore, as Arthur Frank argues: "Narratability means that events and lives are affirmed as being worth telling and thus worth living" (2002, p. 111). For the participants the group created a safe space where their stories and need for telling could be validated: if it was the need for addressing cancer experiences or other facets of life—the latter also being crucial for many: "we are after all not just a cancer diagnosis." All the participants were grateful for being given the opportunity to participate in the group, and everyone wanted that this should be offered to other cancer patients. The unique combination of writing and reading in a group was deemed helpful as one man explained:

> Listening to the texts, or commenting on texts, being part of the group: It has put me in a 'state of being,' a way of thinking and being. A rhythm that has been reflected directly in the texts I have written. So that has been incredibly helpful.

Conclusion

In *Uses of Literature* (2008) Felski asks the following question: "Under what conditions does literature come to play a mediating role in this drama of self-formation?" And she provides the following answer herself: "Often, it seems, when other forms of acknowledgment are felt to be lacking, when one feels estranged from or at odds with one's immediate milieu" (p. 33). We find Felski's perspective befitting when answering the overarching question we pose in this chapter: How can reading and writing be of help when living with the trauma of cancer? A central theme that runs across the four modes we have explored above is how, for so many of the participants, the writing and reading alleviated the loneliness of the disease. The process of writing and listening in a safe group setting of people living in the same situation could involve an openness towards an exchange of experiences that were not met elsewhere in the health care system. The groups could also function as a safe space outside of family and friends where the writing and the reception of the texts opened for a creative community that surprised the participants, but a community that was deemed necessary once it was experienced. Our experiences from the groups underpin the comments from the participants. The atmosphere in the room could sometimes be playful, and sometimes serious, but we always experienced it as good and trusting. There was a lot of fun and laughter, but also tears. It seemed to us, that the participants deeply empathized with each other, showed great care, and gave constructive comments.

At the heart of this group practice is *poetic language*, a language that in both the participants' and our experiences is productive—it is a world-making endeavor. It is this aspect of literature that Felski sees as fundamental in the act of recognition: not merely as repetition of what is already there but as making something known: "…not just the previously known, but the becoming known. Something that may have been sensed in a vague, diffuse, or semi-conscious way now takes on a distinct shape, is amplified, heightened, or made newly visible" (2008, p. 25). It is precisely this aspect of literature that makes Ricoeur see reading, not as duplication, but as a metamorphosis, in the reader (1976).

The world-making phenomenon of poetic language might be especially important related to different kinds of traumatic experiences and in a situation of serious illness. In his book *Poetry as Survival* (2002) Gregory Orr argues for the sense-making and stabilizing powers of lyric poetry in the face of trauma. But Orr also acknowledges the importance of an audience. As he writes in a recent reflection: "To create a poem or story in itself affirms its writer's individual dignity and identity, but to present that writing to an appropriate and appreciative audience ushers the ... author even further out of isolation and back into the human community" (2023, p. xiv). We are also here reminded of Arthur Frank's remark that a crucial goal for narrative ethics is "to help people generate new imaginations that can restart dialogues." (Frank, 2014, p. 17). Echoing Orr and Frank, we argue that creative writing and reading are encouraging interventions for processing and transforming traumatic life experiences that might facilitate community as well as life-affirming openings.

Reference List

Blumer, H. (1954) 'What is wrong with social theory?' *American Sociological Review,* 19(1), pp. 3-10. doi: https://doi.org/10.2307/2088165

Bundesen, B. et al. (2020) 'REWRITALIZE: Participatory creative writing groups led by authors in collaboration with mental health care professionals for people experiencing severe mental illness,' *Nordic Journal of Arts, Culture and Health, 2*(2), 140-147. doi: https://doi.org/10.18261/issn.2535-7913-2020-02-05

Caruth, C. (1996) *Unclaimed experience: trauma, narrative, and history.* Baltimore: John Hopkins University Press.

Charon, R., Hermann, N., and Devlin, M. J. (2016) 'Close reading and creative writing in clinical education: teaching attention, representation, and affiliation,' *Academic Medicine: Journal of the Association of American Medical Colleges,* 91(3), pp. 345-50. PMID: 26200577. PMCID: PMC4721945. doi: https://doi.org/10.1097/acm.0000000000000827

Charon, R. et al. (2017) *The principles and practice of narrative medicine.* New York. Oxford University Press. doi: https://doi.org/10.1093/med/9780199360192.001.0001

Costa, A.C. and Abreu, M.V. (2018) 'Expressive and creative writing in the therapeutic context: from the different concepts to the development of writing therapy programs,' *Psychologia,* 61(1), pp. 69-86. doi: https://doi.org/10.14195/1647-8606_61-1_4

Felski, R. (2008) *Uses of literature. Hoboken: John Wiley Sons.*

Frank, A.W. (2014) 'Narrative ethics as dialogical story-telling,' *Narrative Ethics: The Role of Stories in Bioethics,* special report, *Hastings Center Report,* 44(1), pp. 16-20. doi: https://doi.org/10.1002/hast.263

Frank, A.W. (2002) 'Why study people's stories? The dialogical ethics of narrative analysis,' *International Journal of Qualitative Methods,* 1(1), pp. 109-117. doi: https://doi.org/10.1177/160940690200100102

Gillam, T. (ed.) (2018) 'Creative writing, literature, storytelling and mental health practice,' in *Creativity, wellbeing and mental health practice*, London: Palgrave Pivot, Cham, pp. 101-116. doi: https://doi.org/10.1007/978-3-319-74884-9_7

Gorelick, K. (2005) 'Poetry therapy,' in Malchiodi, C.A. (ed.) *Expressive therapies*, New York and London: Guilford Press, pp. 111-140.

Gubar, S. (2016). *Reading and writing cancer: how words heal.* New York: WW Norton & Company.

Hubbard, G. and Forbat, L. (2012) 'Cancer as biographical disruption: constructions of living with cancer,' *Support Care Cancer*, 20, pp. 2033-2040. doi: https://doi.org/10.1007/s00520-011-1311-9

Jurecic, A. (2012) *Illness as narrative.* Pittsburgh: University of Pittsburgh Press. doi: https://doi.org/10.2307/j.ctt5hjr8p

Orr, G. (2002) *Poetry as survival.* Athens: University of Georgia Press.

Orr, G. (2023) 'Foreword,' in Lehmann, O.V. and Synnes, O. (eds.) *A Poetic Language of Ageing*, London: Bloomsbury Academic, pp. xi-xiv.

Randall, W.L. (2016) 'Narrative environments for narrative care: the need to honor people's stories,' *International Journal for Human Caring*, 20(3), pp. 142-145. doi: https://doi.org/10.20467/1091-5710-20.3.142

Ricoeur, P. (1976) *Interpretation theory: discourse and the surplus of meaning.* Fort Worth: Texas Christian University Press.

Ricoeur, P. [1970 (1981)] 'The hermeneutical function of distanciation,' in *Hermeneutics and the human sciences: essays on language, action and interpretation*, translated from the French and introduced by John B. Thomson (ed.). Cambridge: Cambridge University Press, pp. 131-144.

Ricoeur, P. [1975 (2008)] *The rule of metaphor: the creation of meaning in language*, translated from the French by Robert Czerny, Kathleen McLaughlin and John Costello. London and New York: Routledge Classics.

Romm, K.L., Synnes, O. and Bondevik, H. (2022) 'Creative writing as a means to recover from early psychosis – experiences from a group intervention,' *Arts & Health*, pp. 1-14. doi: https://doi.org/10.1080/17533015.2022.2130379

Sedgwick, E.K. (2003) *Touching feeling: affect, pedagogy, performativity.* Durham: Duke University Press.

Synnes, O., Romm, K.L. and Bondevik, H. (2021) 'The poetics of vulnerability: creative writing among young adults in treatment for psychosis in light of Ricoeu's and Kristeva's philosophy of language and subjectivity,' *Medicine, Health Care and Philosophy*, 24(2), pp. 173-187. PMID: 33453017. PMCID: PMC8128797. doi: https://doi.org/10.1007/s11019-020-09998-5

2.2.2

Narrative Redemptions for Post-Traumatic Loneliness: The Therapeutic Potential of Qualitative Research in the Aftermath of Trauma

Jacob Y. Stein

College of Management, Israel

Rivka Tuval-Mashiach

College of Management, Israel

Abstract

The notion that trauma and story are interlinked is anything but novel. Indeed, the literature is rife with theoretical approaches that attempt to delineate the therapeutic qualities of telling one's story. Nevertheless, while narrative research has advanced rapidly in the past decades, it is all too often the case that such advances have not been incorporated into the literature discussing the healing qualities of narrative and narration in the post-traumatic context. In the proposed chapter we aim to explicate one healing attribute that a narrative research sensibility may offer for individuals in the aftermath of trauma. To this end, we elaborate on the nature of the loneliness that may consolidate after trauma and demonstrate how this loneliness is compatible with the fundamentals of narrative research. Specifically, we argue that loneliness in the aftermath of trauma is in essence one of experiential isolation (i.e., the notion that one must confront one's experience and cope with its ramifications alone). Conversely, narrative research methods guided by hermeneutics (the art of understanding) and phenomenology (the investigation of lived experience) may present suitable solutions. Compatibility is demonstrated by juxtaposing the philosophical-methodological underpinnings and practical applications of such methodologies with the intersubjective needs and challenges presented by trauma victims. Trauma researchers are then encouraged to engage in more research endeavors of this kind as an ethical responsibility as well as serving a means to further scientific knowledge.

***

The physical and mental salutary benefits associated with narration and disclosure in the aftermath of traumatic experiences are now well documented (Pennebaker, 1999). Indeed, in the past two decades, trauma focused interventions wherein the act of narration is pivotal have proliferated. These include narrative exposure therapy (Robjant and Fazel, 2010), testimony therapy (McKinney, 2007), and narrative reconstruction (Peri and Gofman, 2014), to name but a few. Charles Hoge (2011, p. 550), has gone as far as stating that narration is "probably the most therapeutic component" in the treatment of veterans dealing with combat related trauma.

Numerous underlying mechanisms may explain this healing effect of narrative in the aftermath of trauma (Pennebaker, 1999). Among these are the understanding that through narration traumatized individuals attempt to share the burden of the traumatic experience so as not to carry it alone. In a similar vein, some argue that following severe traumatic instances, the act of narration generates a circle of witnesses and works to form a sense of communalization (van de Merwe and Gobodo-Madikizela, 2007). Such explanations allude to the realization that trauma irrevocably compromises several intersubjective needs that relate to our innate need for empathic or intersubjective attunement and emotional understanding (Wilson and Thomas, 2004). The culmination of such compromises in the aftermath of trauma is ultimately an agonizing sense of loneliness (Stein and Tuval-Mashiach, 2015).

According to Jacob Stein and Rivka Tuval-Mashiach (2015) this loneliness, which they term *experiential loneliness,* is rooted in trauma victims' strong belief that those who have never experienced the trauma do not and cannot understand what they have gone through or what they have been experiencing since the trauma. They may feel that others do not wish to hear, might fail to believe, or otherwise remain apathetic to their suffering. This loneliness is rooted in the ineffable nature of traumatic experiences, as it involves a conviction that the trauma cannot be adequately conveyed or articulated. Constantly negotiating what Dan Bar-On referred to as *the indescribable and undiscussable* nature of their traumatic pasts (Bar-On, 1999), trauma victims often face the dialectic between the will to disclose and the will to conceal what they have undergone for fear of what such disclosure may entail (Herman, 1992). Furthermore, this loneliness entails an inner desire that others might come to know and share the pain that the trauma fosters. Shrowded in the shadows of their lonely experiences, there may come a need for what Robert Stolorow (2014, p. 81) identifies as *emotional dwelling*, wherein "one leans into the other's emotional pain and participates in it." Nevertheless, at the same time, there exists a persuasion that this may never come to be. Thus, the loneliness at hand reaffirms itself whenever the desire for a shared inner reality fails to materialize. Such failure occurs, in part, because from the trauma victim's perspective, not everyone bears the capabilities necessary for such attunement and not all trauma victims are prepared to give others the opportunity to prove themselves worthy.

The realization then crystalizes, that interpersonal interactions, may result in additional pain in the form of loneliness on the behalf of trauma victims. One such interpersonal interaction is that which is formed within the research dynamics between researcher and participants. Hence, it is imperative to delineate a way of listening that may possibly minimize such a predicament. In the present chapter, we argue that qualitative research methods, especially those grounded in hermeneutics, phenomenology, and narrative sensibilities, offer a comprehensive methodological (i.e., philosophical, procedural, and analytical) foundation that may facilitate the understanding of the traumatic experience from the point of view of the victims, and thus ameliorate their loneliness and foster a potential redemption.

Towards a Narrative Redemption for Post-Traumatic Loneliness: The Three Pillars of Understanding

A wide range of qualitative research methods rely on the above-mentioned foundations of hermeneutics, phenomenology, and narrative—the three pillars of understanding. These may harbor a redemptive nature in regard to trauma victims' loneliness for, as Gergen, Josselson and Freeman note: "In all of these cases there is an abiding sense that our knowledge is not *about* you, but *with* you" (2015, p. 7, italics in the original). Moreover, the fact that such qualitative approaches solicit stories, and are particularly interested in the lived experiences embedded in and revealed by the narratives, may already bear therapeutic properties (Birch and Miller, 2000; Giorgio, 2009). Such endeavors are particularly interested in understanding the depth, richness, and uniqueness of the experiences under investigation (Gergen, Josselson and Freeman, 2015). Qualitative researchers engaged so in the research process, may become emotionally involved in the experiences of their research participants, and thus become witnesses to those experiences:

> Common across all such inquiry is a concern not only with illuminating the lived experience of human beings but also . . . with sensitizing ourselves to their worlds and imagining ways in which they might be encountered with appreciation. (ibid., p. 4)

Such concern in the research participants may breach trauma victims' experiential isolation bolstered by the confinements of a language that cannot covney a traumatic experience. Narrative facilitates an attempt to understand beyond the given words and what is in the text, to go deeper and reveal that which is conveyed between the lines, in the subtext, in the content and the form of utterances (Lieblich, Tuval-Mashiach and Zilber, 1998). A relationally-oriented narrative interviewer would be inclined to inquire empathically into each experience that participants bring forth, while embracing a relational and caring attitude (Josselson, 2013). Hence an opportunity to penetrate one's experiential isolation materializes. Such an approach is philosophically and methodologically rooted in hermeneutics and phenomenology.

Hermeneutics, most simply, is "the art of understanding" (Schleiermacher, 1998, p. 5). Phenomenology, ultimately refers to the investigation of lived experience (van Manen, 1990). The hermeneutist strives to *understand* that which the text or the "Other" reveals and that which it implies, or otherwise what it *means.* The hermeneutist does not aspire to *explain* why this is so (although an explanation inevitably assists understanding). Conversely, phenomenology is an attempt to see things afresh, and focuses on understanding experiences for what they are or how they present themselves to one's consciousness rather than examining them through our preconceived theoretical points of view. Phenomenology, much like hermeneutics, urges the researcher to keep to a descriptive rather than explanatory understanding. A comprehensive and exhaustive delineation of either philosophical tradition is far beyond the scope of this chapter. Below, however, we explicate some aspects of these traditions and their methodological applications that render qualitative the research endeavors constituted on their premises most suitable for addressing trauma victims' loneliness. By juxtaposing the different aspects of these philosophical-methodological approaches with the intersubjective needs and challenges of trauma victims, we demonstrate how these approaches come together as a methodological gestalt that may address these intersubjective needs and work to, at least partially, redeem trauma victims of their sense of loneliness.

Hermeneutics: The Art of Understanding

Hermeneutically oriented researchers assume *a priori* that one does not adequately understand the phenomenon under investigation and must work hard if they are to change that. Moreover, if one wishes to understand, one needs the person who bears the experience to be willing to reveal it. Within the research interaction, the hermeneutically oriented researcher is there to learn from the participant and not the other way around; at least at first. The latter is the expert on the lived experience being investigated, while the former's task is to work rigorously to capture and understand that experience, or faithfully restore it (Josselson, 2004). Recall that for the trauma victim those who have not endured trauma are "out of the loop," so to speak. They are presumed, once again *a priori*, to be in a state of misunderstanding vis-à-vis the traumatic experience (Stolorow, 2014). Hence, somewhat paradoxically, when a researcher asks participants to share their experiences so he or she may understand how it is like from *their* personal perspective, he or she is implicitly conveying the message: "you were there, I was not. You know what it was like, I do not. Please teach me." Such an attitude may correspond with the trauma victim's conviction that those who have not been there cannot understand. Embracing this stance, the researcher then already demonstrates some understanding of what it is like to bear a traumatic experience, and thus may prove him or herself a worthy interlocutor, and potentially a "relational home" for the participants' emotional trauma (ibid.).

A second premise that is cardinal in hermeneutics is that an understanding of the *Other's* language is paramount for understanding the *Other*. Indeed, hermeneutics as an enterprise of the human sciences "is guided by the basic idea that language is a medium where I and world meet or, rather, manifest their original belonging together" (Gadamer, 2004, p. 469). For Hans-Georg Gadamer, this is an essential element of the merging of interpreter-interpreted horizons. Tracing this idea back to Friedrich Schleiermacher (1998), we find that to achieve understanding one must attend both to the language constituting the utterance and to the psychology of the utterer. People use words differently and may mean very different things even when using the same words. To understand an utterance, one must then have an excellent understanding of the language being used, but also a deep and broad understanding of the person who is using it (e.g., his cultural, experiential and political backgrounds). In order to engage in the hermeneutic endeavor, a researcher must then attempt to place oneself objectively and subjectively in the position of the narrator: objectively by learning the language as the narrator uses it, and subjectively by learning about the narrator's life and thinking (Schmidt, 2006). In our case, learning of the trauma at hand.

According to Chris van de Merwe and Pumla Gobodo-Madikizela: "Extreme trauma is 'unspeakable' precisely because of the inadequacy of language to fully convey victims' experiences" (2007, pp. 25-26). There are undeniably additional reasons for trauma to become incommunicable (e.g., Bar-On, 1999), However, the ineptitude of language as a medium for conveying experiential meaning is reminiscent of the hermeneutic endeavor. When trauma victims share their experiences, they hope that their experiences will be apprehended beyond what their words may reveal. From a hermeneutic perspective there comes the recognition that while all utterances are inevitably finite, they all harbor infinite meanings that were not uttered but nevertheless animate by the utterance and are inveterately a part of it (Gadamer, 2004). Therefore, understanding must aim to find what is present between the lines, what the words mean beyond what is presented on the surface, but not in opposition to it (Josselson, 2004). From a hermeneutic perspective, "meaning reduced to what is stated is always distorted meaning" (Gadamer, 2004, p. 464).

Taking into consideration the inevitable differences between the interpreter and the interpreted (e.g., belonging to different cultures, different times, personal backgrounds, etc.). Schleiermacher notes that it may seem that understanding may never take place because narrator and audience inevitably inhabit different psychological states and therefore their languages bear different meanings (1998). However, he argues, if we remember that there *are* differences and make an effort to uncover them, some understanding may yet transpire, even if this understanding may never be complete. Arguably, our capacity to understand one another and overcome the aforementioned psychological gap may first and foremost be attributed to the fact that we all share a general human nature (Schmidt, 2006). Applying this realization to the research practice, analysis is carried out first ideographically (i.e., per participant) and only then meanings are compared between participants' accounts (Josselson, 2013).

Both the guiding premise and its methodical application may prove beneficial for the trauma victim. That is, both the acknowledgment that the participant's experience must be apprehended in its uniqueness (i.e., idiographically) and that at once it also shares common features with the experience of others (i.e., other trauma survivors) may serve to breach the fortifications of experiential isolation. The former validating the participant's notion that he or she has undergone an extraordinary experience, and the latter asserting that they are not the only ones who have undergone such an experience, and thus that some understanding might yet be achieved.

The third aspect of hermeneutics that is of crucial importance is the hermeneutic circle—a theme that runs like a thread through the entire hermeneutic literature (Schmidt, 2006). The concept of the hermeneutic circle relates to the realization that to understand anything we must understand it as a "whole," but we do this by examining the parts that constitute the whole. However, we also understand the parts in light of the preconceived whole. A cyclical transition between parts and whole, therefore, represents a cycle wherein understanding is perpetually refined. Misunderstanding then transpires when our understanding of either whole or parts, or the manner in which they relate to each other, remains for some reason inadequate or significantly lacking.

Returning to trauma, we may then begin to understand why traumatized individuals feel that their experiences are irrevocably misunderstood by those who have not personally experienced the traumatic scene. In their eyes, the latter may never understand what "war," "rape" or "torture" truly mean because they have no access to the smaller particles of these experiences: the smells, the sounds, the sensations, the trepidation, the helplessness, the desperation, the loss of control, the guilt and the shame. The hermeneutic circle then seems to be forever shattered as audiences may only have access to their own preconceptions of these constructs. It is the task of the hermeneutist to seek those lost parts and reconstruct the whole via rigorous work. Implementing such a notion in research is twofold. First, any interpretative endeavor demands an iterative reading of the research materials (Rennie, 2012). Secondly, these iterative readings begin with a reading of the whole and only then a close reading (i.e., analysis) of the parts (i.e., the smallest units of meanings: words, clauses, metaphors, etc.), finally returning to the whole and understanding the relations between the various units of meaning.

Phenomenology: Researching Lived Experience

Invariably, phenomenology is the term used for research focused on lived-experience; and while there are several diverse phenomenological methods, it is this aspect that is the most prominent common denominator of them all (Finlay, 2011). Indeed, whenever a research method claims to possess phenomenological properties, it is claiming to investigate the intricacies and nuances of experience as it is lived-through. To accomplish this, the phenomenologist might attempt to imaginatively transpose her or himself into the other's experience as it is being disclosed (Finlay, 2008; Spiegelberg, 1980). Concomitantly, Edmund Husserl's famous creed that we must return "to the things themselves," is widely reiterated by proponents of phenomenological research (Finlay, 2011; Giorgi, 2009; van Manen, 1990). It is this return to the things themselves, to lived experience as it is and has been experienced, that makes research methods informed by phenomenology some of the most intersubjectively oriented encounters out there.

A governing idea of phenomenology stems from the acknowledgment that we are all initially set in the *natural attitude*, whereby we experience our everyday world in a pre-reflective taken-for-granted manner. Such understanding is invariably distorted by our preconceptions and therefore we cannot see "the things themselves" as they (presumably) *truly are*. From a phenomenological stance, in order to return to the things themselves we must find a way to *bracket* our preconceptions and thus reduce their effects on our perceptual intake of the phenomena we hope to understand (Giorgi, 2009).

Husserl's term for such reductions is the Greek *epoché* (ἐποχή, pronounced: epokhē), meaning *suspension*. Husserl offers several such reductive reflective suspending processes that must be embraced when adopting the phenomenological attitude (Finlay, 2011, pp. 47-49). In an attempt to understand subjective experience one must, according to Husserl, eschew understandings achieved by prior scientific projects (i.e., the epoché of the natural sciences). One should also set aside the most taken for granted assumptions that govern our everyday understanding of the phenomenon at hand (i.e., the epoché of the natural attitude). Additionally, Husserl suggests that one must step aside from one's own subjective experience to see the phenomenon transcendentally. That is, beyond the situational and contingent (i.e., the transcendental reduction). The employment of such bracketing, for trauma victims, may prove to be highly beneficial. Their experiences, examined from such a stance, then become relatively safeguarded from distortion and misunderstanding rooted in preconception.

Hermeneutic phenomenological research attempts to be evocative (Todres and Galvin, 2008; van Manen, 1990, 2014). As such "Sometimes it languages things we already know tacitly but have not articulated in depth" (Finlay, 2011, p. 10). Moreover, when grafted, phenomenology and hermeneutics recognize the Gordian knot-tying experience to language, and hence realize that one has the capacity to ground experience in novel words, word combinations, and neologisms (Freeman and Vagle, 2013, p. 725). This may bring about the realization that "There are no nonverbal experiences, only experiences not yet put into words," and therefore "it is not necessarily language that is limited, but we who fail to see its potentialities" (ibid., p. 734).

This sensitivity to language offers a response to trauma victims' sense that there exists a linguistic gap preventing the conveyance of traumatic experiences. As narrative researchers grounded in phenomenology repeatedly assert (Josselson, 2013), it is through sincere dialog that a breaching of the linguistic divide may become possible. If, as it seems from many trauma narratives (Stein, 2017; Stein and Tuval-Mashiach, 2015), trauma harbors a sense of experiential isolation and a fear that others will not understand, or that others might attempt to fit the experience into their own preconceptions, then embracing the phenomenological attitude may indeed be the antidote. As noted, phenomenologists attempt to understand the experience under investigation by feeling with the participants. Hence:

> Phenomenological research is potentially **transformative** for both researcher and participant. It offers individuals the opportunity to be **witnessed** in their experience and allows them to '**give voice**' to what they are going through. It also open [sic] new possibilities for both researcher and researched to **make sense of** the experience in focus. (Finlay, 2011, p. 10, emphasis in the original)

Such a transformative process culminates in the writing up of the research. Van Manen notes that: "In the reflective process of writing, the researcher not only engages in analysis but also aims to express the noncognitive, ineffable and pathic aspects of meaning that belong to the phenomenon" (2014, p. 240). A researcher attempting to faithfully express the traumatic experience in this manner may truly be of service for a participant struggling for words of his or her own. Hence, the research report may facilitate not only the participants' need for self-understanding, but also serve as a herald that will give voice to the experience. In this respect, phenomenological reports may be of great significance as they take into consideration also the experience and resonance which the text might evoke in its readers (van Manen, 2014).

Working to express the traumatic experience in this way may once again penetrate the confinements of one's posttraumatic experiential and communicative isolation. It is in this way that their suffering may be given a voice, and the communalization of trauma achieved.

> When trauma survivors hear that enough of the truth of their experience has been understood, remembered, and retold – no one who did not experience their trauma can ever grasp all of this truth – then the circle of communalization is complete. (Shay, 2002, p. 144).

Conclusion

It has been argued in the past that therapy and qualitative research share some significant attributes (Birch and Miller, 2000; Bondi, 2013; Giorgio, 2009; Rossetto, 2014). However, most attention in previous works has been given to the act of soliciting stories within the research practice, and very little attention has been devoted to the underlying philosophical premises guiding the research as a whole, or to the link to specific needs of a given population. Thus, the present chapter's contribution to this realization may be twofold. First, that this kind of research is particularly suitable for addressing trauma survivors' intersubjective needs; and second, that the philosophical underpinnings of the research (i.e., hermeneutics and phenomenology), and not only its execution (e.g., the interview), may have a significant role in shaping the researcher-participant relationship, thus contributing to a therapeutic effect. Naturally, to maximize this effect, participants must be to some extent informed of the research process, its guiding premises, and overall approach, as well as receive a copy of the final report, or better yet, be re-contacted and invited once again to engage in dialog concerning the emerging understanding with the researcher.

Finlay asserts that as therapists: "Every time we seek to know and understand more about our service users, we are doing research" (2011, p. 6). Considering the above, we would like to turn this statement around and claim that for experientially isolated trauma survivors seeking an attentive audience, for those struggling for words to represent their experience, and ultimately for those striving to be fully understood, an informed participation in a hermeneutically and phenomenologically orientated qualitative research may be a somewhat therapeutic interaction. Thus, engaging in such research may not only contribute to our knowledge of trauma's work, but also potentially aid the individual trauma survivors participating in the research Though it is imperative to distinguish research from therapy, and researchers must be wary of crossing the lines within research settings, we urge that it is our ethical obligation, especially in a field as dominated by quantitative endeavors as trauma studies, to conduct more hermeneutically and phenomenologically guided qualitative research that delves into the lived experiences of trauma and its aftermath. In so doing we may give voice to those bearing such experiences, and as researchers, we come to learn of their nature and thus become witnesses to them. Nevertheless, as Liz Bondi notes, the hope is "not that knowledge serves as cure but that our work enriches meaning in its honesty about the limits to knowledge and the losses intrinsic to knowledge" (2013, p. 16). Such an approach may also reduce our participants' loneliness.

It is, nevertheless, important to add necessary caveats. While narrative medicine holds promise in regard to the experiential loneliness that may become manifest in the post-traumatic reality, it is by no way a simple route to healing. The pitfalls of silence, including conspiracies of silence (e.g., Danieli, 1984) make the challenge ever so real. Moreover, much like the lack of agreement and limitations regarding the healing processes involved in storytelling (Kaminer, 2006), one may expect limitations regarding the thesis depicted in this chapter. Nonetheless, it is compelling to examine the potential promise of such ideas not only for clinicians (Orange, 2009, 2011) but also for researchers who face experiential loneliness in the aftermath of trauma.

Reference List

Bar-On, D. (1999) *The indescribable and the undiscussable: reconstructing human discourse after trauma.* Budapest: Central European Universities Press.

Birch, M. and Miller, T. (2000) 'Inviting intimacy: the interview as therapeutic opportunity,' *International Journal of Social Research Methodology*, 3(3), pp. 189-202. doi: https://doi.org/10.1080/13645570050083689

Bondi, L. (2013) 'Research and therapy: generating meaning and feeling gaps,' *Qualitative Inquiry* 19(1), pp. 9-19. doi: https://doi.org/10.1177/1077800412462978

Danieli, Y. (1984). Psychotherapist's participation in the conspiracy of silence about the Holocaust, *Psychoanalytic Psychology*, 1(1), pp. 23-42.

Finlay, L. (2008) 'A dance between the reduction and reflexivity: explicating the "phenomenological psychological attitude,"' *Journal of Phenomenological Psychology*, 39(1), pp. 1-32. doi: https://doi.org/10.1163/156916208X311601

Finlay, L. (2011) *Phenomenology for therapists: researching the livedworld.* Chichester, England: Wiley-Blackwell.

Freeman, M. and Vagle, M.D. (2013) 'Grafting the intentional relation of hermeneutics and phenomenology in linguisticality,' *Qualitative Inquiry*, 19(9), pp. 725-735. doi: https://doi.org/10.1177/1077800413500933

Gadamer, H.-G. [1960 (2004)] *Truth and method.* 2nd revised edn. Translated from the German by John Weinsheimer and Donald G. Marshall. London and New York: Continuum.

Gergen, K.J., Josselson, R. and Freeman, M. (2015) 'The promise of qualitative inquiry,' *American Psychologist*, 70(1), pp. 1-9. PMID: 25581004. doi: https://doi.org/10.1037/a0038597

Giorgio, G. (2009) 'Traumatic truths and the gift of telling,' *Qualitative Inquiry*, 15(1), pp. 149-167. doi: https://doi.org/10.1177/1077800408318300

Herman, J.L. (1992) *Trauma and Recovery*, Basic Books, New York.

Hoge, C.W. (2011) 'Interventions for war-related posttraumatic stress disorder: meeting veterans where they are,' *JAMA: Journal of the American Medical Association*, 306(5), pp. 549-551. PMID: 21813436. doi: https://doi.org/10.1001/jama.2011.1096

Josselson, R. (2004) 'The hermeneutics of faith and the hermeneutics of suspicion,' *Narrative Inquiry*, 14(1), pp. 1-28. doi: https://doi.org/10.1075/ni.14.1.01jos

Josselson, R. (2013). *Interviewing for qualitative inquiry: a relational approach.* New York, NY: Guilford Press.

Kaminer, D. (2006) 'Healing processes in trauma narratives: a review,' *South African Journal of Psychology*, 36(3), 481-49. doi: https://doi.org/10.1177/008124630603600304

Lieblich, A., Tuval-Mashiach, R. and Zilber, T. (1998) *Narrative research: reading, analysis and interpretation.* London: Sage.

McKinney, K. (2007) "Breaking the conspiracy of silence': testimony, traumatic memory, and psychotherapy with survivors of political violence,' *ETHOS: Journal of the Society for Psychological Anthropology*, 35(3), pp. 265-299. doi: https://doi.org/10.1525/eth.2007.35.3.265

Orange, D.M. (2009). *Thinking for clinicians: philosophical resources for contemporary psychoanalysis and the humanistic psychotherapies.* York, NY: Taylor & Francis.

Orange, D.M. (2011). *The suffering stranger: hermeneutics for everyday clinical practice.* New York, NY: Routledge.

Pennebaker, J.W. (1999) 'Forming a story: the health benefits of narrative,' *Journal of Clinical Psychology*, 55(10), pp. 1243-1254. PMID: 11045774. doi: https://doi/10.1002/(SICI)1097-4679(199910)55:10%3C1243::AID-JCLP6%3E3.0.CO;2-N

Peri, T. and Gofman, M. (2014) 'Narrative reconstruction: an integrative intervention module for intrusive symptoms in PTSD patients,' *Psychological Trauma: Theory, Research, Practice, and Policy*, 6(2), pp. 176-183. doi: https://doi/10.1037/a0031965

Rennie, D.L. (2012) 'Qualitative research as methodical hermeneutics,' *Psychological Methods*, 17(3), pp. 385-398. PMID: 22823104. doi: https://doi.org/10.1037/a0029250

Robjant, K. and Fazel, M. (2010) 'The emerging evidence for narrative exposure therapy: a review,' *Clinical Psychology Review*, 30(8), pp. 1030-1039. PMID: 20832922. doi: https://doi.org/10.1016/j.cpr.2010.07.004

Rossetto, K.R. (2014) 'Qualitative research interviews: assessing the therapeutic value and challenges,' *Journal of Social and Personal Relationships*, 31(4), pp. 482-489. doi: https://doi.org/10.1177/0265407514522892

Schleiermacher, F. D.E. (1998 [1828-1829]) *Hermeneutics and criticism: and other writings*. Translated from the German by Andrew Bowie (ed.) Cambridge: Cambridge University Press.

Schmidt, L.K. (2006) *Understanding hermeneutics*. Durham: Acumen Publishing.

Spiegelberg, H. (1980) 'Putting ourselves into the place of others: toward a phenomenology of imaginary self transposal,' *Human Studies*, 3(2), pp. 169-173.

Shay, J. (2002) *Odysseus in America: combat trauma and the trials of homecoming*. New York, NY: Scribner.

Stein, J.Y. (2017) 'The meaning of 'loneliness' for traumatized veterans: a semiotic investigation of veterans' written narratives,' *Journal of Veterans Studies*, 2(2), pp. 121-139. doi: https://doi.org/10.21061/jvs.v2i2.19

Stein, J.Y. and Tuval-Mashiach, R. (2015) 'Loneliness and isolation in life-stories of Israeli veterans of combat and captivity,' *Psychological Trauma: Theory, Research, Practice and Policy*, 7(2), pp. 122-130. doi: https://doi.org/10.1037/a0036936

Stolorow, R.D. (2014) 'Undergoing the situation: emotional dwelling is more than empathic understanding,' *International Journal of Psychoanalytic Self Psychology*, 9(1), pp. 80-83. doi: https://doi.org/10.1080/15551024.2014.857750

Todres, L. and Galvin, K.T. (2008) 'Embodied interpretation: a novel way of evocatively re-presenting meanings in phenomenological research,' *Qualitative Research*, 8(5), pp. 568-583. doi: https://doi.org/10.1177/1468794108094866

van de Merwe, C. and Gobodo-Madikizela, P. (2007) *Narrating our healing: perspectives on working through trauma*. Cambridge: Cambridge Scholars.

van Manen, M. (1990) *Researching lived experience: human science for an action sensitive pedagogy*. New York: State University of New York Press.

van Manen, M. (2014) *Phenomenology of practice: meaning-giving methods in phenomenological research and writing*. Walnut Creek: Left Coast Press.

Wilson, J.P. and Thomas, R.B. (2004) *Empathy in the treatment of trauma and PTSD*. New York, NY: Brunner-Routledge.

2.2.3

Narrative and the Mental Health System: Removing Horror from Mental Health Experiences and Environments

Emma McKenzie

York St John University, England

Abstract

How do stories impact the way in which we define ourselves in the world? What does the environment that we are placed in speak about us? How does it feel to be an in-patient in a mental health care system, or in fact to be a person working in that same system? In this chapter, I will discuss the way in which narrative structures can be used to examine the systems and processes within mental health care settings, as a way of highlighting the need for humanity to be a core component of all mental health care delivery in the West. The current environments in which we are placed in to recover, can become an intrusion into our inner stories, delving into un-narrated episodes of trauma in settings that reinforce binary opposition, where unhealthy power dynamics are played out between roles. Using extracts from a Practice Led PhD in creative writing to illustrate stories from mental health care settings, I aim to highlight the need for new stories to be created in the delivery of mental health care. One where humanity and community are a central focal point of support. The extracts of writing used within this chapter draw on autoethnographic research and my experience of working as an occupational therapist in the mental health care system in Britain over the last twenty years. This chapter highlights how principles of narrative medicine can be used to reimagine mental health care to inspire positive cultural change in places of recovery.[1]

***

[1] Throughout this article I have used extracts of autoethnographical work, taken from developing themes and stories for the practice-led part of my PhD. The final result will be the creation of a fictitious novel that conveys the experience of using and working within mental health care systems. All work has been anonymized to protect the identity of patients and staff that I have worked with in various health settings. Extracts taken from autoethnographical and creative practice are written in italics.

> Your arm aches. The right side of your body hurts. Your wrist is bruised where it has been turned behind your back. Your eyes roll. Your mouth gapes and is dry, sucked of moisture. You run your tongue along dry teeth and reach for a glass. You take it in your hands, realizing it is unfamiliar, a hard plastic tumbler. You slowly bring the rim to your lips. You sway, your head hurts. You stutter as the water reaches your throat.

I recently conducted a lecture to twenty occupational therapy MSc students, discussing traditional models of practice in mental health care. I asked them to identify the social and environmental triggers that can lead to a mental health breakdown, and what resources they would use if this happened to them. Many of them spoke about getting help from family and friends, some mentioned the therapeutic nature of their pets, some discussed getting outdoors into nature to help soothe themselves. I asked them to imagine that they were at the point of a breakdown and how they would feel if I told them not to worry, because a health professional was coming to take them to a psychiatric hospital, where they could stay as long as they needed to recover. I was met with horror, one student said that she felt like running from the room. Another student said that the thought of being out of control of her life terrified her, another related her gut feeling to being told that she was being sent to prison.

> Mental illness haunts us, frightens us, and fascinates us. Its depredations are a source of immense suffering and often embody threats, both symbolic and practical, to the very fabric of social order. Ironically, the stigma that surrounds those who exhibit a loss of reason has often extended to those who have claimed expertise in its identification and treatment. (Scull, 2022, p. xi)

The fear expressed by my students represents a cultural fear linked to the stories that we hear about mental health illness experiences. Stories which are reinforced through the history of mental health care, the culture that surrounds it and the way that mental health illness is portrayed within the media.

Current Experiences of Mental Health Illness

> I read the notes of a girl who has had several casual relationships while she was unwell. Her illness had led her to be disinhibited and over-sexualised. She has an STD and crabs (pubic lice). She sits weeping in her room. She is fragile, hollow. She has not sought the help that she needed, because she was too ashamed. When she goes into therapy she confesses a history of sexual abuse, she is both revulsed by her body and yet finds she can't remove herself from unsafe situations. She tells us that this is the only way that she has known human contact. She is trapped in an unhealthy pattern of behavior linked to trauma and replaying the

> same story that defines her expectations of herself, of who she has been told that she is in the world.

Many of the patients that I have encountered in my career have viewed confinement in hospital as a removal from society and punishment for actions related to mental health illness experiences. Nick Rowe writes of Converge, a project set within York St John University, where university students and people experiencing mental health illness (Converge Students) are brought together to learn from each other in a mutual learning partnership, he writes:

> Recently a Converge student told me that when she had been admitted to a mental health hospital it was like being in quarantine. She felt as if in some way she was contagious and needed to be separated from her own community and from more "normal" health care. (2015, p. 133)

The following images were created by Louise Metcalfe. Louise accessed the same project, Converge, to receive support to complete a Media/Make-up foundation course at York College. Louise used visual media to tell a series of narratives about mental health illness experiences.

Figure 2.1. The hidden pain of mental health.

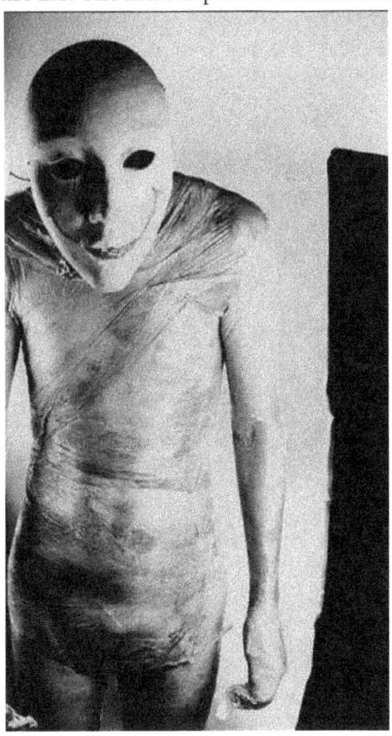

A visual representation of schizophrenia. The model is bound in material that represents the inability to escape the inner pain and symptoms of mental health illness, whilst still having to put on a smile for the world. Reproduced with permission from Louise Metcalfe.

Figure 2.2. Depression.

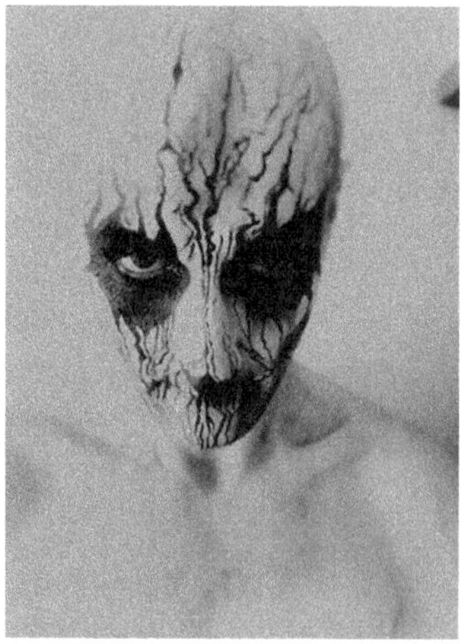

The image illustrates that when we are suffering from depression, we often feel compelled to present a perfect image to the outside world. The black marks represent the feelings of depression seeping through how we present ourselves to the world. Reproduced with permission from Louise Metcalfe.

Figure 2.3. The horror of mental health illness.

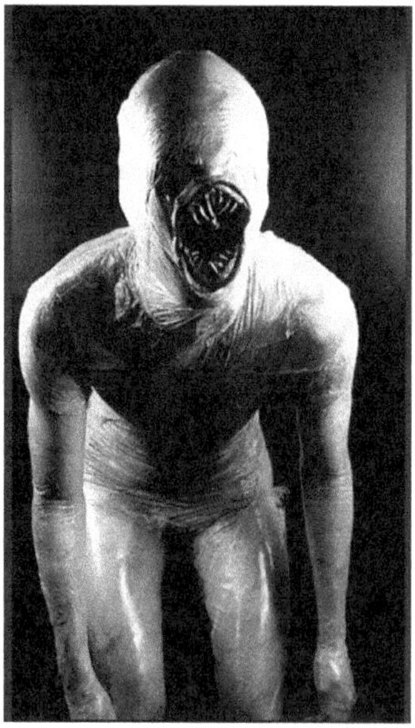

The image illustrates the horror experienced inwardly when suffering from mental health illness. The mouth represents a silent scream, when we are unable to convey what is happening to us to the outside world. Reproduced with permission from Louise Metcalfe.

Images 2.1 and 2.3 are a visual representation of schizophrenia. The models are bound in cling film to represent the inability to be able to escape hallucinations and upsetting thoughts. The mouth screaming in image 2.3 represents the horror of the feelings being experienced. The sodden cling film represents a lack of interest in physical appearance and hygiene when unwell. The masks in images 10.1 and 2.3 also represent the inability to be able to show emotions and expressions. Image 2.2 represents an interpretation of depression. Louise informed me that the darkness (depression) forming around the eyes was her way of showing the inability to see a happy future, to see a life without feeling worthless.

Stories such as these equate the hidden experience and trauma of mental health illness. Using narrative medicine to delve into the inner world and experience of mental health illness enables us to see first-hand the isolation and challenges that patients experience. Mental health illness is often triggered as a result of trauma. Feelings of isolation and low self-worth are reinforced by the stigma and shame of a mental health illness which can result in the loss of roles, employment and community. This is further compounded by the isolation of mental health care settings in our communities. This is described in the book *Circle of Dolphins* written by Clare Roskilly. Roskilly details the frightening experience of being taken to a psychiatric hospital for the first time and the unfamiliarity of the setting.

> The grounds were huge and surrounded by fields with a fence or wall in places to keep us all in. I didn't have a clue that this place existed although it was only twenty minutes from the city and I'd lived in the region for sixteen years out of the twenty two years I'd been on this ear. (Roskilly, 2010, p. 6).

Roskilly goes on to describe the breakdown of her social network, the trauma and the trauma and isolation of being admitted to a psychiatric hospital. This included her suspicion and fear of the nurses and the violence she experienced from other patients alongside the strange and uncanny events of experiencing symptoms of schizophrenia. These are stories that do not surprise me and stories that I have encountered many times in my career as a health professional. Unfortunately, many of these stories are unspoken and unheard due to the fear of being stigmatized and deemed incapable by society.

In narratology the term anti-narratable refers to stories that are deemed shouldn't be told because they are taboo or go against social convention. The stories conveyed in this chapter demonstrate the difficulty in communicating inner turmoil and experiences of mental ill health. In clinical settings, narrative reasoning is used to focus on re-building identity, roles and values in such an environment. This is discussed by Cheryl Mattingly who describes the way in which a therapist uses story making as a way to consider the phenomenological aspects of a patient's life. "Therapists think with stories in two distinct, but equally important, ways through storytelling and story creation" (Mattingly, 1991, p. 998). This can include an understanding of what was previously unnarratable, helping to explore difficult experiences and to re-define a patient's future. "Shifts in the category of the unnarratable are, I would say, significant indicators of generic change itself, and they both reflect and constitute their audiences' developing senses of such matters as politics, ethics and values" (Warhol, 2005, p. 221). This, however, can be very difficult when a therapist can view the potential of a person, but lacks the opportunities and resources to enable recovery due to the way that a person is viewed and treated by society. An additional challenge created by the fear that surrounds mental health illness, as discussed in the opening of this chapter, is the fear of the health professionals trying to provide care, who are often treated with suspicion and fear. This is unfortunately reinforced by negative news stories. A recent example can be seen in the BBC documentary *Undercover Hospital: Patients at Risk* (2022) directed by Joe Plomin. The documentary portrayed the cruel and undignified circumstances of a secure psychiatric hospital in Manchester. Undercover footage shows patients being abused and tormented by health care staff and separated from their families and society.

"Stigma is defined as a sign of disgrace or discredit, which sets a person apart from others" (Byrne, 2000, p. 65). If we can reduce stigma by changing how we treat people on a human level, we can increase our cultural understanding of mental health illness. We can begin to make progress in the stories that define mental health illness experiences and take them from the anti-narratable to the narratable, free of taboo and stigma and full of compassion and empathy. The remaining parts of this chapter will explore the use of narrative medicine and narrative theory to show how examining mental health care settings with a narrative lens may help lead to a different sort of future for mental health care systems.

Using Narrative Structures to Examine Mental Health Care Experiences and Settings

Narrative medicine has a long history of examining stories that people tell about their illness experiences to help build compassion, empathy and understanding between health practitioner and patient. Ethically this helps health practitioners to put the patient's experience at the core of service delivery. This can be challenging in settings that are under pressure due to a lack of finances or resources. However, ethics should be at the heart of every health care practitioner and integrated into their daily practice no matter what the circumstances that they find themselves in. "The alternative is passive acceptance of what we're told, and unthinking adherence to rules and checkboxes that have been handed down to us, just because this is easier." (Seedhouse, 2017, p. 147).

Narrative theory can help us to identify the failings of current mental health care settings. This includes not only relationships between staff and patients, but also the systems and environments that impact on these relationships. For example, mental health care environments are littered with examples of binary opposition that highlight the power imbalance between patients and staff. In the memoir *Out of Me* Fiona Shaw writes of her interactions with a psychiatrist in an acute mental health ward:

> Dr A., my psychiatrist, arrived unannounced a day or so after my arrival. She sat down opposite me and started asking questions. I liked her but was daunted by her. She was intelligent, with her own kind of wit, but never before had I met another woman on such unequal terms: severely depressed patient meets consultant psychiatrist. It was not an equal contest. Her self-confidence was palpable from the first, while my self-esteem had now entirely gone. (2001, p. 40)

In *Narratives: The Basics* (2016), Bronwen Thomas discusses the uses of cluster sets to convey characters and narrative identity through symbolism rather than dialog. For example, writing about punk culture this would be conveyed by including visual cues such as safety pins, ripped jeans and tartan. One of the first things I noticed about ward environments when I wrote about them, was that it was very easy in most instances to define who were staff and who were patients. The signifiers between the groups of staff and patients stood out dramatically:

> In the ward round, two male staff nurses are wearing black suit trousers and sensible shoes, they both wear shirts (one pale lilac, the other blue), neither wear a tie, this is not permitted for safety. Each man has a thick gold wedding band. The patient is called in. He is offered a drink of tea or water. He chooses tea and takes the (half filled) cup in a shaking hand. I notice that his fingers are stained yellow from tobacco. He hasn't shaven, a week's stubble grazes his chin. He has large dark circles under his eyes and his hair is dishevelled.

It is unfortunate that "over time binary oppositions come to seem natural or obvious to us and it takes a new approach to remind us that the meanings attached to them are arbitrary" (Thomas, 2016, p. 33). By examining a mental health ward through the act of story making, we are reminded of the clear divide between staff and patients, a reminder that makes us confront why there is a divide and ask what kind of mental health care setting would bridge this divide? A place that recovers identity, as well as treating symptoms of mental health illness. An environment where a person is seen as more than their illness and supported more widely by the community to integrate back into society.

In narrative theory "description is a privileged site of focalisation, and as such it has great impact on the ideological and aesthetic effect of the text" (Bal, 2009, p. 35). Descriptions of mental health experiences and environments can help to unpick a larger story and to understand mental health in a broader social context. The example of binary opposition demonstrates that narrative structures can be used to examine many components of a system. This type of examination creates an opportunity for narrative medicine by showing us the aspects of systems that are working against individuals in their recovery, rather than with them. We can learn from these stories and structures to begin to re-story the setting, to create new components that create healthier dynamics and relationships within.

The Broader Picture: Examining Story Tropes and Genres to Investigate Mental Health Care Settings

> I was instructed to wear clothes that did not make me vulnerable, nothing tight fitting, nothing that exposed shoulders or knees. High heels must not be worn, only flat sensible shoes that were suitable for running. I was not allowed to wear jewellery that could be used to choke me, or could be torn from my ear lobes. I must wear my lanyard at all times, and must only use the NHS design, with quick release snaps should someone try to use it to restrain me or throttle me. I must not go into the upstairs corridor alone, nor may I see a patient alone in their room.

Drawing on autoethnographical writing and reflecting on the stories that I have heard repeated many times over my career as a health professional, I was able to stand back from the day to day business of my work and uncover an emerging theme of horror within my writing. This was unexpected. As a health practitioner, I had become blind to the system that I worked in. So familiar had I become with stories of trauma within unusual settings, that I had not fully accepted that the links to horror were being reinforced by the modern systems and cultures in mental health care environments. In the book *Folk Horror: Hours Dreadful and Things Strange*, Adam Scovell (2017) identifies the key elements of folk horror. Scovell outlines that folk horror stories are traditionally set in places isolated from mainstream society, places that have their own sets of rules outside of societal norm, places where strange and uncanny events happen to those within the system (often against their will) and where people held within the environment are cut off from trusted relationships.

It is possible to see the parallels within traditional mental health care settings in relation to folk horror story tropes. Andrew Scull has extensively researched the development of psychiatry in Western health care over the twentieth century. His book *Desperate Remedies* (2022) uncovers the practices often used to try and treat mental health illness, as the very practice that has created stigma and horror around mental health environments. Places where people were removed from society and all manner of treatments performed as dreadful as lobotomy, isolation rooms, ice baths and unfortunately a place where hidden from the world all manner of abuse could happen.

As we learnt from Roskilly, mentioned earlier in this chapter, traditionally mental health care hospitals have continued to be set in their own grounds, away from the general population of a town. Mental health care systems follow their own time schedules and routines separate from usual societal norms. The staff gets to decide when a patient is allowed contact with the outside world. There is a separation between patients and staff, different areas to eat, different toilet facilities, areas where patients are not allowed. People can be kept against their will. An environment full of people experiencing psychotic and delusional beliefs will be one of uncanny events and encounters.

There is a disconnect between these environments and local communities. Many health professionals are also treated with the same fear and stigma as their patient's experience (as mentioned at the start of this chapter). This often creates a barrier to delivering positive mental health care, there is a need to find connection and understanding within health care services and the communities they serve.

What Happens When We Change the Story? Linking Mental Health Care with the Community. Stories of Hope and Recovery

Alongside collecting stories of trauma and mental ill health, I have also been collecting stories of hope and recovery. In 2019 I was fortunate enough to visit Trieste in Italy, as described by Roberto Mezzina (2014), a city where mental health care has been revolutionized. In-patient acute hospitals have been abolished and instead replaced with community houses, where individuals experiencing mental health can seek support at any time. Trauma and harm are averted in favor of engaging the community in the support and care of those struggling with mental health illness. Outside the grounds of the old hospital, there is now a statue of a horse (Figure 2.4), representing a model of a real horse (named Marco Cavallo) made by patients of the asylum when it was abolished in 1973.

Figure 2.4. A statue of Marco Cavallo, the Blue Horse of Trieste.

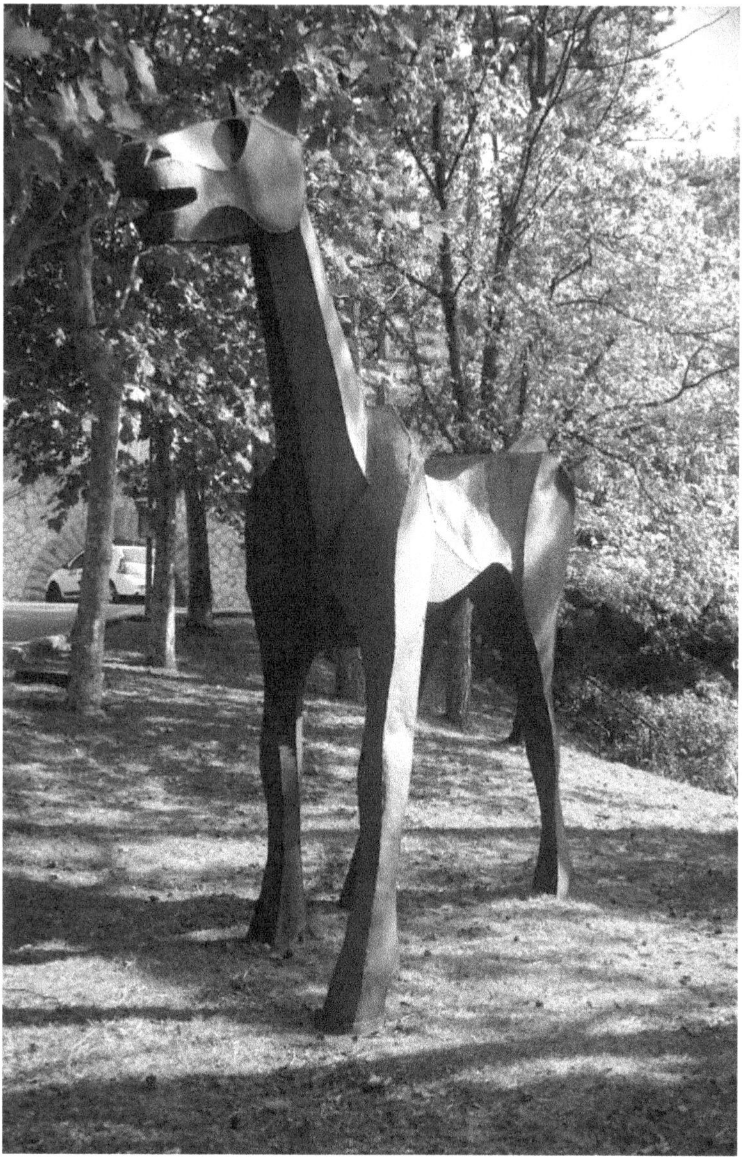

A statue of the original model of 'Marco Cavallo', a horse that came to represent the revolution of the mental health care system in Trieste. Photo taken by the author.

Figure 2.5. The original artwork, Marco Cavallo.

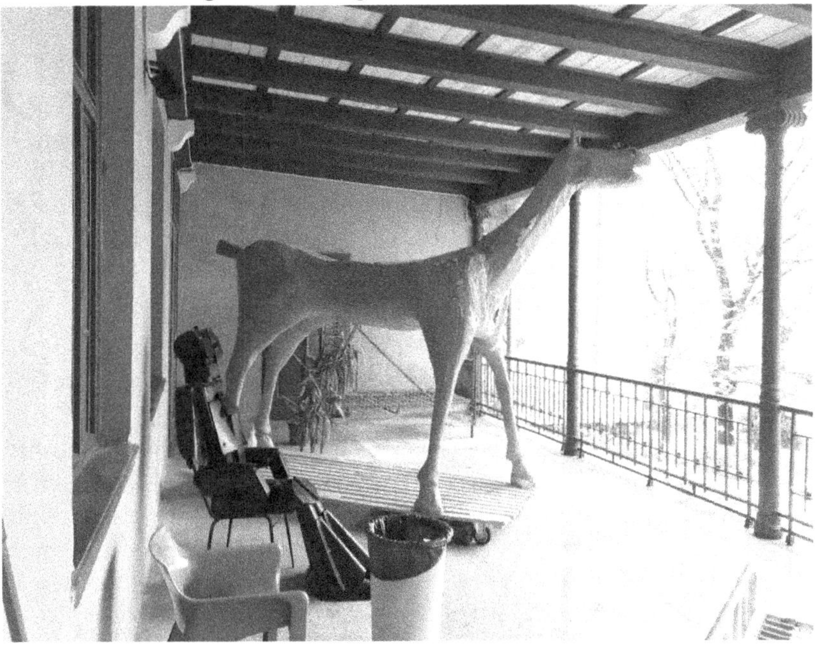

The original model of the horse, Marco Cavallo, made by patients of the abolished asylum in Trieste. Photo taken by the author.

The original model (see Figure 2.5) was made from wood and "...due to Marco Cavallo's sheer height of more than three meters, an opening in the asylum's perimeter wall had to be cut ..." (Schwarz, 2023) in order to get the model out of the hospital grounds. When the asylum was closed the model of Marco Cavallo was paraded through the streets and came to represent the freedom and reform of psychiatric treatment system in Trieste. A permanent statue (Figure 2.4) representing the original model is now a focal point of recovery looking out over the city. The whole community is now invested in preventing and recovering people from mental ill health. In the general hospital in Trieste there are only a couple of beds because people don't reach the same state of acute mental ill health. This is due to treatment and support of mental health illness being delivered swiftly and integrated into the local community. Instead of being kept behind closed doors, a person might stroll down to the seafront with their psychiatrist, to discuss over coffee the symptoms that are troubling them.

This type of story is reflected in a project called Storying Sheffield. Storying Sheffield has brought opposing communities of people together to share stories to create connection and community and to build positive relationships. They comment on the use of physical space and how influential this can be to a person:

> Indeed, physical space can itself represent or 'tell' a kind of narrative, and ... is influenced by the idea that human beings can change the spaces in which they live, both through physical actions, and through acts of re-imagination. Closely allied to these ideas, is the recognition that everyday life is worthy of study and creative engagement, and that through such activities we can learn a great deal about our culture and ourselves. (Storying Sheffield, 2023).

Conclusion

"Playing with language allows us to construct our own world, and question some of the ways in which reality is normally percieved" (Smith, 2005, p. 3). By working with the repeated stories of patients' experiences and re-working them into fictitious stories I have been able to start to look at mental health care settings from a different viewpoint. The strength of this approach is not relying on one individual story or account which may be biased according to experience. By examining repeated themes within stories created through narrative medicine we can begin to build a larger more objective picture. Contrasting stories and comparison with other cultures can engage our imagination in the possibilities available to us to deliver health care with a deeper focus on humanity.

"Narrative fiction provides a controlled wilderness, an opportunity to be and to become the Other" (Morrison, 2017, p. 93). Creating new stories that share the human side of mental health illness provides a way of helping to convey that we all have the capacity to experience mental health illness, that to discriminate and to reinforce the "Other" is to deny humanity to anyone experiencing a severe or enduring mental illness.

Narratology has given me a vehicle to convey the unspoken, to demonstrate the feeling of being inside mental health environments and the trauma that is experienced by people using and working within restrictive systems. This is an opportunity to use narrative medicine to help people experiencing mental health illness convey the trauma behind their experiences and recover their true identity. The act of storytelling between people using and working within mental health care can support the re-shaping of a larger cultural understanding of mental health illness. Nick Rowe (2015) refers to the need to heal the fracture between people that experience mental health illness and their communities describing the fracture as "deepened by medicalization and professional power, the scars of which still remain." He goes on to define the fracture as "not merely that of people who identify as having mental health problems, but of a social and cultural fracture that is revealed in the stigma and shame that still surrounds their experience" (2015, p. 122).

A piece of thought-provoking literature that engages the reader in a human experience will add a voice to those challenged by stigma and stereotyped by the system. This type of literature and storytelling can act as an opening to re-think stereotypes. "If we come to believe that we are the problem and that there is something wrong with us, then it becomes very difficult to take action. All we can do is take action against ourselves" (Denborough, 2014, p. 25). If instead we can use principles of narrative medicine and narrative theory to see not a problem, but something to be healed and addressed by society, then we can shift attitudes and culture, to help prevent further trauma and to begin to remove horror from the mental health care system.

Reference List

Bal, M. (2009) *Narratology: introduction to the theory of narrative.* 3rd edn. London: University of Toronto Press.

Byrne, P. (2000) 'Stigma of mental illness and ways of diminishing it,' *Advances in Psychiatric Treatment,* 6, pp. 65-72. doi: http://dx.doi.org/10.1192/apt.6.1.65

Denborough, D. (2014) *Retelling the stories of our lives: everyday narrative therapy to draw inspiration and transform experience.* New York: W.W. Norton & Company. doi: https://doi.org/10.1002/anzf.1082

Mattingly, C. (1991) 'The narrative nature of clinical reasoning,' *American Journal of Occupational Therapy,* 45(11), pp. 998-1005. doi: https://doi.org/10.5014/ajot.45.11.998

Morrison T. (2017) *The origin of others.* Cambridge, Massachusetts: Harvard University Press.

Mezzina, R. (2014) 'Community mental health care in Trieste and beyond: an 'open door - no restraint' system of care for recovery and citizenship,' *The Journal of Nervous and Mental Disease,* 202(6), pp. 440-445, PMID: 24840089. doi: https://doi.org/10.1097/nmd.0000000000000142

Plomin, J. (2022) *Undercover hospital: patients at risk.* Directed by Joe Plomin. UK: BBC Panorama Undercover. Available at: https://www.bbc.co.uk/programmes/m001ckxr (Accessed: 27 August 2023)

Roskilly, C. (2010). *Circle of Dolphins.* Peterborough: Spiderwize.

Rowe, N. (2015) 'Creating a healing campus: a partnership between a university and a provider of mental health services,' in *University Partnerships for Community and School System Development Vol 5,* Emerald Group Publishing Limited, pp. 119-134. doi: https://doi.org/10.1108/S2055-364120150000005007

Schwarz, J. (2023, September 29) *Cavallo, Marco: sculpture symbolising the psychiatry reform in Italy.* Retrieved from Bia-Psy: Biographical Archive of Psychiatry. Available at: https://biapsy.de/index.php/en/9-biographien-a-z/151-cavallo-marco-e#:~:text=The%20horse%20thus%20symbolised%20%E2%80%9Ca,San%20Vito%20festival%20in%20Trieste (Accessed: 27 August 2023).

Scovell, A. (2017). *Folk horror: hours dreadful and things strange.* Leighton Buzzard: Auteur Publishing.

Scull, A. (2022) *Desperate remedies: psychiatry and the mysteries of mental illness.* London: Penguin Books Ltd.

Seedhouse, D. (2017). *Thoughtful health care: ethical awareness and reflective practice.* London: Sage Publications.

Shaw, F. (2001) *Out of me: the story of a postnatal breakdown.* Foreword by Adam Phillips. Edinburgh: Virago Press.

Smith, H. (2005). *The writing experiment: strategies for innovative creative writing.* Australia: Allen and Unwin.

Storying Sheffield (2023) *Storying Sheffield: telling untold tales.* A project by the School of English at the University of Sheffield. Available at: http://www.storyingsheffield.com/about/principles-and-ideas/ (Accessed: 27 August 2023).

Thomas, B. (2016) *Narrative: the basics.* London: Routledge.

Warhol, R.R. (2005) 'Neonarrative; or, how to render the unnarratable in realist fiction and contemporary film,' in Phelan, J. and Rabinowitz, P.J. (eds.) *A companion to narrative theory.* Oxford: Blackwell Publishing, pp. 220-231. doi: https://doi.org/10.1002/9780470996935.ch15

Part 3:
Studies of Aesthetic Trauma Narratives

3.1 Therapeutic Objective

3.1.1

Healing Narratives: Disclosure Relationships and the Ritual of Storytelling in Michaela Coel's *I May Destroy You*

Ssanyu Birigwa

Columbia University, US

Molly Lindberg

Columbia University, US

Abstract

Often, disclosure of trauma is described in the context of a witness/survivor testimonial dyad, as in Dori Laub's work, but little attention has been given to the narrative choices surrounding disclosure which are impacted by the survivor's relationship with the witness. Using examples of disclosing personal trauma in Michaela Coel's 2020 HBO/BBC One series, *I May Destroy You*, we formulate a new paradigm which recognizes disclosure as necessitating and building relationships that cultivate healing. This series recounts a fictionalized version of Coel's personal experience with sexual assault, centering the challenges of how to tell one's trauma story. Following the work of Sayantani DasGupta, sharing trauma stories is a brave and externalizing act of intentional self-reflection and self-critique. In this chapter, we argue that Coel uses scenes of incomplete and unsatisfactory witnessing to highlight the difficulty and rareness of healthy disclosure/witness encounters. We will show how the episodic telling of *I May Destroy You* is indicative of the complex healing potential of repeated storytelling.

In many cultures worldwide, sitting around a fire, listening to the wisdom and knowledge of the elders, was a common and ritualized healing practice. In the survivor/witness relationship, each participant brings their own history and emotional past to the encounter of disclosure. The repetition of telling trauma stories becomes a ritual, and the use of narrative tools can be supportive and nourishing to both the survivor and witness. The potential for storytelling to address mental wounds stems from the power of sovereignty. Healing for the individual and community is possible, as revealed through the layers of narrative in *I May Destroy You.*

***

Healing is a non-linear journey, one that *I May Destroy You* makes explicitly clear, as we are taken on a journey of realistic messiness. The HBO/BBC One series from 2020 follows Arabella (Michaela Coel) a young woman living in London who is trying to rebuild her life after a traumatic event. Coel, who created, wrote, and starred in the series, tells a semi-autobiographical account of her own experience with trauma. Each episode deals with themes of consent, trauma, and the complexities of modern relationships and friendships. As viewers, we are guided through a portal of tonal changes that feel jarring and upsetting. We are taken from one uncomfortable moment to another, watching Arabella and her friends cope with trauma, reminding us of the importance of sovereignty in healing oneself. This means having agency and autonomy in making decisions about one's own care, rather than relying solely on external sources or experts to dictate the path of healing. This approach we observe Arabella taking can be empowering and can lead to a deeper understanding of oneself and one's trauma. Additionally, being sovereign in healing can also mean being open to different forms of healing, as we also witness through the healing journeys of Arabella's friends, Terry (Weruche Opia) and Kwame (Paapa Essiedu), all avidly searching for a healing process/ritual to combat their individual traumas.

Disclosure Theory

In this chapter, we use the terms "rape and "sexual assault" to refer to the legal definitions of these crimes in the UK, the context in which this show takes place. "The legal definition of rape is when a person intentionally penetrates another's vagina, anus or mouth with a penis, without the other person's consent" (Metropolitan Police). Rape falls under the umbrella of "sexual assault," but the difference is clearly described in this definition: "sexual or indecent assault is an act of physical, psychological and emotional violation in the form of a sexual act, inflicted on someone without their consent. It can involve forcing or manipulating someone to witness or participate in any sexual acts" (ibid.). In this chapter we follow the survivor's descriptions of their own experience, defaulting to "sexual assault" when it is unclear. This chapter will weave together scenes from *I May Destroy You* with theory from trauma experts and practitioners.

Dori Laub, an Israeli-American psychiatrist who has extensively studied the importance of witnessing and testimony in the context of the Holocaust, explains: "This imperative to tell and to be heard can become itself an all-consuming life task. Yet no amount of telling seems ever to do justice to this inner compulsion. There are never enough words or the right words, there is never enough time or the right time, and never enough listening or the right listening to articulate the story that cannot be fully captured in thought, memory, and speech" (1991, p. 63). In this chapter, we argue that Coel uses scenes of incomplete and unsatisfactory witnessing as a way to highlight the difficulty and rareness of healthy disclosure/witness encounters. Coel provides examples of negative disclosures, in situations where the survivor lacks agency, the witnessing is unsatisfying to the survivor, or the disclosure leads to victim-blaming.

Laub's previously quoted article "Truth and Testimony" discusses the complexities and challenges of testimony in the context of traumatic events and survivors of trauma, he prompts readers to reflect on the nature of truth and memory, particularly in relation to traumatic experiences. He also raises questions about the ethics of listening and bearing witness to testimony, and the importance of validation and respect for survivors' experiences (ibid., p. 85). In the dynamic nature of the testimony process, a witness may also feel a sense of empathy and understanding towards the survivors of trauma and the difficulties they face in telling their stories; a sense of responsibility towards active listening and bearing witness, where "this joint responsibility is the source of the reemerging truth" (ibid., p. 86).

Laub argues that the act of bearing witness to traumatic events is crucial for survivors in the process of coming to terms with their trauma, as it allows them to share their experiences and make meaning out of them (ibid., p. 87). He also notes that this witnessing process can be healing, as it can help survivors feel less alone and more understood. In addition, Laub suggests that being witnessed also means that the survivor's testimony is taken seriously and respected, and that the listener is actively engaged in the process of understanding and interpreting the survivor's experiences (ibid., p. 88).

"Knowing one's real truth, however, can also be very costly," Laub notes that testimony can be complicated and challenging, as survivors may struggle to find the words to describe their experiences or may have difficulty remembering or processing their traumatic memories (ibid., p. 88). As Rita Charon, a pioneer in the field of narrative medicine, explains, "To bear witness, is to also radically listen, which is the effort to be present, and to listen without your biases and assumptions. It's about curiosity, not judgment" (Bohanon, 2019). Narrative medicine is the practice that emphasizes the use of storytelling and narrative to improve the communication and understanding between healthcare providers and patients. Charon argues that "narrative medicine simultaneously offers physicians the means to improve the effectiveness of their work with patients, themselves, their colleagues, and the public" (2001, p. 1897).

The act of witnessing and being witnessed helps promote empathy and understanding which can foster deeper connections and relationships. Furthermore, witnessing others can also help to promote a sense of purpose and meaning, as it can provide an opportunity to offer support and assistance to others in need, "the idea that one person can understand what another person says or means is the deepest part of science and the deepest part of art. This idea is the groundspring of language, of beauty, of knowledge, of government, of culture, and of love" (Charon, 2016, p. 176). We argue that it is also the basis of healing through ritual.

Episode 2: "Someone Is Lying"

These rituals and disclosure settings will be the focus of our close reading of the second episode of *I May Destroy You.* Episode 2, entitled, "Someone Is Lying," is a slow revelation decoding the previous night. Arabella begins in a state of confusion, wondering how she smashed her phone, and why she has an image in her head of a man in a toilet stall, blocking the door and making a thumping sound. When she confides this to her best friend, Terry, the viewer and Terry begin putting together the pieces before Arabella does. In her attempts to follow her path from the night before, Arabella realizes that her drink was "spiked," as was the woman's she was with. Arabella goes straight to the police station with her friend, Kwame, ready to report that someone tampered with her drink. At the police station, she and Kwame meet with two policewomen. The women gently ask Arabella about what happened.

Officer Funmi, the Black policewoman, discloses Arabella to herself. By taking the "images in her head" seriously and reading them through a lens of trauma responses, Funmi calls her experience "assault" before Arabella does. Even then, Arabella is hesitant, knowing this word is dangerous, especially in a police station, aware of its implications. Officer Funmi gently insists. In what seems to be a sight of anticipation of being told her story back to her, Arabella pulls her shirt up to cover her face in horror and sobs when Officer Funmi asks her to recall the scene of her assault "Can you see his eyes? Who is he looking at?" When Arabella realizes that she is the answer to the question and the object of the man's gaze, she understands that she was raped. Arabella listens intently to the officers' explanation of what happened and what happens next. The audience, us, bears witness to Arabella's story becoming no longer hers. The survivor story we hope to hear is never told.

The scene is interspersed with flash-forwards to Arabella providing forensic evidence in the Sexual Assault Referal Unit. This obvious foreshadowing means that Arabella will accept Officer Funmi's reading of her story. The control of who she shares her story with and how it is shared has been denied to her. It is not clear that Arabella even understood what it meant to go to the police station to report her assault or the potential risks and benefits of sharing her story—so as to have a plan in place for how to cope with any negative reactions or triggers that may arise. Michaela Coel shows the ritual of accompaniment as her friends join her in encounters with law enforcement. Receiving good or bad news can be an emotionally taxing experience. In later episodes, either Terry or Terry and Kwame are with Arabella, and not just for practical reasons, but as a source of moral support, that can help a survivor like Arabella feel more empowered and in control of the situation. They can also help to advocate for the survivor, making sure that their needs and concerns are being heard and addressed, something that was lacking for Arabella when she first encountered the police, even with Kwame present.

Without consent from Arabella, the plot of her story, of assault, becomes medicalized, disfigured from the actual, felt events. In this context, where Arabella doesn't know what happened to her, narrative humility can't occur. Sayantani DasGupta explains in *"The Art of Medicine, Narrative Humility,"* "narrative humility acknowledges that our patients' stories are not objects that we can comprehend or master, but rather dynamic entities that we can approach and engage with, while simultaneously remaining open to their ambiguity and contradiction, and engaging in constant self-evaluation and self-critique" (2008, p. 981). When Officer Funmi tells Arabella her story, she usurps the narrative, making it impossible for Arabella to tell her own story.

Another example of poor narrative humility is in the scenes where Arabella has to strip down into a medical gown to undergo examinations, so evidence can be gathered of the assault, which we are led to believe can be used in her potential criminal investigation or trial. We see Arabella retraumatized during the examination. Perhaps we see her moving through a sense of guilt or responsibility for the assault as the camera pans closely in as the clinician puts a swab in her mouth to gather saliva and says after Arabella winces, "oh yes, looks like you have a little cut in there"—there is no acknowledgment by the healthcare provider of what she has undergone. Arabella is retraumatized by the process of being swabbed, bruises photographed, bodily fluids taken. In the scenes of gathering forensic evidence from Arabella's body, Arabella suddenly becomes a patient in a hospital gown. Her body is separated into zones, as the camera pans and zooms in, following the movements and audible "clicks" of the clinician's camera, taking pictures of the cut on her head and the bruises on her hip bones. The clinician takes samples, and Arabella complies, opening her mouth and holding her gown for the photos. This process is cold, performed in a sterile room with harsh lights. The viewer can see the tear lines on Arabella's face, but she remains calm.

The clinician follows protocols, a check-list, an order of operations. Arabella isn't so lucky, she doesn't know sexual trauma's looping, disjointed path. Perhaps her patient story isn't hers, co-opted by this clinical encounter, but her trauma story remains her own. Arabella didn't intend to be a patient, but this marks the beginning of a process of coming to terms with what happened, of remembering and relating her story to others.' She begins to pull together threads that will help her on her way to recovery. These threads serve as guidance in her journey of healing, and in the center are her relationships with others, and to the culture of showing and telling a curated life online to free herself from feeling and/or seeming vulnerable.

Episode 5: "...It Just Came Up"

The scenes in the police station of Episode 2 pair well with scenes of disclosing trauma in the fifth episode. Episode 5 is titled "...It Just Came Up," and it centers around Arabella's experiences with Zain (Karan Gill) and Kwame's decision to report his own sexual assault. Zain is a writer her agents recommend to Arabella to help her finish her manuscript. They meet in Episode 4 and have a rocky start due to Zain's condescension about Arabella's education (he went to Cambridge), and her hyper-vigilance resulting from her recent rape. They have sex partially because Arabella doesn't want to be alone with her thoughts in the aftermath of her rape. The first time they have sex, Zain removes the condom without Arabella noticing, and continues, finishing inside her. When Arabella confronts him afterwards, he claims that he thought she knew, and agrees to buy her Plan B.

In Episode 5, Arabella listens to a podcast which exposes this act of removing a condom during sex as an act of rape which has happened to many women. Arabella immediately leaves Zain's apartment, and, in a meeting later that day with her publisher, agents, and Zain, she discloses that she was recently raped. She begins a pattern of gas-lighting Zain by bringing his name up whenever she mentions her rape, and she ends the episode by exposing him during a public event as a rapist. Interspersed into this story are scenes of Arabella trying to tell Biagio (Marouane Zotti), her Italian lover, that she was raped and that she needs him to go to the police station in Italy to provide DNA samples to compare with those found on her body and clothing. Biagio immediately accuses her of not being careful and not watching her drink. This escalates when he learns the whole story, especially because, as a drug dealer, Biagio doesn't want to give his DNA to the authorities. Arabella reaches out to Biagio under the guise of practical reasons, but she deeply wants him to take charge and save her from the destruction of her trauma. His lack of compassion for Arabella and what she is going through is echoed by Zain's efforts to get Arabella to open up to him, even after he raped her. Arabella's decision to publicly out Zain, which occurs only after another woman intimates her own negative experience with him, also seems like a response to her first rape, especially because she doesn't know the name of her first rapist.

Arabella's whirlwind of action is contrasted in this episode by Kwame's efforts to report his own sexual assault. Kwame was sexually assaulted by a man who agreed to host a threesome with him and Damon, his crush. Kwame had consensual sex with the host, but, after Damon (Fehinti Balogun) left, the man pulled down his pants and violated Kwame when he tried to leave. After accompanying Arabella to the station with Terry for an update on her case, Kwame googles whether what happened to him was rape. He goes back to the police station to report the crime alone. The policeman blames Kwame for what happened to him. He doesn't say those words, exactly, but they are felt. He asks about the man's name, unable to imagine the anonymous casual sex environment that is Grindr. He ignores Kwame's repeated insistence that he has the man's address, a lead, instead zeroing in on the username "hornyman808" for its titillating potential. He doesn't ask Kwame to leave, but leaves him waiting, while he "talks to a superior." He tells Kwame that there's "a big difference between rape and sexual assault," but in the end, Kwame asks to leave without giving forensic evidence, and, even then, he must wait for someone else to show him out. The legal system grants legitimacy, but the way they treat Kwame only dimly shadows blame. It's not Biagio, screaming on the phone that Arabella ruined his life with the rape he clearly believes to be her fault. "If you watched your drink, you wouldn't have been raped," he tells her. Both sly and overt forms of victim-blaming can retraumatize a survivor and cause them to question the benefits of disclosing trauma.

Disclosure and Victim-Blaming

In Episode 5, disclosure isn't satisfying for the survivor or the witness, and multiple examples lead to the survivor being retraumatized by their attempts to connect. Both Arabella's and Kwame's stories in this episode focus on efforts to obtain recognition and support for their experiences. While Kwame tries to do this through reporting his assault to the police, Arabella looks to the public for support and validation. This is especially evident at the end of Episode 5, when Arabella is crying in bed after outing Zain, but wipes away the tears to take a selfie with her fist raised in a gesture of empowerment and solidarity. Isolated from her friends and community, she turns to the anonymous online masses for likes on her Instagram. This ending shows that, while she tries to heal through hours of yoga, the numbing presence of others, and performative acts of agency and power, she still has a long way to go in terms of dealing with the realities and complex ramifications of living through/with trauma. The following few episodes echo these themes, focusing on the commodification of online presence and the problematic exploitation that occurs there.

Arabella finds meaning in exploring many modes of potential healing. She attempts to "transport herself to a place of joy self-care" in authentic and water-downed ways. These methods seem authentic in the scene where she attends a group meeting with other survivors of assault, all sitting in a circle, re-telling their stories in what seems to be a supportive and non-judgmental environment, receiving and giving words of acknowledgment, validation, and support, or in her attending therapy sessions. Yet, her methods are water-downed as we see in her obsession in filming her recovery and sharing it over social media. Her authentic acts of self-care and reflection have the potential to improve her quality of life, a necessity in early trauma recovery. This helps her begin to alleviate feelings of isolation and disconnection, while depicting the hideously real and fraught feelings resulting from sexual trauma. As we watch Arabella choose the "items" to put into and use from her "self-care toolbox," the narrative shifts, from self-actualizing healing to realizing she has not become familiar with the emotional and physical parts of herself that feel and have memorized the harm done through her consecutive rapes.

Interestingly, in these episodes, positive moments of disclosure between friends often happen off-screen. For instance, in Episode 7, Terry tells Kwame that he needs to tell Arabella that he was sexually assaulted, and by the beginning of Episode 8, it is clear that Arabella knows, but there is no scene of disclosure. This choice feels purposeful, either because of the difficulty of portraying disclosure in a way that captures the vulnerability and trust shared between friends, or because this omission works to maintain the privacy of the characters who are otherwise so often required to tell or show all, for the police, for the public, or for the audience.

Throughout the series, best friends Terry and Arabella repeat to one another, "My birth is your birth. My death is your death," with conviction, suggesting the two share a deep sense of unity and solidarity with one another and that the current, shared moment or experience is significant to them. As viewers, we witness this phrase used repeatedly, and we know that they are not alone, that Arabella and Terry are authentically one another's support system. In this repetition, ritual is created. And in this ritual of affirming their solidarity to one another, they too are healing.

"My birth is your birth," the friends intone, but birth is complicated and messy. It suggests that they are connected to one another on a shared spiritual journey or path, both playing a significant role in helping one another cope with trauma, whether their own or the other's. Using the phrase is also a way to acknowledge victories and triumphs within their lives. The extension of the phrase "your death is my death" creates a continuum of shared experiences and connections that spans from birth to death, and that encompasses not only physical experiences but also emotional, spiritual, and cultural experiences.

This repeated promise is one of accompaniment, the act of walking beside someone in life and sharing their highs and lows. It means "I am with you, we are in this life together," but it doesn't mean that they always know how to be there for one another, how to love each other in the ways they need to be loved. They are born into this trauma story together, but they also can't go through things for one another. They have one story, but also multiple, interweaving their lives in this chosen family. "My death is your death." The effort is there, even when it's not the perfect friendship. They show up for one another, saying the same words, even when their needs differ from one another's and each means something slightly different. This relates directly to how Laub describes the importance of the witness, encapsulated in the "sense that you are not alone any longer – that someone can be there as your companion – knowing you, living with you through the unfulfilled hope, someone saying: "I'll be with you in the very process of you losing me. I am your witness'" (1991, p. 74). Infusing their friendship with this ritual of witnessing means incorporating the act of listening and validating one another's experiences and emotions. This ritual promotes self-awareness and reflection for Arabella and Terry, key components for creating a sense of safety and trust that will facilitate the healing process.

Conclusion

In many cultures worldwide, sitting around a fire, listening to the wisdom and knowledge of the elders, was a common and ritualized healing practice. The community would come together to restore safety and empowerment because re-establishing safety is the first and most central step in healing and recovery for a survivor of trauma and supporting healthy communities. In this ritual, there is room to experience feelings and emotions that are acknowledged and validated by another, which is the act of being witnessed.

Trauma at its core affects a person's capacity to be self-compassionate, and vulnerable. Its isolating effects can deceive a survivor into thinking they are alone in their experience. Through sharing trauma stories, survivors see that they are not alone, and this telling can have ritual significance. Describing what happened during the traumatic event is one thread of the mosaic that is being assembled in *I May Destroy You.* This mosaic has many layers, one being the emotional layer, where the survivor describes their feelings. Another is a symbolic layer, which describes the meaning and significance of the event in the survivor's life. Lastly, there is a cultural layer, which we experience as we traverse these layers along with the character of Arabella. Identifying the impact of cultural and societal factors on the survivors' experience through therapeutic, resiliency, and advocacy layers helps us not only see the threads of the mosaic more clearly but experience them along with Arabella.

The miracle of this show is that it doesn't run away from complexity. There isn't a straightforward message. *I May Destroy You* leans into the ambiguity of trauma and recovery as the characters bring their guilt, their complex flaws, to their efforts at "healing," though this word means something different for different characters. The show reveals a survivor's deep-set need for disclosure, and the difficulty of having this need met. Because Coel writes from her own experience, the show is also the result of a meaning-making process for her own traumatic past, which allows a viewer to hope for the possibility of healing and the integration of traumatic memories. The show is a node of connection between characters, as well as between Coel and her audience. In *I May Destroy You,* the viewer experiences a fractured, nuanced, fraught world that still has room for hope.

Reference List

Bohanon, M. (2019) 'The evolving field of narrative medicine reaches the "core of the human condition,"' *Insight Into Diversity.* Available at: https://www.insightintodiversity.com/the-evolving-field-of-narrative-medicine-reaches-the-core-of-the-human-condition/ (Accessed August 27, 2023)

Charon, R. (2001) 'Narrative medicine: a model for empathy, reflection, profession, and trust,' *JAMA: Journal of the American Medical Association,* 286(15), pp. 1897-1902. doi: http://doi.org/10.1001/jama.286.15.1897

Charon, R. (2016) 'Close reading: the signature method of narrative medicine,' in Charon, R. et al. (eds.) *The principles and practice of narrative medicine.* New York: Oxford University Press, pp. 157-179. doi: https://doi.org/10.1093/med/9780199360192.003.0008

DasGupta, S. (2008) 'The art of medicine: narrative humility,' *The Lancet,* 371(9617), pp. 980-981. doi: https://doi.org/10.1016/S0140-6736(08)60440-7

I May Destroy You (2020) Directed by M. Coel. Available at: HBO Max (Accessed: February 1, 2023)

Laub, D. (1991) 'Truth and testimony: the process and the struggle,' *American Amigo: Psychoanalysis, Culture and Trauma,* 48(1), pp. 75-91.

Metropolitan Police (no date) *What is rape and sexual assault?* Available at: https://www.met.police.uk/advice/advice-and-information/rsa/rape-and-sexual-assault/what-is-rape-and-sexual-assault/ (Accessed: August 27, 2023)

3.1.2

Narrating Trauma in Contemporary Literature: The Cases of António Lobo Antunes and Patrick McGrath

Ricardo Rato Rodrigues

Uniwersytet Marii Curie-Skłodowskiej w Lublinie, Poland

Abstract

Literature has been, for centuries, a useful outlet for certain emotional realities that are otherwise difficult to express or to frame. The realities of trauma, which have been deemed as unnarratable (Caruth, 1996), have naturally been a subject of literary representation, albeit with difficulty. The twentieth century, with its harsh events (two world wars, the holocaust, other smaller wars, the fall of communism, etc.), has been particularly fertile in producing accounts of trauma across several countries and historical experiences.

Several writers have tackled the issue, in a myriad of different approaches. This chapter aims to focus on two of them: Portuguese psychiatrist and novelist António Lobo Antunes, whose novels, particularly the early ones, have delved into the realities of the Portuguese colonial war and its traumatic aftermath, articulating it with the world of mental institutions in post-war Portugal; and British novelist Patrick McGrath, whose work has returned to the topic countless times, with particular importance in his novel *Trauma* (2008), which is centered on Post-Traumatic Stress Disorder (PTSD) cases as narrated by an American psychiatrist.

The chapter will explore how the two writers have narrated trauma, highlighting their similarities and the literary (and ethical) strategies employed in the process of narration. Furthermore, the chapter will argue the importance of literature for the formation of narratives centered on and surrounding the realities of trauma, as well as its powerful therapeutic role.

***

Throughout the twentieth and the twenty-first centuries, the scientific fields concerning the study of the human mind have advanced greatly and the human capacity to understand its own inner ailments has become greater and a great deal more articulated in its expression. Fields such as Psychology or Psychiatry have evolved in leaps and bounds since the years when Jean-Martin Charcot (still in the nineteenth century) and Sigmund Freud decided to turn their gaze not outwards, but inwards into the human psyche. However, as often it is the case, scientific advancements still have to play catch-up with that older, much older reality—human experience. For all the extraordinary progresses in identification and diagnosis, the truth is that mental ailments continue to pose a challenge, whether is terms of treatment and actual understanding, to medical practitioners, patients and society in general. It is then inevitable that in order to better understand the human dimension of mental illness, an older area than psychiatry has been called into play—literature. For what is literature other than the expression of human emotion, of human insight? Accordingly, the relationship between literature and the medical sciences has been, albeit not entirely peaceful, quite a close one.

This has been particularly notorious in the case of trauma, given the gruesome historical events of the twentieth century and the better understanding of the mental and physical consequences of war and violence. Trauma, perhaps like no other diagnostic category, has gone through a significant evolution, as Cathy Caruth highlights:

> In 1980, the American Psychiatric Association finally officially acknowledged the long-recognized but frequently ignored phenomenon under the title "Post-Traumatic Stress Disorder" (PTSD), which included the symptoms of what had previously been called shell shock, combat stress, delayed stress syndrome, and traumatic neurosis, and referred to responses to both human and natural catastrophes. (1995, p. 3)

This development has been a very important step into the recognition of trauma as a sort of powerful diagnostics umbrella term that has been "so powerful that it has seemed to engulf everything around it" (ibid.), that is, it has expanded to contain realities as diverse as child abuse, rape and other forms of violence, thus permitting a wider assessment of human suffering and its potential damage.

However, and as Caruth also identifies, this development has "provided anything but a solid explanation of the disease" (ibid.). In fact, she explains:

> The impact of trauma as a concept and a category, if it has helped diagnosis, has done so only at the cost of a fundamental disruption in our received modes of understanding ... and a challenge to our very comprehension of what constitutes pathology. (ibid.)

In other words, even though the ability to diagnose and identify has become more accomplished, it has also made things more complex and therefore pushed the ethical and ontological boundaries around the experience of trauma to its limits in what concerns its dimension as a diagnosis. It is here that literature and literary insight can (and indeed do) contribute. Quite unconcerned with the wider theoretical debates going on in medical philosophy, literature continues to (as it has always done) catalog the human experience in a variety of voices, perspectives, and dimensions. Trauma, a pervasive experience in human history, both individually and collectively, has been a recurring topic throughout the history of literature. There are a plethora of texts and authors that have dealt with the topic of trauma, but for the purposes of this chapter, I will focus on two writers, Portuguese novelist António Lobo Antunes (b.1942) and British novelist Patrick McGrath (b.1950), in particular their novels *Conhecimento do inferno (Knowledge of hell)* (2010) and *Trauma* (2008), respectively. The reasons behind this choice are various and have as much to do with their similarities as with their differences, but it was mainly a certain shared standpoint, an attitude of radical questioning and of human involvement that ultimately defined them as case studies.

António Lobo Antunes and Patrick McGrath

Before exploring these two authors and their works in more detail, it is nevertheless necessary to reflect on the problem of representation of trauma, as it is crucial to understand the type of ethical considerations surrounding psychiatry and how these shape the ability to narrate trauma without breaching ethical commitment. As expected, psychiatry is bound by the ethical coordinates "provided by the principles of bioethics applicable to all fields of medicine" (Radden, 2002, p. 52), which at face-value seems to be a well-defined framework. But according to Sidney Bloch and Stephen Green, the matter is more complicated:

> The task, however, is complicated by the lack of a coherent framework or ethical decision-making, a conclusion buttressed by two observations. First, rationales and methods used to resolve ethical questions differ radically. Indeed, competing ethical theories may so contradict one another as to generate irreconcilable tensions for the clinician. (2006, p. 7)

The ethical difficulties are many and, since medical sciences deal with real-life patients, such considerations need to be taken seriously. It is, then, reasonable to approach any attempt to narrate a traumatic experience with a high degree of care and reserve. But even with these caveats in mind,

> [t]he clinician is, however, not obliged to perch on an elevated moral pedestal. The latter serves as a flexible framework in which ... the

> opportunity is provided to examine the "ethical nuts and bolts" of the clinical context through sound moral reasoning. (ibid., p.12)

It is precisely here that literature can have its biggest contribution to the matter. Not restraint by the same ethical rules (representations can be disguised under anonymity or a different name or simply fictionalized altogether), it can help clinicians navigate through and inform their moral reasoning without having to risk crossing the ethical boundaries that could endanger real-life patients, not to mention the fact that it could widen their perspectives and understanding of the human dimension behind what (and who!) is being diagnosed. In fact, the necessity of including literature as an element of psychiatric training has already been very well documented by several sources, such as Paul Crawford and Charley Baker:

> An argument can be proposed that is specifically relevant to the reading of fiction in psychiatric training – one that goes to the heart of the practice of psychiatry. Psychiatry as a discipline is increasingly focused on biological causes of mental illnesses – at times to the exclusion of other relevant discourses – yet it is a study that focuses on the mind. The human mind is too complex and unique to be reduced to a series of chemical and electrical responses. Merely knowing that serotonin levels affect depression does not induce any level of understanding in a professional regarding the experience of depression, for example. (2009, p. 239)

This brings us to the two authors selected for this chapter and how their works could contribute significantly to the narration of trauma as a wider phenomenon. It is relevant, but by no means a necessity, that both authors have a personal connection to Psychiatry. Lobo Antunes is a psychiatrist himself and has practiced for many years before living exclusively of his literature; Patrick McGrath, albeit not being a doctor himself, had close contact with the realities of mental illness and psychiatric care, as his father was the medical superintendent at the famous Broadmoor Hospital, in England. Their personal experiences have undoubtedly shaped their writings about the realities of trauma, even though their perspectives and styles are radically different. However, regardless of their differences in style and content, both successfully place their narrations of trauma on a more egalitarian level, by enmeshing the figure of the doctor as an active participant in the ethical dialog of the realities of trauma, a participation that it is not coming from above (from a moral pedestal) but one that exists within traumatic realities in themselves.

Psychiatrist, Novelist and War Veteran: The Perspective of António Lobo Antunes

In Lobo Antunes' novel *Knowledge of hell,*[1] the last part of a trilogy that revolves around the experiences of a young psychiatrist in his work at a psychiatric hospital and his experiences at war (the Portuguese Colonial War, 1961-1974), we are presented with a cynical and caustic narrator who, as a psychiatrist, seems to detest the world of psychiatric confinement but at the same time manifest an immense understanding for the humanity of his patients. As it has been written elsewhere, "Lobo Antunes writes against the grain of the medical outlook, an outlook, a gaze, that reduces the multiplicity of human experience (especially the multiplicity of suffering and pain)" (Rato Rodrigues, 2021, p. 99), and this is what is visible in the novel. A psychiatrist, working at the Miguel Bombarda psychiatric hospital in Lisbon, deals with the day-to-day life of his patients whilst he himself wrestles with his own traumatic memories from the war. Highly autobiographical, the novel is animated by an antipsychiatric ethos. In a powerful passage towards the end of the novel, the narrator reaches the conclusion that the only possible solution would be the destruction of the hospital:

> The only thing to do was to destroy the hospital, physically destroy the hospital, the leper walls, the cloisters, ... the sinister concentrational organization of madness, the heavy and hideous bureaucratization of anguish, and start from the beginning, elsewhere, in another way, to fight suffering, anxiety, depression, mania. (Lobo Antunes, 2010, p. 185)[2]

The symbolic act of destruction is also (in the eyes of the narrator), an act of purification and liberation that would permit society (and humanity in general) to start anew the reassessment of madness and trauma. Such conclusion comes from the narrator's own suffering and the juxtaposition of his war memories, and the reality of the mental institution influences his idea of the abolition of this place of confinement by realizing it upon the rest of society. By this way of narrating trauma—his own, the narrator's, the mental patients,' the collective trauma of Portuguese post-colonial war society—Lobo Antunes is doing several things at once. On the one hand, he is indicating that psychiatry, as a discipline,

---

[1] For the purposes of this chapter, I have used the original Portuguese version of the novel, *Conhecimento do Inferno*. All the translations are mine.

[2] a única coisa a fazer era destruir o hospital, destruir fisicamente o hospital, os muros leprosos, os claustros, ... a sinistra organização concentracionária da loucura, a pesada e hedionda burocratização da angústia, e começar do princípio, noutro local, de uma outra forma, a combater o sofrimento, a ansiedade, a depressão, a mania. (Lobo Antunes, 2010, p. 185)

needs to confront itself with its own origins and do an honest appraisal of its potential, in order to attain integrity as a discipline and to truly be useful in the treatment of trauma (Szasz, 1974). Here, it is easy to see that literature can not only be used to further the knowledge about trauma and its human dimension, but also as a powerful tool of reflection about the institutional, theoretical, and material apparatus surrounding the problem of trauma and other mental ailments. This is a crucial aspect to maintain a healthy and productive dialog between psychiatry and society at large and Lobo Antunes, by placing himself in the position of intermediary, is simultaneously narrating and reflecting upon trauma.

Lobo Antunes's novel is a descent to hell, a journey that aims to give the readers the knowledge of hell (as the title indicates), calling for the readers' participation and commitment but above all, it is a howl of discontent and a call for a new way to approach trauma. Trauma, for Lobo Antunes, is not a fascinating topic for literature, quite the opposite. This can be seen as a tearing down of the romantization of trauma and madness that sometimes can be found in certain artistic representations. In this aspect, Lobo Antunes is aligned with Robert Musil, who in his novel *The Man Without Qualities* (1930), describes the main character's view of an asylum he walks by:

> Hell is not interesting, it is terrifying … It is precisely the bare idea of an unimaginable and thereby inescapable everlasting punishment and agony, the premise of an inexorable change for the worse, impervious to any attempt to reverse it, that has the fascination of an abyss. Insane asylums are also like that. They are poorhouses. They have something of hell's lack of imagination. (1995, p. 1070)

On the other hand, Lobo Antunes is abolishing the ethical pedestal of psychiatrists by presenting us with a psychiatrist who is, himself, traumatized and therefore at the same level as his patients and with this, he is implying that trauma is not only pervasive and its origins diverse, it is also a common experience that rather than being committed within the walls of a mental institution, it rather requires another type of commitment—a personal, societal and human commitment from psychiatrists themselves and from society at large. This goes in line with what Thomas Szasz has also identified, that "whereas the so-called madman is one who characteristically *commits* himself, the psychiatrist is one who characteristically remains *uncommitted.*" (1974, p. 9). For Lobo Antunes, a possible solution is indeed that the psychiatrist becomes more committed, in a process that becomes *dialogical*, where the psychiatrist (and ultimately the reader) confronts his/her own traumas and embarks upon a journey of self-discovery and betterment or, ideally, healing.

Troubled Doctors: The Perspective of Patrick McGrath

In the work of Patrick McGrath, we also find a similar act of commitment. Quite often in his novels, the narrators and main characters are physically and/or mentally troubled doctors who are confronted with their own failings or the negative consequences of their actions, normally motivated by their ailments. The settings of his works are spread through several historical periods, but the novel that merits our attention for the purposes of this chapter is one set in the contemporary world—the Unites States of post-Vietnam war.

The novel *Trauma*, first released in 2008, deals with a psychiatrist, Charlie Weir, who is struggling with reconciling his professional and personal decisions, particularly his perceived failure in helping Danny, the brother of his wife Agnes. We meet Charlie several years after his experiences of unsuccessfully treating Danny (who would eventually commit suicide), a veteran of the Vietnam War who had been traumatized and as a result committed some unspeakable act of violence (which is never spelled out for the reader, but that is heavily hinted at as acts of cannibalism). Moreover, as we progress in the novel, we also gradually discover that Charlie himself suffers from trauma, resulting from child abuse at the hands of his mother, which is not revealed to us until the very last pages but that it is hinted at throughout. The result and manifestation of his trauma is the constant failure in his close relationships, be it with his brother, his father, or romantic partners. Once again, just like in Lobo Antunes' novel, we have a troubled psychiatrist dealing with his own trauma, once again an act of inclusion, commitment and blurring of the boundaries between patient/doctor.

However, there are crucial differences between the two. Lobo Antunes' narrators are earnest, but their voices are confused, nuanced, delivered in a stream-of-consciousness way, an inner flow that gives us access to the interior worlds of characters through fragmented, dispersed images. Patrick McGrath's narrators are, on the contrary, unreliable but logical, displaying (as doctors) ordered and methodical thoughts.

The importance of the unreliable narrator in narratives of trauma has been identified by Paul Crawford and Charlie Baker:

> Unreliable narration is a fact of life as well as literature – rarely do we admit to anyone (including ourselves) the deeper, painful and sometimes darker sides of ourselves. The literary device of unreliable narrator can serve clinically as a reminder to gather a multitude of known and establish able facts about individuals, as well as listening to self-interpretation and accounting in order to enable a wide-ranging perspective. Ultimately, this particular literary device indicates that the

> manner in which we narrate ourselves can speak volumes about who we inherently are. (2009, p. 243)

In McGrath's novel, Charlie Weir is indeed an unreliable narrator, and it takes yet another act of commitment, this time from the reader, to explore what lies in those "darker sides," thus accessing the traumatic locus. Nevertheless, Charlie Weir is also a very "ordered" human being and his narrative voice, far from Lobo Antunes' meandering stream-of-consciousness, is a clear, highly rational one. As Christine Ferguson has written about the author's narrators:

> In each case, the reader is constantly aware of the deleterious effects of trauma upon the speaker's testimony. One might argue that McGrath has indeed followed in his father's footsteps, devoting a career to the observation, documentation and attempted explication (for do not all acts of fiction constitute acts of explication?) of mental disease. (1999, p. 234)

These observations (his novels) are indeed almost pedagogical. In *Trauma*, for example, Charlie describes accurately the therapeutic process of his patients and the psychiatric theoretical framework that accompanies it. When describing the working assumption behind his treatment of Danny and his fellow veterans suffering from PTSD, he offers this insight:

> The most potent charge of emotion weakens over time, unless it is repressed. Then it can wreak havoc in the psyche for years to come, which was what had happened to Danny and his buddies. Their buried material was throwing up nightmares and other symptoms, and would continue to do so until the trauma could be translated into a narrative and assimilated into the self … (McGrath, 2008, p. 29)

By sharing the thought process of his main character, McGrath is also revealing how the supposedly highly scientific mind of a doctor processes the therapeutic endeavor. Besides the obvious pedagogical value (not only for medical students) in sharing how psychiatric thinking works, McGrath is also doing something more subversive—inverting the gaze. In Ferguson's view: "In McGrath's fiction, however, this paradigm is reversed; it is the world of health and reason which becomes subject to the scrutinising gaze of madness" (1999, p. 235).

In another significant insight, Charlie Weir tries to subject Danny to "immersive therapy" by accompanying him to a bar and forcing a drunken dialog with the man, so he confronts his trauma. Danny does get drunk, and his trauma comes back to him, forced out by Charlie's questions. The result is devastating; Danny storms out of the bar, disappearing into the night. Later, after unsuccessfully looking for Danny, Charlie finds him at home, where he had committed suicide. The effects of this discovery are very impactful for

Charlie and serve as a trigger for his own traumatic memories to resurface, damaging his personal life.

Slowly, the reader discovers Charlie's humanity beyond his role as a psychiatrist, his vulnerabilities, failures and trauma. The scrutinizing gaze of madness and trauma is turned to a failing and ailing psychiatrist, whose descent into the darkness of his own trauma cannot be stopped by him, a tried and tested psychiatrist, supposedly armed with the relevant knowledge but still impotent against his own trauma. Could it be that McGrath is placing the responsibility in the reader? Could it be that he is inviting the reader into a participative role in the process of not only individual but of collective care and healing? Whether or not that is the case, the benefit of tacking trauma in such a way has enduring potential. As Femi Oyebode states:

> Whether psychiatrists read these fictional accounts or not, the accounts will undoubtedly influence how wider society perceives mental illness, how they react to it and, ultimately, how governments respond by way of policy. Novels are revealing insofar as what is implicit in them, the unexplained and unexamined context, tells us something about the assumptions that cultures make about mental illness. Fictional literature is an attempt to create and reflect, using the imagination, the world we as psychiatrists know well. It gives us the opportunity to stand back from that world, to contemplate it, before once again immersing ourselves in it, for better or worse. (2004, p. 145)

Conclusion

Therefore, the novels and authors here presented, a mere selection amongst hundreds of potentially "useful" works are, in my view, the best examples of how trauma not only *can* be narrated (if literally or not, that is another matter) but also how these narrations offer a leap in imagination, a necessary step to overcome ethical concerns and to hold an entire discipline, an entire society into account and scrutiny.

They do so by offering what Ruth Leys identifies as the "participatory account" (2000, p. 87), where the patient's account was an inseparable element of the therapeutic process, against the "surgical account" (ibid.), which is the accepted mode in most Western societies, where the patient's contribution and collaboration is irrelevant to the whole process. Furthermore, both McGrath and Lobo Antunes seem to be widening the call for participation, not only by including the patient's perspectives and by blurring the differences between patient/doctor, but also by including the reader in the participatory therapeutic process, asking for his/her critical judgments, engaging attention and, more importantly, by providing imaginative leaps from which the reader can access knowledge and experience about diverse traumatic experiences.

The imaginative leap is, then, an essential element. If trauma is inherently *literal*, that is, imprinted in our minds as something that cannot be narrated *as truth*, then other strategies must be devised to somehow access the traumatic region and to enable cure, or at least betterment. Cathy Caruth has reflected upon this difficulty:

> Trauma seems to be much more than a pathology, or the simple illness of a wounded psyche: it is always the story of a wound that cries out, that addresses us in an attempt to tell us of a reality or truth that is not otherwise available. This truth, in its delayed appearance and its belated address, cannot be linked only to what is known, but also to what remains unknown in our very actions and our language. (1996, p. 3)

This is a difficulty that affects both the medical sciences and literature, for, as Anne Whitehead has advanced in her work about trauma fiction: "Trauma carries the force of a literality which renders it resistant to narrative structures and linear temporalities. Insufficiently grasped at the time of its occurrence, trauma (...) acts as a haunting or possessive influence" (2004, p. 5).

Nevertheless, such a difficulty does not prevent writers from trying to present their narratives, to bridge the gap, to overcome the hole that trauma presents in their (as it does for patients, doctors, society) path. It is precisely the imaginative leap they take when narrating that permits them not to be literal, but *lateral*, and to creatively find ways to still tackle the narratively slippery concept of trauma. Paradoxically, this is also the path that those suffering from trauma must find in their therapeutic process, the path to resilience.

This is certainly not an easy or straightforward path. It is, on the contrary, full of hardships and obstacles which need to be overcome. For the traumatized person, the way to resilience is a broken and sinuous path. It is the capacity to be creative that will permit the person to overcome the hole, the precipice that they will inevitably find along the way, thus becoming resilient. For non-traumatized people, creativity may come as a choice. But for those carrying the burden of trauma, it is not a choice, but a necessity. "The normal walker may become creative; the resilient person is forced to" (Cyrulnik, 2005, p. 100).

Lobo Antunes and McGrath are writers whose work goes beyond the narrow concern of trauma studies but whose contributions are, nevertheless, essential for furthering our understanding of the realities, consequences, dilemmas, and wider questions of trauma. They forged their creative paths, tackling various dimensions of trauma (the personal, the collective, the ethical, the institutional) so that our way into understanding trauma is, if not an easy ride, at least somewhat smoother.

Reference List

Bloch, S. and Green, S.A. (2006) 'An ethical framework for psychiatry,' *The British Journal of Psychiatry: The Journal of Mental Science*, 188, pp. 7-12.

Caruth, C. (ed.) (1995) *Trauma: explorations in memory*. Baltimore and London: Johns Hopkins University Press.

Caruth, C. (1996) *Unclaimed experience: trauma, narrative, and history*. Baltimore and London: Johns Hopkins University Press.

Crawford, P. and Baker, C. (2009) 'Literature and madness: fiction for students and professionals,' *The Journal of Medical Humanities*, 30(4), pp. 237-251. PMID: 19789966. doi: https://doi.org/10.1007/s10912-009-9089-1

Cyrulnik, B. (2005) *The whispering of ghosts: trauma and resilience*. New York: Other Press

Ferguson, C. (1999) 'Dr McGrath's disease: radical pathology in Patrick McGrath's neo-Gothicism,' in Byron, G. and Punter, D. (eds.) *Spectral Readings: Towards a Gothic Geography*, pp. 233-243.

Leys, R. (2000) *Trauma: a genealogy*. Chicago: The University of Chicago Press

Lobo Antunes, A. (2010) *Conhecimento do inferno*. Lisboa: Dom Quixote.

McGrath, P. (2008) *Trauma*. London: Bloomsbury

Musil, R. (1995 [1930]) *The man without qualities*. Translated from the German by Sophie Wilkins. London: Picador.

Oyebode, F. (2004) 'Fictional narrative and psychiatry,' *Advances in Psychiatric Treatment* 10(2), pp. 140-145. doi: https://doi.org/10.1192/apt.10.2.140

Radden, J. (2002) 'Notes towards a professional ethics for psychiatry,' *Australian and New Zealand Journal of Psychiatry*, 36(1), pp. 52-59. doi: https://doi.org/10.1046/j.1440-1614.2002.00989.x

Rato, R. (2021) 'Doctor, soldier, writer: António Lobo Antunes as Portugal's pathographer,' in Sarkar, J. and Basu, J. (eds.) *The portrait of an artist as a pathographer: on writing illnesses and illnesses in writing*. Malaga: Vernon Press, pp. 95-110.

Szasz, T. (1974) *Ideology and insanity*. Harmondsworth: Penguin Books.

Whitehead, A. (2004) *Trauma fiction*. Edinburgh: Edinburgh University Press.

3.1.3

Narrative Medicine and Holistic Healing: An Ethics of Cure

T. S. Kavitha

Banaras Hindu University, India

Mahesh Sharma

Central Institute at Higher Tibetan Studies, Sarnath, India

Abstract

In 2001, at the intersection of various fields such as humanities, health care, arts and clinical practices, a new discipline called "narrative medicine" emerged at Columbia University. Siddhartha Mukherjee, a faculty member in the Department of Medicine at Columbia University in the Division of Hematology/Oncology, permeates into the historical, cultural, political, medical, and metaphorical journey of cancer in his book *The Emperor of All Maladies: A Biography of Cancer*. As a text, this book follows narrative features present both in narrative text and narrative medicine as defined by Rita Charon (Charon, 2006, 2008). It situates itself at the crossroads of biographical research of cancer as a "*someone*," a feature of a narrative text, and narrative medicine, where the historical clinical practice of cancer originating from the ancient Egyptian civilization to the present day, is "informed by the theory and practice of reading, writing telling and receiving of stories" by clinical practitioners such as Galen, Sydney Farber, Halsted and Mary Lasker among others.

However, the stories by the physicians, rather than being an encounter and intersubjective exchange between human patient and doctor, is a discourse between doctor/researcher and cancer as (a) someone replacing the human. The encounters reveal a mode of ethical practices vis-à-vis cancer in an attempt, on the one hand, to find methods to treat cancer patients and, on the other, to find a cure at the root of the illness. Through the analysis of John Green's novel, *The Fault in Our Stars,* this aspect of healing and curing will be understood in a rather concrete manner. The encounter with the incomprehensible (here cancer), at the heart of Levinasian ethics, is firmly at play in *The Emperor of All Maladies* as well as in the novel. A medical decision should not be taken solely to heal the body. The ethics behind decision-making must value health rather than healing the illness, which becomes possible with strong interhuman bonds. This chapter argues that for ages, physicians have tried to understand the ethics of care/cure through medical and scientific research, and narrative medicine is not only "recognizing, absorbing, interpreting and being moved by the stories of illness" through intersubjective discourses but moving towards a holistic form of healing that will reveal *the Other* in a new light.

***

The history of cancer is an amalgamation of multiple narratives. Cancer, as an illness or a pathology, creates a scientific and medical narrative; as an experience, it creates personal narratives; as the "emperor of all maladies," it establishes narratives of hope and despair; as a disease, it gives birth to narrative medicine. Siddhartha Mukherjee, in his book *The Emperor of All Maladies: A Biography of Cancer* (2010), has woven together all these various forms of narratives that establish both the dark sides of cancer research through the depiction of egomania, arrogance, corruption, fraud and clashes between research groups. On the other hand, it shows the long way cancer has come along, showing its healing success in some forms of cancer. As the title suggests, cancer has not only been treated as a research subject in medicine but as something that has had a life of its own, as something living, with human characteristics. In medicine, curing cancer does not indicate that cancer is being cured but rather that the patient with this disease is being cured. Our objective in his chapter is to show that *The Emperor of All Maladies* permeates into the historical, cultural, political, medical, and metaphorical journey of cancer. As a text, this book follows narrative features present both in narrative text and narrative medicine as defined by Rita Charon, situating itself at the crossroads of biographical research of cancer as a someone. For a comprehensive understanding of this form of narrative, we will first begin by analyzing the methodology Mukherjee uses to recount the biography of this disease, written in semi-historical and semi-fictional manner. Further, we will analyze a fictional cancer narrative, i.e. John Green's novel *The Fault in Our Stars* (2012). Analyzing this novel will enhance our understanding of the narratological aspect of narrative medicine. To illustrate this further from an ethical perspective, we will attempt to see how the incomprehensibility of this disease can be dealt with through the lens of Emmanuel Levinas's understanding of ethics of care. Finally, the concepts of care and cure, two sides of the same coin, are mutually exclusive processes in the healing process. Taking into account the varieties of cancers, healing is not finding a cure for the disease in general but rather taking care of the patient with the disease as exclusive individuals with exclusive cancer. In light of the complexity of cancer and its long history, within the rhetoric of illness and cure, care for the patient as a human being should be the focus of research rather than setting the patient simply as a case or a patient X and, in later research, as a case study for further investigation.

Writing The Emperor of all Maladies

Mukherjee is a doctor-writer who published his first book, *The Emperor of All Maladies*, in 2010. In the New York Times magazine, it was listed as one of the top 100 non-fiction books of the year. Having won several awards and been translated into many different languages, the book remains a milestone achievement in the domain of medical research as well as narrative medicine. Adopting a comprehensive and honest approach to cancer and its history of cancer research reveals that acquiring knowledge is not always pleasant. The book traces the history of cancer from ancient Egypt till 2010, indicating the permanence of the disease while the attitudes and approaches towards cancer have changed immensely. Mukherjee speaks about his experience treating cancer by providing a unique insight into the ongoing fight against "our desperate, malevolent, contemporary doppelganger" (2010, p. 52), which is cancer. The approach he adopts towards writing about cancer in this book is by treating it as a "someone" rather than a "something" which means a living entity with human characteristics rather than a scientific object for research:

> In writing this book, I started off by imagining my project as a "history" of cancer. But it felt, inescapably, as if I were writing not about something but about someone. My subject daily morphed into something that resembled an individual – an enigmatic, if somewhat deranged, image in a mirror. This was not so much a medical history of an illness but something more personal, more visceral; its biography. (ibid., p. 53)

The personification of cancer as "someone" remains enigmatic even today as so many still suffer from this illness and clinical trials continue putting patients at risk through experimentation (although the patients enter the clinical trials willingly). The biography of cancer is an ongoing one and will continue to write history and be written about for years to come.

In writing a book, the author must always remember what comes between the solitary act of writing and the solo act of reading, such as the editors, publishers, etc. This process is very similar to the practice of medicine. The course of treatment takes place primarily between the doctor and the patient. All that lies in between, such as tests, scans, medications etc., are essential components of the medical narrative that can neither be avoided, neglected, nor forgotten. The parallel between these two practices is storytelling. The patient recounts his disease and symptoms to the doctor in a narrative form.

The doctor must create his diagnosis in response to this individual, creating a subjective narrative. For example, if a patient goes to the doctor with a recurrent cough, say how often it has taken place in the last few days or months. The doctor then asks the patient to provide his whereabouts, his diet, his activities, his (workplace) environment, etc. After careful examination, the doctor might pinpoint the source of the cough as his being surrounded by smokers at his workplace or whatever the diagnosis may be. A constant exchange of narratives occurs at both ends, communicating between two people through a story. Medicine, according to the author, "begins with storytelling. Patients tell stories to describe illness; doctors tell stories to understand it. Science tells its own story to explain diseases" (ibid., p. 428).

In her book *Narrative Medicine: Honoring the Stories of Illness*, Charon focuses on this practice of exchanging stories through the study of techniques of narratology to understand the relationship between patient and doctor. She defines narrative medicine as "a clinical practice informed by the theory and practice of reading, writing, telling and receiving of stories" (Charon, 2006, p. viii). What drove her to develop such a field of study was to bridge the gap between professional health caregivers and their patients and a lack of sympathy and empathy towards the patients. As Mukherjee mentions in his book promotion at the Harvard bookstore, the average time of listening to patients before giving their diagnosis is about 18 seconds, indicating a lack of listening skills on behalf of the healthcare practitioners. Using techniques of narration such as reader-response theory, ethical criticism etc., Charon, in a way, creates a training platform to improve doctor-patient relations and dialog.

In order to transform a medical text or medical experience into literature, one needs narrative tools and techniques such as the use of metaphors, etc. The device Mukherjee uses in writing the book is looking for the stories of the patients, the stories of the scientists involved in the research of cancer as well as the stories of the places, cities and storytellers such as Herodotus. While the stories of the patients remain central to the writing, all the science that comes along is secondary, a secondary achievement. The author does not follow a linear form of writing; he switches back and forth in time, moves between characters, etc. However, some crucial questions remain – how is a medical text written in a scientific language converted into literature? How are medical reports of patients and case studies transformed into stories? How is a science immersed in its past, a practice that very often lacked ethical practices as shown in the book, today become part of a field of study called literary studies, in particular, incorporated into the rather moral field of narrative medicine?

Storytelling, as a practice and element in science, can answer all these questions. One such example is the case of Arthur Aufderheide, a pathologist who specialized in mummies from archaeological sites. Mukherjee describes one of the graves as follows:

> The graves contain the mummified remains of members of the Chiribaya tribe. The Chiribaya tribe made no effort to preserve their dead, but the climate is almost providentially perfect for mummification. The clay leaches water and fluids out of the body from below, and the wind dries the tissues from above. The bodies, often placed seated, are thus swiftly frozen in time and space. (2011, p. 56)

This description of the grave has no scientific or technical terminology that could define the text as being scientific. Metaphorical words such as "providentially," "leaches," and "frozen in time and space" give the impression of reading a story, a literary text rather than a site of scientific research. This particular research incident spans over four pages in the book and includes imagination, metaphors, and descriptions of the wind and the terrain, it goes back in time from 1990 to 1914 and further back to 4000 BC.

In his book from 1988 *The Illness Narrative*, Arthur Kleinman differentiates three critical terms, illness, disease and sickness, from one another. He defines an illness experience as "always culturally shaped" (2020, p. 32) and distinctive from patient to patient; disease as "what the practitioner creates in the recasting of illness in terms of theories of disorder" (ibid., p. 33); and sickness as "the understanding of a disorder in its generic sense across a population in relation to macrosocial, (economic, political, institutional) forces." (ibid., p. 35). Like Kleinman, Mukherjee also indicates the cultural component of illness when he claims that "the names of ancient illnesses are condensed stories in their own rights" (ibid., 60). He then explains the origins of several illnesses and their names, such as "typhus," "influenza," and "tuberculosis." Even the word "cancer" is culturally motivated; that is, it originates from the Greek word "karkinos," which means "crab," while the word "oncology" has its origins in the Greek word "onkos," which was often used to denote a tumor. Understanding the history and origin of a word is important because it is accompanied by a cultural and historical understanding of a phenomenon, especially a complicated one such as cancer.

The central character in Mukherjee's book is Sydney Farber, who discovered a chemo-therapeutic drug called Aminopterin, an antifolate for children with acute lymphoblastic leukemia, that proved to be at that time a hundred percent lethal. One of the children, who died during this drug experimentation, was Robert Sandler (RS). However, his twin brother grew up to be healthy. In the book presentation at the Harvard bookstore, Mukherjee expresses Sandler's mother's reaction to the publication. The author discovers that the book's writing brought a sense of closure to RS's mother and reconciliation with herself and the decision she had made to give up her dead son for an autopsy to advance the research. Ironically, these multiple autopsies were a source of the follow-up drug used to treat this cancer prevalent in children. The book mentions this positive result of autopsies performed, among which was RS, that brought the 87-year-old story of this mother to a close. This is one such incident where books and narratives could prove therapeutic.

To convert RS's case study into a story, a single page of a medical report written by the doctor or the researcher was described in great detail, including metaphors of emotions, and terminology of healing and expanded to a narrative covering several pages. Transforming case studies and specific research into stories gave rise to a cancer story, which, as the book's subtitle says, is *A Biography of Cancer*. Throughout the book, Siddharth expresses the importance accorded to finding a cure by researchers and medical practitioners, very often, especially through medical trials, directly experimenting on the patients unaware of the consequences of the experiment. The novel *The Fault in Our Stars* seems the most appropriate example to illustrate the kind of psychological impact a positive attitude towards cure can have. Given the fictional category, in the following section, we will analyze the extremely unique narrative technique used by the author to foreground the importance of cancer narratives.

Intimate Narratology in *The Fault in Our Stars*

One of the best ways to interpret and witness the functionality and utility of narrative medicine is to analyze *The Fault in Out Stars* by Green in this context. The novel narrates the story of the struggle of two young cancer patients, Hazel Grace Lancaster and Augustus Waters. Hazel suffers from thyroid cancer affecting her lungs whereas Augustus struggles to live through osteosarcoma with the loss of one leg already.

Both meet at a weekly cancer support group which is a place to narrate and supposedly share the pain and suffering to a group of co-sufferers in the absence of a doctor. The group meets in the basement of a church where the friendship of Hazel, Isaac and Augustus thrives. The novel makes fun of the act of smoking by using it as an implied metaphor of death and the experience of dying. "It's a metaphor, see: You put the killing thing right between your teeth, but you don't give it the power to do its killing" (Green, 2012, p. 24). Ironically, almost in the end of the novel, the same desire to buy cigarettes turns out to be nemesis for Augustus in a tragic incident at the gas station.

The inevitability of death is also postponed in the novel by the intense desire to know the ending of a narrative *An Imperial Affliction* as the novel written by the Dutch author Peter Van Houten ends in mid-sentence. The trace of the novelist, the desire to know the ending connects the suffering of Hazel and

Augustus together in a form of mission. The narratives of suffering coalesce and collide at various intersections in the novel. The novel should be praised as giving space to the sufferings of the family as well as colleagues. Both Hazel's mother and Lidewij Vliegenthart also narrate the pain as co-sharers. The costly wish to visit the author in Amsterdam is finally granted by a charitable foundation that funds the dreams of sick children. Ironically, Augustus exhausts his wish to take Hazel on the tour. The way the doctors understand the importance of the final wish of Hazel given to her critical condition also adds up to the value attached to the doctor-patient relationship.

Though the search to find the appropriate ending to the novel ends tragically for both Hazel and Augustus as they are appalled to find a chaotic and incoherent reception by the author. The episode opens up the novel to interlink more narratives of trauma as the dejected young lovers visit Anne Frank House as well as Augustus' promise to write the ending to the unfinished narrative.

The romantic date between the young lovers in Amsterdam has another ominous yet strange revelation about the "death suit" of Augustus. He had planned his own funeral and rituals associated with it. The capacity of the author to reveal the black humor in all these instances makes the novel quite interesting and disturbing at the same time. After the first sexual encounter of the central characters, Augustus first time narrates the instance of reappearance of Cancer back in his body, which also portrays the intense human desire to fight and win over a deadly disease like Cancer with the sense of narrative intimacy and companionship. The suffering of Isaac, Hazel's mother also has intense episodes of revelation of feelings every now and then in the novel.

One of the very touching incidents of intimate narratology is when the almost-dying Augustus calls both his best friends to recite his own eulogy at the same church where they used to share feelings of suffering in a close support group. The weird idiosyncrasies of Augustus—chewing a cigarette between his teeth, buying his death suit, making people read his own death eulogy etc. save his character from being a type of cancer patient. Humanely enough, Hazel narrates the life story of Augustus differently from her original eulogy which she has narrated to Augustus when he was alive. The final chapters show a kind of culmination of narratives within the grand cancer narratives. The failed attempt to narrate the ending of the story by the Van Houten symbolizes a very big thing in the novel. It is the unforgivable atonement, which is not granted by Hazel. It is the cryptic ending of every cancer narrative, which should not be sought after for fruition. Cancer appears metaphorically like an "imperial affliction" here, which is very close to Mukherjee's book *The Emperor of All Maladies.* The intimate narratives of two patients win over the "imperial affliction or emperor of all malady" emotionally, though physically they lose the battle.

One of the ways the dead can relive in the form of a written memory is presented in the form of a narrative to a different narrative in the novel. Augustus tries to give his ending to *An Imperial Affliction*. The care given by the different characters of the novel such as the patient-protagonists' parents, friends, colleagues is an essential aspect of narrative medicine. An approach of empathy, patience, and understanding towards the patient as well as the disease remains central to this form of narrative.

Let us now turn to the aspect of "ethics of care," a key theme of study in medical humanities as well as narrative medicine. One of the pioneering theorists of this form of care is Levinas, who examines the altruistic aspect of care through responsibility for *the Other*, in the face of *the Other*. An evaluation of this form of ethics will help the field of medicine build empathy and function as a moral guide to build healthy and ethical interpersonal relations.

Care for *the Other* in view of Levinas's "Ethics of Care"

Curing through care is the primary responsibility of doctors; what is expected of them is an altruistic attitude. Understanding the pain of *the Other* is undertaken by allotting sufficient time to listen to the plight of *the Other* through their narration, sympathy as well as sensitivity and openness to their stories. By examining Levinas' ethics of *the Other*, we will try to show that cure and care for the patient are two sides of the same coin.

Levinas is a well-known philosopher of ethics, but his approach to ethical questions and problems stands him out as one of the forerunners of the philosophy of "interconnected cosmopolitanism." Having belonged to the Continental philosophical tradition, he does not propose any universal formula of right and wrong. For him, the first and foremost aim of ethics is to establish the intersubjective relationality between Self and *the Other*. The ethical is the precondition for the existence of the power politics of self and *the Other* where his notion of ethical relationship is always guided by the notion of responsibility. In other words, before the doctor even meets the patient the first time, the practitioner should be repleted with a sense of responsibility towards *the Other*. Caring for *the Other* in this sense, ennobles not only professional ethics but also establishes a sense of security in the mind and body of the person who is suffering. This unique relationship also keeps the narrative of suffering in the circle of faith.

Moreover, unlike other traditional theories of ethics, Levinasian ethical framework emphasizes more on the physical embodiment of the human with alterity, in the sense that the self gets its ontological meaning only in relation to *the Other*. By doing so, the European notion of the medical self as a knowledgeable self gets its fruition only while encountering with the patient-other. The ethical self, in this case, the medical practitioner is formed by coming face to face with *the Other.*

Standing on the shoulders of his predecessors like Husserl (1969) and Heidegger (1967), Levinas puts forward the notion of "totality of being" in relation to philosophical terms like alterity and exteriority. In medical sciences, investigation plays a very important role, but narratology is the first act that situates the diseased in the relationship with the practitioner. It is with the art of listening and the craft of analyzing, that the self welcomes the exteriority of *the Other,* not to throttle but to nurture and embrace.

Borrowing the Levinasian model of ethics in medical humanities serves one more purpose. It allows alternative medicine practices like Ayurveda and Tibetan Sowa-Rigpa as more ethical practices based on touch where the self feels the pain of *the Other* by sensing the nerve. It is the relationship of healing, caring and curing at the same time which defies the European notion of a totalitarian attitude towards *the Other.*

If "Self" and "Other" both are deemed to be single entities, then the chances of a narratological relationship are reduced because both categories exude totalitarian power and contest each other. If we consider these categories as radically different from each other, we risk objectifying them. Considering these intricacies, Levinas proposes a reconciliatory approach, a middle path where the notion of "Same" and "Other" can be understood properly without falling prey to any grammar of totality. He molds the whole philosophical problem anew by understanding the "Self" as being constitutive of the "Other" without sacrificing its ontological essence. Levinas is not falling prey to romanticizing the relationship between "Self" and "Other" as a utopian condition, rather, he is aware of the innate tension between "Self" and "Other" and aims to smoothen out the clash by considering the radical alterity of the "Other." When the doctor listens to the suffering of *the Other,* he/she comes in full play as an operative self; he/she learns and improves based on the experience and exteriority of *the Other.*

The model of Levinasian ethics injects the rhetoric of care and responsibility of listening and responding to *the Other.* It avoids the egocentric attitude of the self if it fails to respect the narrative act of the patient. One of the ways to break the vicious power politics in the relationship between the self and *the Other* is to understand the infinity of the act of responsibility towards *the Other* without asking for it in return. In other words, doctors should exercise their act of responsibility without demanding it back from the patients. The act of listening, responsibility and the desire to cure is not an obligation for a doctor, but rather it should be part of their ontological self. It is what makes them who they are.

One more advantage associated with the model of the Levinasian framework of ethics is that it also dismantles and deconstructs the aporia in the relationship between doctor and patient when they are in communication. There are unavoidable points of crises while the patient narrates the pain and suffering caused because of trauma and the incapability to speak properly. The diagnostic is based mostly on the "said" by the patients, however, Levinas prioritizes the "saying" over "said" as an ongoing process of listening and interpretation. To acknowledge the silences, trauma and the act of saying of the patients and the family members is also an act of medical ethics. The practitioner should never try to interpret or summarize the "saying" in the form of "said." Saying is infinite, as the suffering and the narratives of suffering.

The recent development in postmodernism seems to rob the agency of the human being and declares the death of humanity, which has given rise to the study of post-subjectivity. One form of this post-subjectivity can be sought out in the works of Levinas, for whom the subjectivity gets its energy in the form of being "responsible for the other." Responsibility is not a burden here, but ethically a choice that relates the "me" to *the Other* and helps both to thrive. If the communication takes place in this ethical framework, the journey of cure and care can be visualized in a holistic way which is informed by an ethical framework which enables medical humanities to solve various problems.

Reference List

Charon, R. (2006) *Narrative medicine: honoring the stories of illness.* New York: Oxford University Press.

Charon, R. (2008) *Psychoanalysis and narrative medicine.* Albany: State University of New York Press.Green, John (2012) *The fault in our stars.* New York: Penguin Young Readers Group.

Heidegger, M. [1927 (1967)] *Being and time.* Translated from the German by John Macquarrie and Edward Robinson. Oxford: Blackwell.

Husserl, E. (1969) *Formal and transcendental logic.* The Hague: Nijhoff. Kleinman, A. (2020) *The illness narratives: suffering, healing, and the human condition.* London: Hachette UK.

Levinas, E. [1961 (1979)] *Totality and infinity: an essay on exteriority.* Translated from the French by Alphonso Lingis. The Haag, Boston and London: Martinus Nijhoff Publishers.

Levinas, E. and Nemo, P. (1985) *Ethics and infinity.* Pittsburgh: Duquesne University Press.

Levinas, E. [1974 (1998)] *Otherwise than being, or, beyond essence.* Translated from the French by Alphonso Lingis. Pittsburgh: Duquesne University Press.

Levinas, E .[1995 (1999)] *Alterity and transcendence.* Translated from French by Michael B. Smith,New York: Columbia University Press.

Levinas, E. [1991 (2006)] *Entre Nous: thinking-of-the-other.* Translated from French by Michael B. Smith and Benjamin Harshav. London: A&C Black.

Mukherjee, S. (2010) *The emperor of all maladies: a biography of cancer.* London: Fourth Estate.

3.1.4

Ta(l)king Away the Trauma: Verbo-Visual Testimony and Narrative Humility in Psychiatric Treatment

Preeti Puri

National Institute of Technology Hamirpur, India

Shefali

Dr B R Ambedkar National Institute of Technology, Jalandhar, India

Abstract

The hegemonic stance of healthcare institutions on mental illness often marginalizes the patients' experience. Their suffering which is caught between physical and emotional distress defies linguistic processing. In this context, verbo-visual mode of storytelling emerges as an important touchstone of Narrative Medicine to integrate the fundamental aspects of illness, suffering, and healing. To reflect this, the chapter investigates the ways in which Bastien, the narrator of Espé's *The Parakeet* (2021), employs verbo-visual language and chronicles his mother's psychological trauma when she conceives before marriage. The thought of getting an abortion and losing her child makes her vulnerable to the extent that after giving birth to Bastien she slips into depression. However, the invisible scar of trauma which exacerbates her mental health and induces the course of "bipolar disorder with schizophrenic tendencies" in her psyche is largely ignored by the clinicians as they remain focused on the visible signs of illness on her body. Owing to this, Bastien depicts those traumatic aspects of his mother's suffering that may be difficult to put into words. Through verbal and visual metaphors, his narrative fortifies the importance of understanding patients' perspectives and restoring compassion during the clinical diagnosis of mental illness. Apropos to this, the chapter discusses how art-based interventions like verbo-visual narratives can facilitate trauma patients to testify their suffering and assist the doctors in strengthening Sayantani DasGupta's principle of "narrative humility" in medical treatment. The objective of the chapter is to do a close reading of

Bastien's narrative as a therapeutic practice that can help trauma patients to overcome isolation through the visual depiction of body. In doing so, it draws theoretical insights from Elisabeth El Refaie's idea of "pictorial embodiment" in illness narratives and probes the text as a valuable resource which challenges the conventional boundaries of psychiatric treatment.

***

Given that psychiatrists diagnose mental illness based on symptoms, it would be reasonable for patients to form a narrative to explain their experience to the doctor. However, the hegemonic stance of healthcare institutions on mental illness hinders patients' attempts to interact freely and share insights into their past experiences, due to which a significant barrier gets created between the doctor and the patient. The prevalent psychiatric discourse views the afflicted person primarily as an abnormal being with a disturbed psychological balance that can be stabilized using psychopharmaceutical drugs and medicalized treatment. Against this supremacy of a medicalized system of knowledge, Narrative Medicine with its patient-centered approach in healthcare, calls for the creation of a novel space in which subjective narratives, relating to illness, "give voice back to patients, fragile people, and persons who had no right to speak and claim how they lived their disease" (Marini, 2015, p. 13). However, it might be difficult for a patient to find appropriate words and express their mental illness inflicted by a traumatic event. The challenge that trauma places before the sufferer is that of representation through language, as "language fails in the face of trauma, and that trauma mocks language and confronts it with its insufficiency" (Gilmore, 2001, p. 6). To quote Gabriele Schwab: "How then do we write what resists representation?" (2006, p. 102). How does one articulate the experience of psychological trauma, emotional distress, and the resulting mental illness that defies linguistic processing?

In case of trauma and psychological suffering, "literary verbalization" argues Geoffrey Hartman "remains a basis for making the wound perceivable and the silence audible" (2003, p. 259). However, a lot of narratives that attempt to convey a subjective perspective of traumatic suffering fall short of depicting the actual experience. Many find memoirs as a way to tell the personal story of their experience, but it is worth noting that the verbo-visual mode of storytelling used by artists in comics and graphic narratives can emerge as an important touchstone of Narrative Medicine to integrate the fundamental aspects of illness, suffering, and healing. In fact, the ability to showcase psychic suffering in a verbo-visual format creates a counter-discourse through which one unearths the "real" and invisible side of mental illness. We elucidate these claims through a close reading of Espé's graphic novel *The Parakeet* (2021), in which Bastien, the narrator employs verbo-visual language and chronicles his mother's psychological trauma, which exacerbates her mental health and induces the course of "bipolar disorder with schizophrenic tendencies" in her psyche. Furthermore, to interrogate the problems as well as the possibilities of communicating the experience of trauma in a clinical setting, we turn to Sayantani DasGupta's concept of "narrative humility" and formulate a productive critique of the need for clinical empathy in psychiatric treatment. To build onto these aforementioned ideas, the chapter draws conceptual insights from Elisabeth El Refaie's idea of "pictorial embodiment" in illness narratives, and probes *The Parakeet* as a valuable resource which can aid in ta(l)king away the trauma.

The Invisible Presence of Trauma

From the shock of a sudden disaster to the repeated experience of emotional anguish or psychological abuse, trauma can take many forms. One often thinks of trauma as something that is beyond our ability to describe and comprehend because the effect of a traumatic "event is not assimilated or experienced fully at the time, but only belatedly, in its repeated *possession* of the one who experiences it." (Caruth, 1995, p. 4, emphasis in original). In other words, trauma manifests itself through a repetitive perception of memory and flashbacks that "disrupts the previous ideas of an individual's sense of self" (Balaev, 2008, p. 150). The victim's inability to move out of it is largely because of the fact that it does not restrict itself to one specific moment in time, but "returns to haunt the survivor later on" (Caruth, 1996, p. 4). Its invisible presence "shocks the system, be it the mind or body" (Eyerman 2019, p. 42) and makes the person an object of suffering. This sense of trauma, as a psychological injury inflicted on a sufferer's mind, is reflected in *The Parakeet* wherein Bastien recounts his mother, Marie Laporte's mental illness and connects it to her trauma of psychological abuse, that she faces when she conceives before marriage. Her sense of identity disintegrates when her father forces her to undergo an abortion. The process of cultural othering by her relatives and community becomes a significant contributor to her mental breakdown. In actuality, the stigma that she faces, for being an "unwed mother" (Espé, 2021, p. 19), makes her vulnerable and far more emotionally sensitive.

An agonizing ordeal of these incidents traumatizes her to the point that even after giving birth to his son, Bastien, a persistent fear of losing him invades her mind. Marie's friends recommend her to start working again but she gets worried for Bastien. They assure her that her family will take care of him, but her mind registers the memory of losing Bastien: "They'll take Bastien from me!" (Espé, 2021, p. 36). A slightest mishap "or later situations that repeat or echo the original" (Luckhurst, 2008, p. 1), not only causes an irreversible psychic rupture but also puts her at risk for post-traumatic stress and depression. Marie's inefficiency in explaining her situation to her father: "I... I... I can't help it... All I want... is just... to die... die!" (Espé, 2021, p. 14), signals the difficulty of describing her own psychic perspective to others. A conflicted discussion about her condition with her friends: "Maybe... Yes... I am sick... I... I don't know..." (ibid., p. 35) reflects how the need to speak about herself has been ignored by her family and friends. In the section "The Shirt with the Belts," Bastien recounts an episode of his mother's mental breakdown. He narrates how her voice "sounded like a hurt animal" (ibid., p. 6), while her body writhed in pain around the bush side area of the house. To control her, two medical professionals "put her in a big white shirt with belts on it" (ibid., p. 9) to take her to the psychiatric facility. The consternation that follows manifests itself through a fragmentation in her speech, as the "experience severs the connection between the memory of the event and the language that would and/or could describe it" (Rodrigue, 2012, p. 39). Marie's inability to deal with trauma and mental illness bruises her mind while her inefficacy to process her feelings leads to emotional outbursts which her family calls by the name "episodes." The invisible presence of illness makes it difficult for her family to understand her condition. For instance, while illustrating his grandpa's frustration with Marie's illness, Bastien writes: "When he is mad. He shakes mama really hard...like she's one of the plum trees in the garden...Maybe he wants to shake the rotten fruit out of her head" (p. 15). A visual representation of the grandfather shaking the tree—a metaphor for Marie's body—portrays his anger towards Marie's invisible illness that has taken roots inside her body.

Further, describing an object associated with the memory of his mother in the final part of the narrative, titled "Parakeet," Bastien recounts another episode of her mental breakdown when on returning from the psychiatric hospital she is unable to find him at home. She behaves so violently that her family sends her again to the psychiatric facility in Lavaur, where she hangs herself. Here, her suicide, in many ways, indicts her family for its failure to save her. This incident is related to Marie's fear of losing connection with Bastien that tears the fabric of her current reality because "trauma cannot simply be consigned to the past: it is relived endlessly in the present through repeated painful re-enactments, nightmares, hallucinations, and flashbacks" (Robson, 2004, p. 11). As a witness to his mother's failure to survive the illness, Bastien "comes to be a participant and co-owner of the traumatic event: through his very listening, he comes to partially experience trauma in himself ... [and] comes to feel the bewilderment, injury, confusion, dread and conflicts" (Laub, 1992, pp. 57-58) that his mother has gone through. To re-establish empathy, he portrays her everyday experience by reconfiguring the representation of psychological suffering in sequential panels of comics. Through verbo-visual representation, he demonstrates her intense struggle to come to terms with psychiatric treatment.

Verbo-visual Testimony of Psychological Suffering

One cannot deny that "accurate representation of trauma can never be achieved without recreating the event since, by its very definition, trauma lies beyond the bounds of "normal" conception" (Tal, 1996, p. 15). The memory of a traumatic event is difficult to be "organized on a linguistic level and this failure to arrange the memory in words and symbols leaves it to be organized on a somatosensory or iconic" (van der Kolk and van der Hart, 1995, p. 172). However, as Valerie Raoul and colleagues contend, trauma "cannot be removed or remedied" but "a supportive environment where the effects of such experiences are acknowledged and literally taken into account can allow a new story of healing to begin" (2007, p. 204). Arnold-de Simine also observes that '"[t]rauma cannot be contained by verbal exegesis but spills out in uncontrollable images and is part of a fragmented and cyclical temporality" (2018, p. 141). Accordingly, Bastien brings into representation the gaps of silence between Marie's unspoken trauma "by mimicking its forms and symptoms" (Whitehead, 2004, p. 3). Following the observation of her unspeakable trauma and emotional blunting, Bastien expresses: "I think that if grandpa had gotten what he wanted... Mama wouldn't have gotten sick because of me" (Espé, 2021, p. 20). He makes clear that what begins as a case of internalized trauma for Marie by the consequence of social ostracism becomes a manifestation of mental illness. To a significant extent, his incisive insights challenge the standardized medical discourse that homogenizes Marie's subjective feelings. His verbo-visual testimony dismantles the limit of linguistic depiction of a traumatic memory and provides "a process of constructing a narrative, of reconstructing a history and essentially, of *re-externalizating the event*" (Laub, 1992, p. 69, italics in original). Through visual cues Bastien tells the reader that his mother looks normal like people in the street, but her "illness is invisible. Silent. Shameful" (ibid., p. 66); following behind her in the form of scary black creature (Figure 3.1).

Figure 3.1. Mental illness as an invisible scary monster that follows Marie.

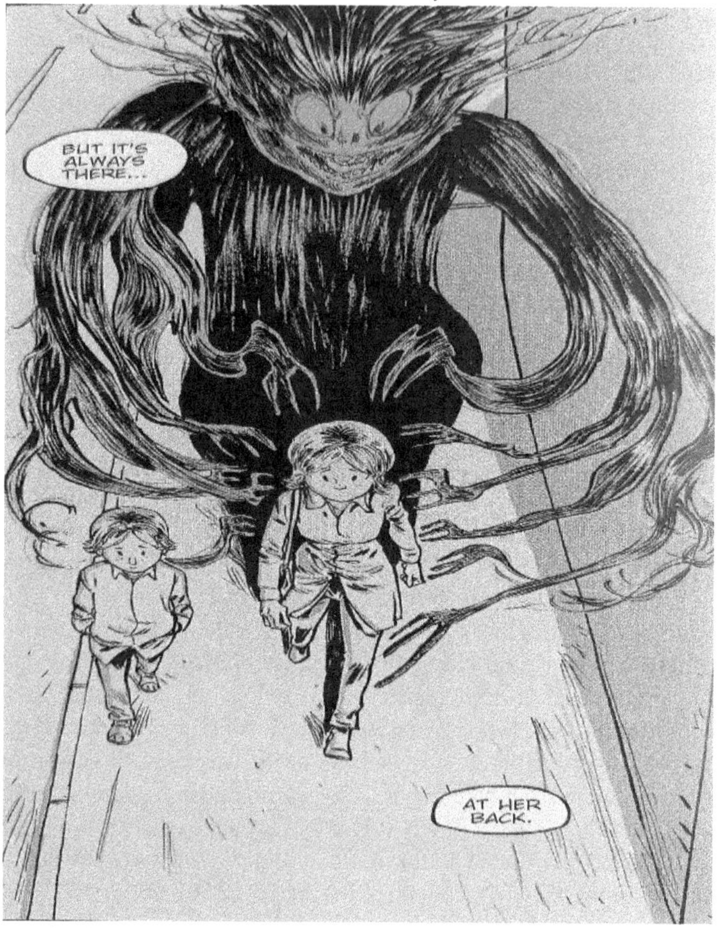

From Espé's *The Parakeet*, p. 66. Image reproduced with permission from the publishing house, Graphic Mundi, an imprint of The Pennsylvania State University Press, © 2021.

Offering a child's eye-view of her suffering he states: "Mama's like Jean Grey in the X-Men. She might explode any moment! But no one knows...except me" (p. 67). Further, he uses the visual register of a tightrope walker (Figure 3.2) to represent Marie's struggle to navigate through the tribulations casted by mental illness. He pictures her off the rope, "lost between two worlds... off balance... about to tumble into the dark depths of her illness" (ibid., p. 81). Illness worsens her mental state to the extent that she descends into a state of self-destructive behavior. In the section "Wallpaper," Bastien pictures Marie's emotional fragility by comparing it to a candy jar. Through image (Figure 3.3), he externalizes the psyche of Marie breaking like a candy jar, while the transition in colors—from sap green to burning red—serve as a visual language for representing the chaotic realm of her mind during one of the episodes.

Figure 3.2. Marie's struggle to navigate through life.

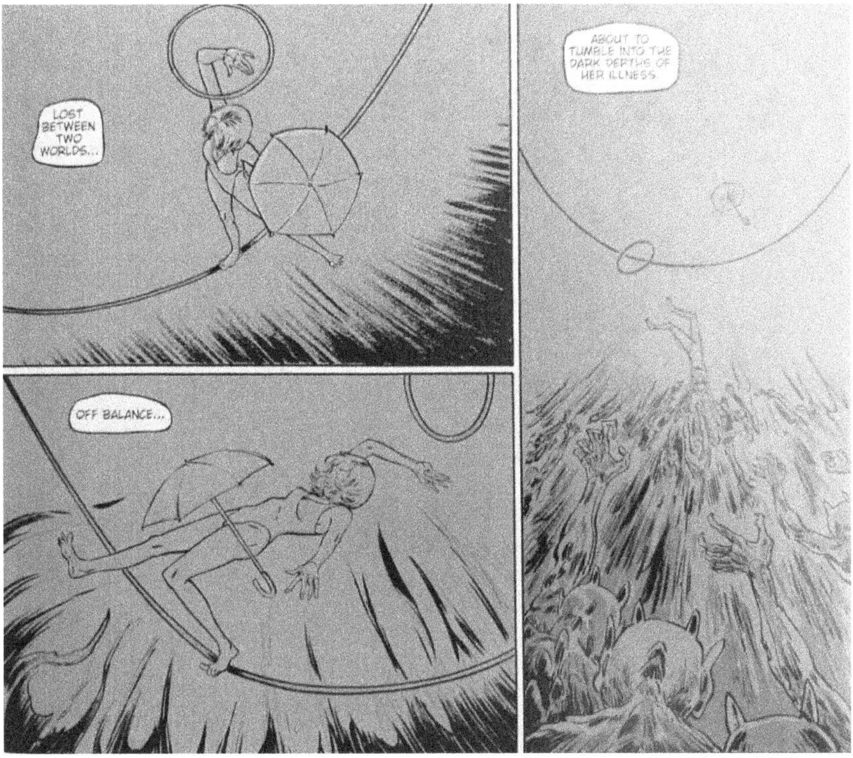

From Espé's *The Parakeet*, p. 81. Image reproduced with permission from the publishing house, Graphic Mundi, an imprint of The Pennsylvania State University Press, © 2021.

Figure 3.3. Marie's nervous breakdown.

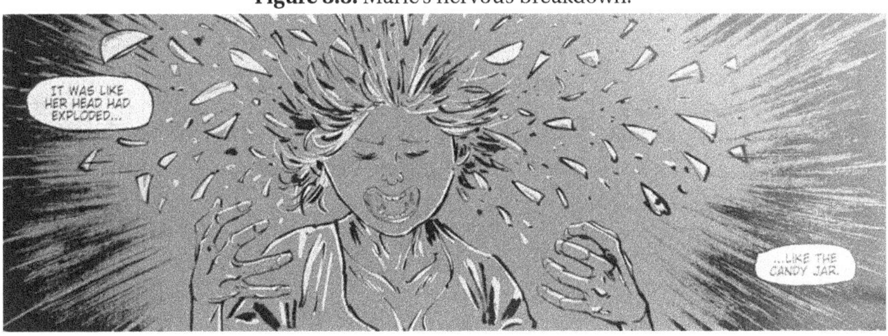

From Espé's *The Parakeet*, p. 85. Image reproduced with permission from the publishing house, Graphic Mundi, an imprint of The Pennsylvania State University Press, © 2021.

Figure 3.4. Burden of psychiatric medicines.

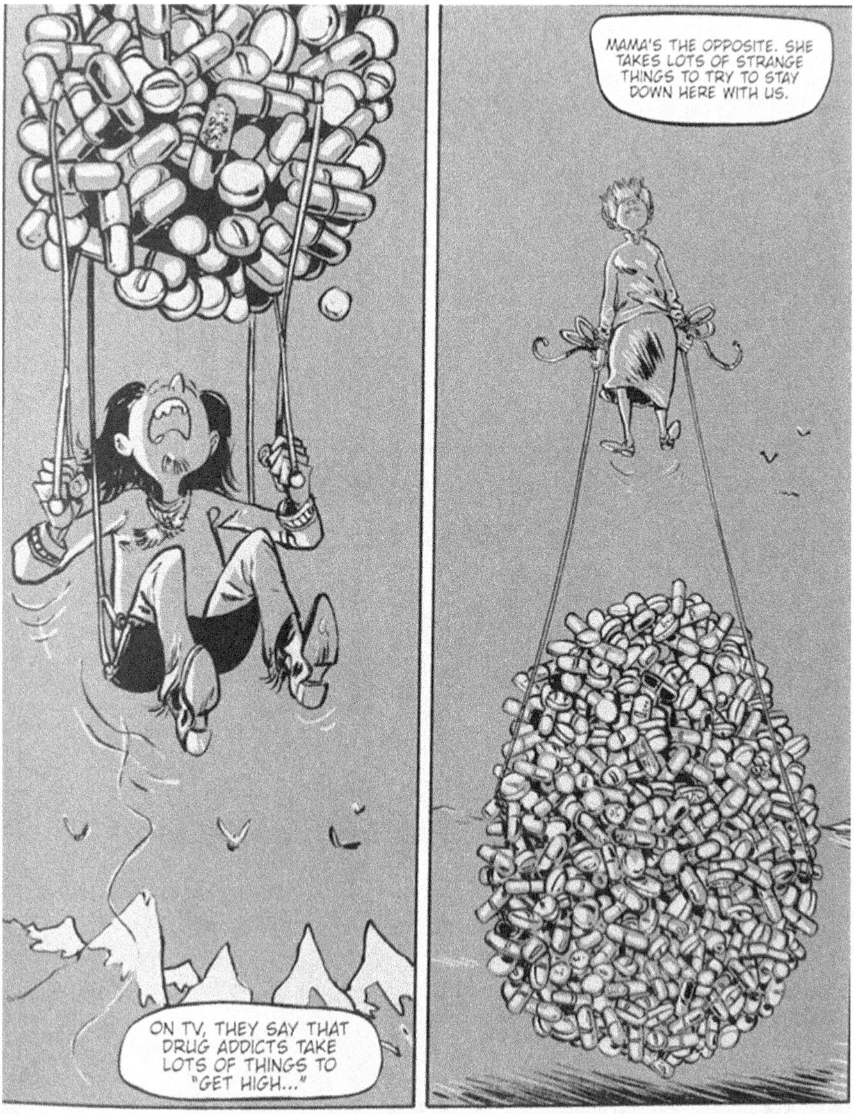
ON TV, THEY SAY THAT DRUG ADDICTS TAKE LOTS OF THINGS TO "GET HIGH..."
MAMA'S THE OPPOSITE. SHE TAKES LOTS OF STRANGE THINGS TO TRY TO STAY DOWN HERE WITH US.

From Espé's *The Parakeet*, p. 123. Image reproduced with permission from the publishing house, Graphic Mundi, an imprint of The Pennsylvania State University Press, © 2021.

When a social security inspector arrives to check on Marie for being on prolonged leave, her husband, Francis, tells him that she suffers from severe depression and had an episode the night before. The officer with a notepad in his hand with the most apathetic expressions states: “I’ll make up my own mind once I’ve seen the ‘patient’ with my own eyes” (Espé, 2021, p. 71). His cold and clinical stare indicates a general disinterest in the patient, as he responds to Francis’ statement by saying: “My, my... depression, the modern affliction. If you knew how many ‘depressive patients’ I assess who turn out to be perfectly fine...” (ibid., p. 71). Later, however, when Marie gets there, she is clearly on the verge of a nervous breakdown. The visual representation of her ghost-like body and blank eyes, with a deep void in them, embodies how the dark force of depression has taken control over her mental faculties. She expresses her psychological suffering vociferously before the officer and states: “There are shadows trapping me in the room... They’re raping me... You must help!!! Doctor you must help!!!” (ibid., p. 73). In a fit of emotional outburst, Marie loses control of herself, attacks the officer, and breaks everything lying around the room. After witnessing the whole incident, the officer calms Marie down by administering tranquilizers, and has a completely “different expression and tone of voice” (ibid., p. 75). He tries to shows compassion by telling Francis to stay strong, but the real person in need of compassion is Marie, whose cry for “help” from the officer reflects her plea to privilege her narrative voice that has been ignored for years.

Breaking the Barrier: Integrating Narrative Humility in Psychiatric Treatment

When a social security inspector arrives to check on Marie for being on prolonged leave, her husband, Francis, tells him that she suffers from severe depression and had an episode the night before. The officer with a notepad in his hand with the most apathetic expression states: “I’ll make up my own mind once I’ve seen the ‘patient’ with my own eyes” (Espé, 2021, p. 71). His cold and clinical stare indicates a general disinterest in the patient, as he responds to Francis’ statement by saying: “My, my... depression, the modern affliction. If you knew how many ‘depressive patients’ I assess who turn out to be perfectly fine...” (ibid., p. 71). Later, however, when Marie gets there, she is clearly on the verge of a nervous breakdown. The visual representation of her ghost-like body and blank eyes, with a deep void in them, embodies how the dark force of depression has taken control over her mental faculties. She expresses her psychological suffering vociferously before the officer and states: “There are shadows trapping me in the room... They’re raping me... You must help!!! Doctor you must help!!!” (ibid., p. 73). In a fit of emotional outburst, Marie loses control of herself, attacks the officer, and breaks everything lying around the room. After witnessing the whole incident, the officer calms Marie down by administering tranquilizers, and has a completely "different expression and tone of voice" (ibid., p. 75). He tries to show compassion by telling Francis to stay strong, but the real person in need of compassion is Marie, whose cry for "help" from the officer reflects her plea to privilege her narrative voice that has been ignored for years.

This calls to attention the ways in which empathetic listening can be restored in psychiatric treatment to navigate the process of diagnosis and treatment alongside patient's complex reality of illness. In the context of Narrative Medicine, physicians consider "storytelling as a germinal part of the care itself" (Irvine and Charon, 2016, p. 129), as narratives have the power to "connect patients and health-care providers and link evidence-based medicine and medicine based on narrative, as well as clinical sciences and human science" (Marini, 2015, p. 8). While recognizing the value of such an approach to foster an authentic understanding of patient's perspective, Sayantani DasGupta puts forward the concept of narrative humility. Narrative humility strengthens physicians to practice "empathic witnessing that enters into narratives rather than dissects them" (Shapiro, 2011, p. 71), because a patient's story belongs to him or her. DasGupta (2008, p. 981) acknowledges that the narratives which patients share are not objects to be mastered, "but rather dynamic entities" to be approached with ethical and emotional understanding. Bastien's verbo-visual testimony of Marie's illness, in its unique self, "holds elements that are unfamiliar—be they cultural, socioeconomic, sexual, religious, or idiosyncratically personal" (ibid., p. 981). And these elements can only be understood through a "mutual investment, reciprocal clarity, and affiliation" (Charon, 2016, p. 157) between the patient and the physician. Instead of relying on established models for diagnosis and therapy, narrative humility facilitates the physician to "restore the pivotal role of the patient's own story in the healing process (Langer and Ribarich, 2008, p. 61). Bastien's narrative provides enough evidence that it can be used to humanize psychiatric treatment. It gives the impression that if physicians imbibe the aspect of verbo-visual storytelling during the diagnosis of mental illness, it will strengthen the notion of narrative humility and therapeutic healing in psychiatric treatment. In clinical practice, by equipping the healthcare professionals with "practical wisdom" (Charon, 2006, p. vii), such narratives can guide the healthcare professionals to listen to the narratives of psychological trauma and mental illness.

Taking a Closer Look: The Idea of Pictorial Embodiment

Verbo-visual representation of an individual in the graphic narratives, involves some process of engagement with the body in relation to its social, cultural, and political context. One "cannot avoid engaging with the sociocultural models that underpin body image, including categories of sex, gender, health, and beauty" (El Refaie, 2012, p. 73). Mental illness becomes visible through the pictorial embodiment of body as artists "are obliged to engage with the role of body in constructing and maintaining a person's identity" (El Refaie, 2018, Kindle location p. 56). Also, pictorial embodiment "provide[s] entirely novel ways of understanding the body, both for the graphic memoirist him-or herself and for the wider reading public" (El Refaie, 2012, p. 91). In *Parakeet,* one can see that illness affects all aspects of Marie's being, however, it is her body that bears the brunt of its effects and appears to be fragile, weak, and powerless throughout the narrative. For instance, delineating upon the effect of psychiatric treatment upon her body Bastien states: "When she comes back from the centers, she's a vegetable. Like a turnip... round... weak... limp... on the outside... and on the inside." (Espé, 2021, p. 59). The treatment disturbs her mental equilibrium as "she doesn't react... has no feelings... no wants" (ibid., p. 60). She is unable to engage her body in any kind of activity be it even walking. Although doctors think that this state is good for her, but for Bastien she is already dead, lying in a coffin just like his grandfather's mom. Bastien's portrayal of her mother as a superhero (Figure 3.5), when she undergoes electroshock therapy, is a clear example of how his penchant for comic superheroes, such as Wolverine and Iron Man, allows him to present her body in this particular manner. Through drawing his mother as a superhero, Bastien imagines the manner of his mother's endurance of electroshock therapy. Elsewhere, when his father brings Marie back from the psychiatric hospital he draws her as a comic character on a page, with button-like dead eyes wherein the physical outlook of her body finds its representation in the emotionally dull figure of a cartoon that stands in contrast to her living body. So, instead of cultural or social variabilities, the aspect of pictorial embodiment in *The Parakeet* depends upon Bastien's eye-view of his mother's mental illness. The visual language plays a central role in the narrative, as rather than just relying on words or narration, Bastien uses the vocabulary of comics to convey the experience of his mother's treatment process. Through verbo-visual storytelling, he is able to externalize her emotions and experiences, which have robbed her of words.

Figure 3.5. Bastien imagining his mother as a superhero.

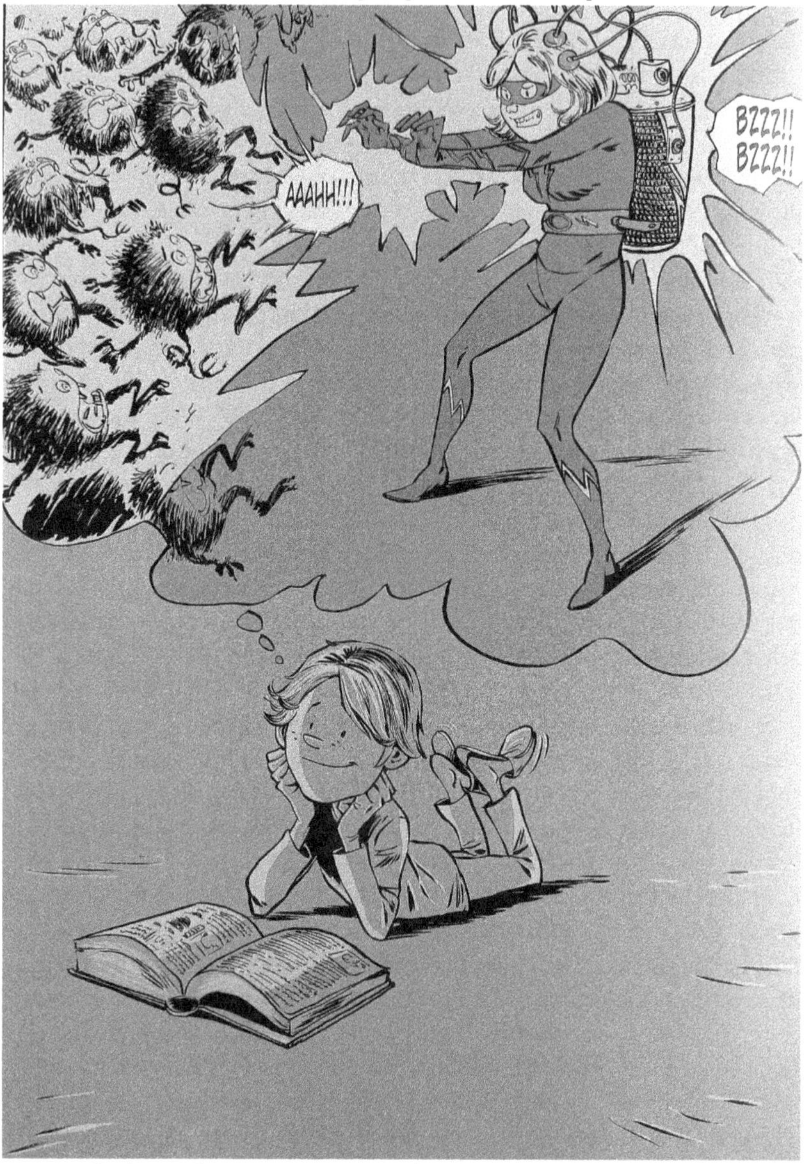

From Espé's *The Parakeet*, p. 44. Image reproduced with permission from the publishing house, Graphic Mundi, an imprint of The Pennsylvania State University Press, © 2021.

As we have seen over the course of this chapter, the verbo-visual medium of *The Parakeet* provides a way to improve mental health care by offering "a unique opportunity to examine the dynamics of disease from the point of view of those directly involved" (Marini, 2015, p. 29). Bastien's narrative, through a portrayal of his mother's trauma and mental illness, places strong emphasis on the lack of empathetic understanding during the clinical diagnosis of her illness. While, as DasGupta (2016, p. 148) contends, all aspects of her story "will necessarily be unfamiliar or unknowable," the narrative provides an access point into her psychic-scape enabling the physician to practice contemplative care with narrative humility. To conclude, Bastien's verbo-visual testimony illustrates the complex and multifaceted nature of trauma and its relation to mental illness. Along with this, the creative expression of verbo-visual metaphors that he uses acknowledges the pain of patients undergoing psychiatric treatment and provides a forum for them to share their suffering. In contrast to the standardized approach of clinical diagnosis, the visual depiction of patient's experience can further our understanding of the complexities of trauma-related experience. By moving beyond the politics of official medical discourse, the verbo-visual narratives can act as a window into how patients can depict their trauma. In essence, through the intersection of verbal and visual text, it prompts that patients can configure their bodies in their own way. In so doing, they will be able to articulate the invisible aspect of trauma and psychological suffering through drawings and metaphors that promote therapeutic healing and function as an alternate discourse to stigmatizing images that socially exclude patients with mental illness.

Reference List

Arnold-de Simine, S. (2018) 'Trauma and memory,' in Kurtz, J.R. (ed.) *Trauma and literature.* Cambridge: Cambridge University Press, pp. 140-152.

Baleav, M. (2008) 'Trends in literary trauma theory,' *Mosaic: An Interdisciplinary Critical Journal,* 41(2), pp. 149-166. Available at: http://www.jstor.org/stable/44029500 (Accessed: August 27, 2023).

Caruth, C. (1995) 'Introduction,' in Caruth, C. (ed.) *Trauma: explorations in memory.* Baltimore: Johns Hopkins University Press, pp. 3-12.

Caruth, C. (1996) *Unclaimed experience: trauma, narrative, and history.* Baltimore: Johns Hopkins University Press.

Charon, R. (2006) *Narrative medicine: honoring the stories of illness.* New York: Oxford University Press.

Charon, R. (2016) 'Close reading: the signature method of narrative medicine,' in Charon, R. et al. (eds.) *The principles and practice of narrative medicine.* New York: Oxford University Press, pp. 157-179. doi: https://doi.org/10.1093/med/9780199360192.003.0008

DasGupta, S. (2008) 'Narrative humility,' *The Lancet,* 371(9617), pp. 980-981. doi: https://doi.org/10.1016/S0140-6736(08)60440-7

DasGupta, S. (2016) 'The politics of the pedagogy: cripping, queering and un-homing Health Humanities,' in Charon, R. et al. (eds.) *The principles and practice of narrative medicine.* New York: Oxford University Press, pp. 137-153, doi: https://doi.org/10.1093/med/9780199360192.003.0007

El Refaie, E. (2012) *Autobiographical comics: life writing in pictures.* Jackson: University Press of Mississippi.

El Refaie, E. (2014) 'Looking on the dark and bright side: creative metaphors of depression in two graphic memoirs,' *a/b: Auto/Biography Studies*, 29(1), pp. 149-174. doi: https://doi.org/10.1080/08989575.2014.921989

El Refaie, E. (2019) *Visual metaphor and embodiment in graphic illness narratives.* [Kindle edition] Oxford: Oxford University Press.

Espé (2021) *The Parakeet.* Translated from the French by Hannah Chute. United States: Pennsylvania State University Press/Graphic Mundi.

Eyerman R. (2019) *Memory trauma and identity.* Palgrave Macmillan.

Gilmore, L. (2001) *The limits of autobiography: trauma and testimony.* Ithaca and London: Cornell University Press.

Hartman, G. (2003) 'Trauma within the limits of literature,' *European Journal of English Studies*, 7(3), pp. 257-274. doi: https://doi.org/10.1076/ejes.7.3.257.27984

Irvine, C., and Charon, R. (2016) 'Deliver us from certainty: training for narrative ethics,' in Charon, R. et al. (eds.) *The principles and practice of narrative medicine.* New York: Oxford University Press, pp. 110-134. doi: https://doi.org/10.1093/med/9780199360192.003.0006

Lakoff, G., and Johnson, M. (2003) *Metaphors we live by: with a new afterword.* Chicago and London: The University of Chicago Press.

Langer, N., and Ribarich, M. (2008) 'Using narratives in healthcare communication,' *Educational Gerontology*, 35(1), pp. 55-62. doi: https://doi.org/10.1080/03601270802388930

Laub, D. (1992) 'Bearing witness or the vicissitudes of listening,' in Felman, S, and Laub, D. (eds.) *Testimony: crises of witnessing in literature, psychoanalysis, and history.* New York and London: Routledge, pp. 57-74.

Luckhurst, R. (2008) *The trauma question.* London and New York: Routledge.

Marini, M.G. (2015) *Narrative Medicine: bridging the gap between evidence-based care and medical humanities.* London: Springer.

Raoul, V. et al. (eds.) (2007) 'Introduction: metanarrative politics and polemics,' in *Unfitting stories: narrative approaches to disease, disability, and trauma.* Canada: Wilfrid Laurier University Press, pp. 203-208.

Robson, K. (2004) *Writing wounds: the inscription of trauma in post-1968. French women's life-writing.* Amsterdam and New York: Rodopi.

Rodrigue, T.K. (2012) 'PostSecret as imageText: the reclamation of traumatic experiences and Identity,' in Amihay, O. and Walsh, L. (eds.) *The future of text and image: collected essays on literary and visual conjunctures.* United Kingdom: Cambridge Scholars Publishing, pp. 39-68.

Schwab, G. (2006) 'Writing against memory and forgetting,' *Literature and Medicine*, 25(1), pp. 95-121. doi: http://doi.org/10.1353/lm.2006.0026

Shapiro, J. (2011) 'Illness narratives: reliability, authenticity and the empathic witness,' *Medical Humanities*, 37(2), pp. 68-72. doi: https://doi.org/10.1136/jmh.2011.007328

Tal, K. (1996) *Worlds of hurt: reading the literatures of trauma.* United Kingdom: Cambridge University Press.

van der Kolk, B. A., and van der Hart, O. (1995) 'The intrusive past: the flexibility of memory and the engraving of trauma,' in Caruth, C. (ed.) *Trauma: explorations in memory.* Baltimore: Johns Hopkins University Press, pp. 158-182.

Whitehead, A. (2004) *Trauma fiction.* Edinburgh: Edinburgh University Press.

3.2 Analytical Objective

3.2.1
The Trauma of Illness: Reading and Teaching Sarah Manguso's *The Two Kinds of Decay*

Mona Baie

University of Heidelberg, Germany

Abstract

Illness, especially severe and chronic illness, has for a long time been recognized as a "biographical disruption." Following from that, certain illness experiences can be considered traumatic: A disease presents itself as a sudden, unexpected, and overwhelming force, it radically alters a person's life course, and its repercussions can be felt long after the "actual" event of (physical) sickness. This paper looks at a recent American memoir, Sarah Manguso's *The Two Kinds of Decay* (2008), in which the protagonist falls ill with a rare, severely debilitating neurological condition at the age of only 21. It argues that considering this autopathography through the lens of trauma theory allows for new insights for both literary scholarship and narrative medicine. From the perspective of literary studies, it opens the genre of illness writing to ways of interpretation that focus less on the physical, acute realities of disease, but on its psychological, long-term effects. *The Two Kinds of Decay*, as I illustrate, uses narrative strategies such as montage and an oscillating temporal structure to explore the traumatic experience of illness as well as the (im)possibility of its representation through language. From the perspective of narrative medicine, the text, used in a medical school setting, allows future physicians to explore topics such as illness as biographical disruption, different ways and meanings of "healing," and the ethics of bearing witness.

***

Sarah Manguso's acclaimed memoir *The Two Kinds of Decay* (2008) recounts the author's experience of falling ill with a rare autoimmune disorder that comes to be diagnosed as "CIDP"—short for "chronic inflammatory demyelinating polyradiculoneuropathy." At the age of 21, after a seemingly trivial cold, she begins to feel a tingling in her hands and soon after suddenly loses power and feeling in both arms and legs. The year of the disease's onset she spends almost entirely in hospitals and day clinics, being examined and treated by various specialists. In the years that follow, ongoing treatment and several relapses shape her life as she returns to college, graduates, and moves to New York—all while struggling with severe mental health problems.

While it is stated in the text—in a subtly ironic, self-mocking way, a tone that pervades the book – that "[t]his is the usual sort of book about illness" (p. 183), *The Two Kinds of Decay*, consisting of 81 brief chapters and written in a poetic, often aphoristic language is anything *but* the "usual" book about illness. As Cindie Maagaard points out, the text, with its segmented, episodic form and its morally complex protagonist who claims that illness has made her a bitter, less amiable person runs counter to conventional, normative expectations of illness stories: it refuses to follow a logic of "triumph" over illness, refuses to frame illness as a journey towards self-realization, and instead "embrace[s] ambiguities and contradictions about what illness is and means" (Maagaard, 2020, p. 321).

In this paper, I want to elaborate on the ambiguities and contradictions in Manguso's memoir and offer a reading from the angle of trauma theory. In the following, I first provide an overview of existing scholarship on illness narratives and trauma studies. Secondly, I analyze *The Two Kinds of Decay* in regard to trauma theory, illustrating how narrative strategies such as achronological storytelling and montage are used to explore the traumatic experience of illness as well as the (im)possibility of its representation through language. Thirdly, I reflect on using the memoir in medical education, arguing that it allows its readers to explore topics such as illness as biographical disruption, different ways and meanings of "healing," and the ethics of bearing witness.

Trauma Theory and Illness Narratives

In contemporary trauma studies, even though definitions remain a subject of dispute, traumatic events are generally seen as 'overwhelming' in nature, which means that they exceed an individual's consciousness at the time of their occurrence and are experienced and assimilated only belatedly (Caruth, 1995; 1996). They can result in stress disorders manifesting as "repeated, intrusive hallucinations, dreams, thoughts or behaviors stemming from the event along with numbing that may have begun during or after the experience, and possibly also increased arousal to (and avoidance of) stimuli recalling the event" (ibid., 1995, p. 4). In other words, an event does not stay in the past, but continues to haunt a person's presence, as it returns in involuntary bodily or psychological symptoms such as visual memories ("flashbacks" in psychiatric terminology), or repeated and compulsive behaviors. Moreover, because of its characteristic of exceeding a person's consciousness at the time of its occurrence, the experience of trauma in its fullness resists understanding: there is an "incompletion in knowing," a "traumatic void" that remains in place for the experience and memory of the event itself (ibid., 1995, pp. 5-6; Felman and Laub, 1992).

Certain illness experiences, especially in the case of severe and chronic illness as depicted in Manguso's memoir, can be considered traumatic: A disease presents itself as a sudden, unexpected, and overwhelming force, it radically alters a person's life course (it "disrupts" someone's biography, see e.g. Bury, 1982), and its repercussions can be felt long after the "actual" event of (physical) sickness. While the benefits of giving voice to, of narrating one's "woundedness" (Frank, 1995) are routinely emphasized, representing such experiences through narrative proves rather difficult in practice. Not only is the experience of illness hard to put into words (Scarry, 1985; Conway, 2007); trauma(tic illness) in particular is an experience so overwhelming that it inherently "resists language or representation" (Whitehead, 2004, p. 3), which leaves literature with the paradoxical tasks of trying to speak about the unspeakable as well as ordering the inorderable.

Without dismissing these complexities, I argue that illness narratives such as Manguso's nevertheless "come to function as containers for the trauma of illness" (Winning, 2020, p. 266) and find creative ways to give voice to their characters' experiences. *The Two Kinds of Decay*, as I argue in the following, provides a sense of the protagonist's trauma because the text itself bears signs of trauma in its language and narrative structure. It has what I will call a "traumatic structure," which means that the text does not follow a linear, chronological way of storytelling, but instead is "mimicking its [trauma's] forms and symptoms, so that temporality and chronology collapse, and narratives are characterized by repetition and indirection" (Whitehead, 2004, p. 3). In the following, I analyze how such a traumatic structure is present in the book, both at the level of the plot and at the level of the text's narrative structure.

Trauma and Traumatic Structure in Sarah Manguso's *The Two Kinds of Decay*

It is in the very opening sentences of the book that the attempt to reassemble and give voice to an experience of traumatic illness is introduced as its central theme. Written from the perspective of the present, the narrator states her determination to try to recall the painful, overwhelming events of her illness experience, events she feels she will never be able to fully understand – the best she can do is attempt a tentative grasp at memory:

> The disease has been in remission seven years. Now I can try to remember what happened. Not understand. Just remember. For seven years I tried not to remember much because there was too much to remember, and I didn't want to fall any further behind with the events of my life. (Manguso, 2008, p. 3)

Moreover, the segment goes on: "Sometimes I think the content of those days might not have finished happening ... The events that began in 1995 might keep happening to me as long as things can happen to me." (ibid., p. 4) This phrasing can be read as alluding to a doubly "haunted" presence: That which "might keep happening" stands in for both the physical aspects of disease (one of CIDP's characteristics is that it can recur at any time) and the lasting psychological effects of what she lived through, beginning in 1995.

Regarding its thematic and temporal focus, the book can be divided into two parts. The first, longer part ranges from "The Beginning" to the segment "Tableau Vivant" and traces chiefly the events of 1995, the year of the disease's onset, which, as I argue, represent the text's core trauma. Recounting various stages of that year—the initial cold which possibly triggered the later autoimmune response, the first symptoms, hospitalizations, apparent remissions, and relapses which bring her back to the hospital—it chronicles in often excruciating detail the multiple traumas that constitute the protagonist's illness experience: the feelings of complete horror and helplessness as she experiences neuralgic pains, is unable to move, and fears to die (ibid., pp. 52-53); surgical interventions that leave her covered in her own blood (pp. 36-38; on this see also Sanai, 2011); and seeing others suffer and even die in hospital beside her. Regarding those details, the text plays with the notion of "order." Through consistent cues about time (e.g. "February 1995") and a sequencing of events (e.g. "first" hospitalization, "first" central line, the "second" needle, etc.), the text indicates that it is an attempt to order, structure, and hereby apprehend what felt to be "too much to remember" for many years. The text's overall narrative structure, however, eludes the possibility of such an ordering of the past. The text frequently jumps back and forth in time to scenes and moments from other stages of her life and intersperses the depiction of hospital experience with philosophical reflections on life in general, hereby mirroring trauma's missing neat chronologies and the complexity of its representation.

Similarly, the text constantly emphasizes the "incompletion in knowing" inherent to the experience. Trying to remember and represent what happened in an accurate manner, the protagonist fails repeatedly, and often states this explicitly. "[T]his memory must not be right," she remarks at one point when comparing her recollection of the size of an MRI scanner, which she remembers to be so scarily narrow it made her panic, with the actual sizes in use at the time (p. 59). Another, more indirect strategy to highlight gaps and distortions in memory is montage. In the chapter "Supplies," Manguso seems to employ language stemming from medical writing when she lists a range of supplies needed to care for a central line:

> 1 large red biohazard container; 10 cc syringes; 5 cc syringes; 3 cc syringes; saline vials; heparin vials, vial spikes; needle covers; interlink caps; injection caps; adhesive patches in three sizes; gauze pads; nonsterile rubber gloves; individually wrapped "sterile field" kits, each of which included 1 sterile waterproof paper sheet, 1 pair sterile gloves, 1 sterile surgical mask, sterile gauze patches, alcohol swabs, iodine swabs, adhesive compound swabs, 1 roll sterile plastic surgical tape. (ibid., p. 113)

The list of objects, typographically set off from the rest of the text by its italicization, seems taken from a surgical or nursing handbook, and the technical language clearly shifts away from the poetic style of other passages. Alongside other sections written in medical terminology, this passage can be read as overtly "replacing" faulty personal memories with general, seemingly more "accurate" medical information, thereby illustrating the difficulties of approaching and finding a language for traumatic illness.

With the segment "The Admiral's Nephew" begins the text's second part, which focuses on the years 1996 to 2006, the text's "today" (ibid., p. 131). The most acute episode of the protagonist's illness trajectory—months of severe bodily symptoms, pain, and distress, spent almost entirely in hospital—are over; still under treatment but more physically stable and again able to live by herself she returns to college. However, the notion of a clear cut between the events of 1995 and a presumably healthier state in the present is run counter by the text in various ways that go far beyond the depiction of the ongoingness of certain symptoms or medical check-ups.

To an extent, it is the protagonist's life trajectory and psychological state that illustrates the ongoing impact of a severe, traumatic illness experience on the narrator's present. While still suffering from CIDP relapses over the years—although these are described as less severe than the first major episode in 1995—she starts experiencing mood swings, which she first considers to be mere side-effects of steroids but which soon develop into episodes of severe, suicidal depression. The text details her stay in a psychiatric institution and the various psychotropic medication she takes. At some point, she crashes her mother's car "so everyone would see I wanted to die" (ibid., p. 178). In 2004, the "biggest problem" in her life changes "from CIDP to drinking" (ibid., p. 170). Although the traumatic illness experience and the later depression and substance abuse are never discussed as clearly, causally related, the lingering psychological effects of what the protagonist lived through in 1995 shine through again and again. Many of her life choices seem to still be shaped by the events of that year. She describes, e.g., how since her first experience of long-term hospitalization, of all of a sudden being subject to the dictates of a disease, she lives in a constant state of "relapse anxiety" that prevents her from having a steady job, a serious partnership, or a cared-for home, because "I haven't lost the fear that at any moment I will have to quit my job, say goodbye to my friends, leave my home, and go to the hospital not knowing when, or in what condition, I'll be discharged." (ibid., p. 158) Apart from the anxiety that results from experiencing a sudden, total loss of control, feeling like she has lost a year of her youth has led her to engage in various compulsive, self-harming behaviors such as excessive partying and promiscuous sexual conduct driven by a desire to "catch up" on sex rather than pleasure; it continues to shape her perception of time and productivity in the sense of an urge to always work, always write, never having time to stop (ibid., pp. 180-182).

However the nature of trauma as ongoingness is also mirrored in the narrative structure of the text itself. In the second part, the narrative becomes even more labyrinthic as the text begins to fragment into ever bigger time distances between the single episodes. Assuming an oscillating way of storytelling, the text meanders, constantly blending current events with recollections of her previous life, led by illness, in disruptive ways, hereby evoking a sense of the past and presence as constantly in communication and interdependence. Manguso's use of frequently changing narrative perspectives, switching from focalized, experiential (e.g. segment "Kimiko") to more distanced, stark, at times aphoristic modes (e.g. segment "Uncertainty"), and again intersecting her own voice with that of others through montage (e.g. segments "Mary" and "Memory"), further poses the "narrating I" telling in the "now" as a rather ephemeral and fragile voice—a powerful mode of narration that provides a sense of the effects of (past) catastrophic illness on an individual's present life.

Teaching Narratives of Trauma

As seen, *The Two Kinds of Decay* conveys not only the experience of a once lived, possibly recurring physical ailment, but also the psychological, long-term effects of traumatic illness through both content and form. In the final section of this chapter, I consider the prospects of using this text in medical education drawing on my own teaching experience with an elective seminar at the medical faculty of the University of Heidelberg, Germany.[1] In doing so, I align with a line of research that advocates the use of literature in medical education—most notably among them the work of Rita Charon—perceiving such courses as heightening future clinicians' reflective skills and attention to the perceptions and emotional landscapes of others (Hawkins and McEntyre, 2000; Charon, 2005, 2006; Lembert-Heidenreich and Mildorf, 2013; Bleakley, 2015; for German-speakers Wohlmann et al., 2021). Aware of the persistent contestations of the idea of "literary training" for medical students and health care workers—not least because of the difficulties of measuring such training's effectiveness (Remein et al., 2020) as well as more general doubts about the ability of narrative(s) to convey illness and other medical experiences (Woods, 2011)—I wish to contribute to the conversation by reflecting on an exemplary teaching experience in an exemplary setting, its prospects and its challenges.

In Heidelberg, we discussed *The Two Kinds of Decay* in a two-hour seminar, offered for fourth-year students and above, with no additional examination. Students were required to have read the text beforehand and to have noted down first impressions. Since the seminar was optional, we did not have to follow fixed learning objectives set out by the faculty. The teaching goal was to open a space for close reading, following the notion that this method originating in literary studies enhances attentive listening in clinical practice and deepens affiliation with a patient (Charon, Hermann and Devlin, 2016), as well as offers a learning experience that would differ from their routine classes and spark interest in literature as an alternative, valuable mode of thinking about and for medicine. The session ended with a 15-minute writing exercise in which students were asked to reflect on a short selected passage. In the following, I elaborate on three themes that emerged during the discussion and the exercise.

One was the lived experience of CIDP, which arguably forms the book's contentual mainstay. We started by covering the "medical basics" of this rare neurological disease. Regarding Manguso's text, students were interested in the depiction of a diagnostic and therapeutic process shaped by medical uncertainty, differing specialist opinions, and constantly changing therapeutic guidelines as well as in the various, at times rather unusual neurological symptoms the protagonist exhibits (Manguso, 2008, pp. 27-28). A challenge that presented was to keep a balance between reading the text as illness testimony based on a

---

[1] Two years earlier, while still in medical school, I was lucky enough to read *The Two Kinds of Decay* as part of an interdisciplinary workshop on illness metaphors organized by the German Academic Scholarship Foundation and held by Associate Professor Anita Wohlmann (University of Southern Denmark).The seminar not only sparked my interest in narrative medicine, but also in this particular text, for which I hereby express my gratitude.

person's lived experience *and* as an aesthetic artifact, i.e., to not read the text too "literally" and hereby lose sight of the literary as a construction. It was helpful to discuss passages in the text that explicitly mention the issue of language and lay bare the complexities and limits of language in representing (bodily) experience – one particular section we spoke about, e.g., was the one in which the protagonist describes her difficulties in explaining to friends what it "feels like" to be paralyzed (ibid., p. 50).

Another theme we explored, not dissimilar to what I outline in the analysis above, was the ways in which *The Two Kinds of Decay* explores the long-term effects of severe—possibly traumatic—illness on a patient's life. On a content level, the students, most of whom were of a similar age to the story's protagonist at the onset of her disease, seemed to easily identify with the trauma that comes with having one's everyday life so severely interrupted, and they were particularly interested in her comments on wanting to "catch up" with her peers' biographies. Talking about the narrator's life trajectory after her initial hospitalization and the ongoingness of her bodily and mental struggles then led us to discussions about notions of "recovery," "cure," and "healing" in autoimmune and other chronic illnesses more generally. It was great to see how scholarly arguments dissecting medicine's tendencies to conceptualize health as an absence of all bodily ill and to idealize "cure" over more integrative models of care (e.g., Clare, 2017) showed up in the students' statements, and how they were able to critically assess such normative modes of medical thinking through the shared reading of Manguso's memoir. Again, a difficulty was to not read too "literally" but to try to discern how the text may formally convey the experience of illness and trauma through the use of certain narrative techniques, too. Whenever this was pointed out to them, however, students seemed eager to revisit the text, now from different angles; moreover, my own comments on various technical terms and concepts from literary studies were complemented by one of the students who had studied literature before turning to medicine.

Lastly, and this was the only topic I directed the students to, we discussed the ethical implications of bearing witness to someone else's narrative of trauma—ethics which apply to clinicians listening to patients' stories of illness, too. Scholarship on narrative ethics (Phelan, 2014) backgrounded my guiding of the discussion which focused on the question: What does it mean to read/listen to difficult stories? What we highlighted regarding listening attitudes was to not superimpose oneself on the other's story but instead be attentive and curious towards what the person has—and wants—to tell, to enter the conversation from a position of trust, and to leave space for contradictions and narrative gaps. *The Two Kinds of Decay*, depicting a multi-layered, medically difficult illness process proved to be a very instructive source text. Regarding clinical work as interaction, we touched on the emotional landscape of the caregiver, too. That stories of trauma can themselves be traumatizing for those who listen to them showed up in our discussion; many found Manguso's text "hard to stomach," and related this to encounters already experienced during their clinical rotations. Therefore, in the closing writing exercise we touched on physician's emotional toll in the face of difficult illness stories. I asked students to reflect on a short excerpt from the segment "The Hematologist," in which the narrator ponders the job of one of her specialist doctors who sees chronically and terminally ill patients all day (Manguso, 2008, pp. 34-35). The results were impressive, ranging from a doctor's inner monologue to the fictitious conversation between two visitors' flowers.

Taken together, the range of topics addressed in a single two-hour session was astounding. A huge advantage (and a possible challenge for other such electives) was, of course, that the course was optional and therefore chosen by particularly motivated students. To think through how it could work in other formats—with, perhaps, more teaching hours and an official examination that counts towards the students' degrees—remains a task for the future. Within the scope of this paper, it is sufficient to state that reading *The Two Kinds of Decay* in a medical school setting clearly demonstrated the potential of literature in helping future doctors confront, pay close attention to, and possibly learn to embrace the complexity and ambiguity of human (illness) experience.

Reference List

Bleakley, A. (2015) *Medical humanities and medical education: how the medical humanities can shape better doctors*. London: Routledge.

Bury, M. (1982) Chronic illness as biographical disruption. *Sociology of Health and Illness*, 4(2), pp. 167-182.

Caruth, C. (ed.) (1995) *Trauma: explorations in memory*. Baltimore: John Hopkins University Press.

Caruth, C. (1996) *Unclaimed experience: trauma, narrative, and history*. Baltimore: John Hopkins University Press.

Charon, R. (2005) Narrative medicine: attention, representation, affiliation, *Narrative*, 13(3), pp. 261-270. doi: https://doi.org/10.1353/nar.2005.0017

Charon, R. (2006) *Narrative medicine: honoring the stories of illness*. New York: Oxford University Press.

Charon, R., Hermann, N. and Devlin, M.J. (2016) 'Close reading and creative writing in clinical education: teaching attention, representation, and affiliation,' *Academic Medicine*, 91(3), pp. 345-350.

Clare, E. (2017) *Brilliant imperfection: grappling with cure*. Durham: Duke University Press.

Conway, K. (2007) *Illness and the limits of expression*. Michigan: University of Michigan Press.

Felman, S. and Laub, D. (1992) *Testimony: crises of witnessing in literature, psychoanalysis, and history*. New York: Routledge, Traylor & Francis Group.

Frank, A.W (1995) *The wounded storyteller: body, illness, and ethics.* Chicago: University of Chicago Press.

Hawkins, A.H. and McEnytre, M.C. (2000) *Teaching literature and medicine.* New York: Modern Language Association.

Lembert-Heidenreich, A. and Mildorf, J. (eds.) (2013) *The writing cure: literature and medicine in context.* Münster: LIT Verlag.

Maagaard, C.A. (2020) 'Countering prescriptive coherence in narratives of illness: Sarah Manguso's *The two kinds of decay* and Maria Gerhardt's *Transfer window,* in Lueg, K. and Lundholt, M.W. (eds.) *Routledge handbook of counter-narratives.* New York: Routledge, pp. 321-334.

Manguso, S. (2008) *The two kinds of decay.* London: Granta Books.

Phelan, J. (2014) 'Narrative ethics,' in Hühn, P. et al. (eds.) *Handbook of narratology.* Berlin: De Gruyter, pp. 531-546.

Remein, C.D. et al. (2020) 'Content and outcomes of narrative medicine programmes: a systematic review of the literature through 2019,' in *BMJ Open,* 10(1), doi: https://doi.org/10.1136/bmjopen-2019-031568

Sanai, L. (2011) Poet turned patient. *British Medical Journal,* 342(7795), p. 502.

Scarry, E. (1985) *The body in pain: the making and unmaking of the world.* Oxford: Oxford University Press.

Whitehead, A. (2004) *Trauma fiction.* Edinburgh: Edinburgh University Press.

Winning, J. (2020) 'Trauma, illness and narrative in the medical humanities,' in Davis, C. and Meretoja, H. (eds.) *The Routledge companion to literature and trauma.* London: Routledge, pp. 266-274.

Wohlmann, A., Teufel, D. and Berberat, P.O. (2021) *Narrative Medizin. Praxisbeispiele aus dem deutschsprachigen Raum.* [Narrative medicine. Practical examples from German-speaking countries] Göttingen: Vandenhoeck & Ruprecht.

Woods, A. (2011) 'The limits of narrative: provocations for the medical humanities,' *Medical Humanities* 37(2), pp. 73-78. doi: https://doi.org/10.1136/medhum-2011-010045

3.2.2

Tell Me Your (Counter)Story: Disrupting Dominant Approaches to Narrative(s), Medicine and Trauma

Brooke Covington

Christopher Newport University, US

Abstract

This chapter brings together narrative medicine, trauma, and critical race theory (CRT) in hopes of enriching the work of healthcare educators, researchers, and practitioners. Specifically, this chapter offers CRT's methodology of counterstorytelling as a way to grapple with multigenerational racial trauma by centering the narratives of those who identify as Black, Indigenous, and/or a Person of Color (BIPOC). Moreover, by bringing CRT to conversations concerning narrative medicine and trauma, this chapter seeks to invite (indeed, urge) healthcare practitioners to intentionally examine the ways in which racism, racial trauma, and whiteness negatively impact the clinical encounter and how to mitigate such effects.

Admittedly, narrative medicine has made significant strides in stressing the influence of racism on healthcare, but to move the field forward in a way that prioritizes anti-racism and anti-oppression requires educators, researchers, and practitioners to not only acknowledge but also intentionally incorporate key tenets of CRT and counterstorytelling (Delgado, 1989; Martinez, 2020; Solórzano and Yosso, 2002) into their work. The chapter thus proceeds by situating the aims of narrative medicine within the context of ethno-racial health disparities and theorizations of racial trauma. I then present CRT's counterstorytelling as a potential vehicle to enrich and expand the practice of narrative medicine. Finally, the chapter ends by offering a set of recommendations for how to intentionally incorporate counterstorytelling into a trauma-informed practice of narrative medicine.

***

This piece is written primarily for educators, researchers, and practitioners in the field of healthcare. Because the author is situated within an American context, much of the chapter will focus on structural and racial trauma as it has been witnessed in the United States, particularly among Black Americans. Deeply troubled by the systematic disenfranchisement and mistreatment experienced by Black Americans at the hands of U.S. institutions, the author purposefully draws from narratives that emerge from those who identify as Black and/or African American. Nevertheless, racial trauma is a global phenomenon evidenced by state-sanctioned violence and oppression of BIPOC communities around the globe. Though largely under-researched in trauma studies, racial trauma does impact the research and praxis of healthcare—both at the micro-level of individual patients and caregivers as well as at the macro-level of the system itself. This chapter presents one way in which healthcare workers might attune to the micro- and macro-woundings bred by racial trauma through the study of counterstories. Counterstorytelling is an interdisciplinary CRT methodology that draws attention to the dominant "stock" narratives that organize society while also bringing attention to the stories that run "counter" to those dominant interpretations. Such counterstories can challenge received wisdom about healthcare; expose stereotypes that infect clinicians and caregivers; and draw from BIPOC experiential and embodied knowledge to disrupt racist paradigms, co-create narratives with patients, and improve the quality of care.

To some degree, healthcare has always been infected with systemic and institutionalized racism—and though the links between racism, medicine, and trauma are substantial, such connections are not well-defined in trauma studies (Quiros, Varghese and Vanidestine, 2020). As a white educator committed to the (learning) process of anti-racist pedagogy and practice, I ultimately argue that traditional colorblind approaches to medicine and/or trauma do not adequately prepare practitioners to examine the central role that race, racism, and whiteness play in healthcare systems around the globe, but especially in the US. For the purposes of this chapter, *racism* is defined as "discrimination based on beliefs of racial superiority or differences in attributes and abilities based on race" (Jones et al., 2022, p. 480); whereas *whiteness* "refers to the invisible and hegemonic processes that support and uphold White supremacy and result in differential laws, policies, and practices that most often benefit those who are constructed as White" (Quiros, Varghese and Vanidestine, 2020, p. 160). Distinct from being white, whiteness refers to the normalization of white racial identity, the elevated social status attributed to those who identify as white, and the systemic racism that produces (and sustains) white privilege.

The statistics are grim. According to William J. Hall and colleagues: "disparities based on race and ethnicity persist in access to health care, quality of care received, disease incidence and prevalence, life expectancy, and mortality" (2015, p. 61). In the US, those who identify as Black, Hispanic, and/or American Indian experience higher infant mortality rates than whites (ibid., 2015). When compared to white Americans: "Black Americans die earlier, at higher rates, and suffer more complications of cardiovascular disease, renal disease, lung disease, cancer, and infectious diseases" (Jones et al., 2022, p. 481).

COVID-19 offers a case in point. The pandemic has disproportionately impacted BIPOC communities in terms of delayed diagnoses, longer hospitalizations (Grooms et al., 2022), and rates of mortality (Yancy, 2020). Of course, I hesitate to highlight any of these negative trends, since as Ray points out, "When health professions learners' primary pedagogical experience of Black patients is through statistics, it becomes very easy for them to think of Black people as data points rather than as individuals whose health is often at the mercy of racist institutions" (2021, p. 725).

Beyond evidence of worse health outcomes, such health disparities—particularly when combined with the historical and structural racism experienced by BIPOC populations in the US—can lead to and compound existing racial trauma. Racial trauma "refers to the events of danger related to real or perceived experience of racial discrimination [including] threats of harm and injury, humiliating and shaming events, and witnessing harm to other [BIPOC] due to real or perceived racism" (Comas-Díaz, Hall and Neville, 2019, p. 1). Such "severe psychological and physiological trauma can have intergenerational effects [especially] the cumulative psychological wounds that result from historical traumatic experiences, such as colonization, genocide, slavery, dislocation, and other related trauma" (ibid., p. 2). Shytierra Gaston confirms this point in her analysis of narratives from descendants of US lynching victims, arguing that "cumulative, collective historical racialized trauma and its effects can be experienced over multiple generations… [meaning] that even descendants who did not directly experience the traumatic event can evince trauma-related symptoms and responses" (2021, p. 83).

Racial trauma and poor health outcomes are connected. David R. Williams and Selina A. Mohammed (2013) found that experiences with racial discrimination led to increased chronic stress that directly damages BIPOC health. In light of ethno-racial health disparities *and* the multigenerational psychological and physiological effects of racial trauma, it's clear that "racism must be named as a critical driver of health inequities" (Jones et al., 2022, p. 480), and anti-racist practitioners must "actively confront[s] racism by making deliberate and consistent equitable decisions" (ibid.). In recent decades, narrative medicine has been proposed as a potential corrective to healthcare's purported "colorblindness" by training physicians to provide culturally humble and patient-centered care.

Narrative Medicine

Rita Charon defines narrative medicine as "medicine practiced with the narrative competencies to recognize, absorb, interpret, and be moved by stories of illness" (2005, p. 262). While proponents of narrative medicine claim that close reading, reflective and creative writing, and radical listening "will lead to more humane, more ethical, and perhaps more effective care" (Charon, 2006, p. vii), there is little evidence to prove that absorbing literary or patient narratives will enable physicians to grasp the trauma that comes with (or before or after) illness—much less be compelled to act. Delese Wear and Julie M. Aultman warn that, "a major shortcoming of narrative medicine is the fact that it relies almost exclusively on exchanges between individual entities—readers/listeners and patients/texts – and not on social structures" (2005, p. 1063). As narrative medicine wisens to the harm of phenomenological "bracketing" of identities, practitioners will need tools to confront the messy social contexts from which narratives emerge. As the next section describes, CRT's interdisciplinary method of counterstorytelling provides one possible tool to enrich the practice of narrative medicine by enabling practitioners to attend to the social, historical, and structural contexts from which narratives of the Self and the Other emerge.

Critical Race Theory & Counterstorytelling

As a methodological framework, counterstorytelling emerges from CRT—a school of thought that "challenges the ways in which race and racial power are constructed and represented in American legal culture and, more generally, in American society as a whole" (Crenshaw et al., 1996, p. xiii). CRT asserts that ignoring racial difference preserves and sustains the status quo with all of its deeply institutionalized injustices to BIPOC minorities and insists that diminishing the importance of race will enable racism to continue, even prosper. Of course, this point is supported by traditional colorblind approaches to healthcare that fail to acknowledge (much less eradicate) ethno-racial inequities and mistreatment. Importantly, CRT aims to challenge discussions of race and racism that fail to acknowledge the role of whiteness in American society.

Critical race theory is thus an effort to disrupt the status quo by situating the experiences of people of color as central to understandings of racism and whiteness, particularly in institutions where racial inequities proliferate like healthcare. Daniel Solórzano and Tara Yosso lay out five key tenets of CRT, namely that CRT:

1. Situates race and racism as central to other forms of subordination
2. Challenges dominant ideology, particularly narratives concerning objectivity, meritocracy, colorblindness, race neutrality, and equal opportunity
3. Is committed to social justice and the empowering of subordinated minority groups
4. Recognizes experiential and embodied knowledge of people of color as legitimate and critical to understanding racism
5. Analyzes issues of race, gender, sexual orientation, class, language, and national origin from a transdisciplinary and historical perspective

I share these key tenets because Solórzano and Yosso argue that "a story becomes a counterstory when it begins to incorporate the five elements of critical race theory" (2002, p. 39).

What is a Counterstory?

Richard Delgado, one of the pioneers of CRT, explains that stock stories are narratives told by dominant ingroups, whereas counterstories are narratives that emerge from marginalized perspectives to challenge dangerous hegemonic narratives present in stock stories. "Stock" stories depict a reality that is favorable to the dominant ingroup in order to maintain their privileged status. For example, common American exceptionalism stock stories situate the country as built on "equal opportunity" or "meritocracy." These stock stories have become so naturalized they are often accepted as truth and thus preserve a racially stratified society.

Counterstories aim to disrupt stock stories. Richard Delgado explains that counterstories can appear in several genres: narratives, chronicles, dialogs, parables, and allegories (1989). Counterstories might be autobiographical, biographical, or composite narratives (Solórzano and Yosso, 2002). And because it is both a method and methodology, counterstorytelling can be the research tool used to collect narratives and/or the rationale and approach guiding the research process (the lens through which the narrative analysis occurs). For example, many CRT scholars adopt the "stock story vs. counterstory" methodological approach, where a stock story is directly compared to a counterstory. This approach enables the audience "to first experience a version of the events from a status quo point of view [i.e. the stock story]" before presenting a counterstory "to critique the viewpoint put forth by the stock story while offering alternative possibilities for the audience to consider" (Martinez, 2020, p. 70). By inviting this intentional comparison, audiences may reevaluate their unrealized assumptions, stereotypes, and conflicting viewpoints. In light of these conflicting narratives, audiences consider: "Can my world still stand? What parts of it remain valid? What parts of the story seem true? How can I reconcile the two worlds, and will the resulting world be a better one than the one with which I began?" (Delgado, 1989, p. 2435).

As method and methodology, counterstory enables those practicing narrative medicine to analyze existing stock stories and counterstories, or create their own. Either posture requires a deep understanding of CRT as well as *narrative humility*. According to Sayantani DasGupta, narrative humility "acknowledges that our patients' stories are not objects that we can comprehend or master, but rather dynamic entities that we can approach and engage with, while simultaneously remaining open to their ambiguity and contradiction" (2008, p. 981). Narrative humility admits that any story might have unfamiliar cultural, social, religious, sexual, and socioeconomic elements – and invites readers to remain humble to the fact that our interpretation of the story will always be partial, exploratory, indefinite.

Others have recognized the untapped potential of racially informed storytelling in healthcare contexts. For example, Keisha Ray advocates a form of counterstorytelling she calls experiential race testimonies (ERT), an approach that "1) centers patients, not their illness or the provider; 2) situates Black patients' experiences with health care within the context of racism; and 3) amoralizes Black people's health" (2021, p. 726). Much of what Ray argues aligns with the goals of counterstorytelling.

Beyond amplifying BIPOC narratives, counterstorytelling has the potential to deeply enrich narrative medicine curricula by compelling practitioners to critically interrogate whiteness and its impact on the clinical encounter. Given the statistics surrounding the diversity of physicians in the US, deliberate examinations of whiteness in healthcare are essential. According to the AAMC (2019), data from 2019 indicated that 56% of physicians identified as white, 17% identified as Asian, 5.8% identified as Hispanic, 5% identified as Black or African American, and 1% identified as multi-race (which doesn't account for the 13.7% unknown). In light of these statistics, I join Laura Quiros, Rani Varghese, and Todd Vanidestine in arguing for the importance of "clinicians and leaders in the field, particularly those who are White identified, [to] examine their own positionality and understand the ways their beliefs and actions uphold White supremacy and institutions that support this" (2020, p. 164). CRT motivates learners to do just that, while also calling upon practitioners to speak directly to (and against) racism and whiteness when confronted with it. The following section provides some brief recommendations for how to incorporate CRT's counterstory in narrative medicine curricula.

Counterstorytelling Narrative Medicine Toolkit

This toolkit was built in keeping with Roger Fallot and Maxine Harris's (2009) five key values of trauma-informed care: safety, trustworthiness, choice, collaboration, and empowerment. In the clinical encounter, it's vital for all parties to feel physically and emotionally safe, while also maintaining an atmosphere of trustworthiness through clear articulation of expectations and boundaries. Patients must be seen as partners who have some degree of *choice*, which requires both *collaboration* and sharing of power (*empowerment*). Each of these five values is vital to a trauma-informed approach to narrative medicine that incorporates counterstorytelling as a lens through which to analyze narratives. A trauma-informed approach to narrative medicine thus invites practitioners to pause and consider the role that trauma plays in the lives of those they care for—to consider how they might behave differently, how they might avoid (or at least minimize) the risk of retraumatizing patients, and how they might co-create narratives to help trauma survivors heal.

This toolkit was also built around a commitment to draw from historical and contemporary narratives that are appropriately contextualized, and, whenever possible, curating contemporary stock and counter-narratives that are place-based, meaning that these narratives emerge in close proximity to where practitioners actually are. Such place-based counterstories will help ensure that practitioners reckon with the inequities present in their own backyards, making it more difficult to pass the inequities off as someone or somewhere else's problem. Stock stories are important, too, as a framework to help learners spot master narratives, challenge such interpretations, and disrupt complacency within oppressive paradigms.

My recommendations include Toni Morrison's short story "Recitatif" (2022) as well as *Mend* (2018) by Kwoya Fagin Maples. Another recommended multi-genre text that bridges both historical and contemporary narratives is Claudia Rankine's highly praised *Citizen* (2014), a collection of lyric essays that interweaves visual media and text to expose the macro- and micro-aggressions faced by minoritized populations in the U.S.

Morrison's "Recitatif" traces intermittent meetings of two main characters—Twyla and Roberta—from age 8 into adulthood. The two meet at a children's shelter where Twyla, the focalizer, recalls feeling "stuck in a strange place with a girl from a whole other race" (Morrison, 2022, p. 4). What makes the story a counterstory is that it disrupts expectations of racial narratives by withholding one key detail: the racial identity of the two main characters. By withholding this detail, both the characters *and* the reader are implicated in their assumptions about racial differences. As the reader searches for clues in their attempt to settle the racial identity of each character, they are also forced to reckon with their own racism and the power of racial hierarchies.

Beyond its interrogation of race, "Recitatif" also explores trauma through the symbolism associated with Maggie, a character with multiple disabilities whose racial identity Twyla cannot remember. As a racially ambiguous and presumed mute woman who gets attacked in the apple orchard behind the shelter where Twyla and Roberta first meet, Maggie symbolizes the unspeakable event of racialized trauma. As Cathy Caruth (1996) has theorized, trauma fractures consciousness and destroys the ability to linguistically represent the traumatic experience. Twyla has multiple dreams about Maggie, but cannot recall Maggie's race, if Maggie fell or was attacked, and whether she participated—such symbolic interweavings of race and violence point to the suppressed racial trauma that Maggie represents as a marginalized person with no social power, no agency, and (literally and symbolically) no voice. As an inventive and beautifully crafted counterstory that uses racial ambiguity to centralize race while challenging dominant narratives, "Recitatif" offers multiple points of entry for discussions of trauma, power, racism, and whiteness in the clinical encounter.

Mend by Kwoya Fagin Maples is a collection of poems that captures the "imagined memories and experiences" of Anarcha Wescott, Betsey Harris, Lucy Zimmerman and the (at least) eleven other enslaved women upon whom J. Marion Sims performed his gynecological experiments in Alabama between 1845 and 1849 (2018, p. xi). The Preface to this collection of poems directly invites the reader to "consider how this story relates to now. Presently, in 2018, black women are three times more likely to die after childbirth than white women, regardless of ability to pay and regardless of prenatal care" (ibid., p. xi-xii). *Mend* offers an example of counterstorytelling in the composite genre, in that Maples draws on real contexts and characters to provide "imagined memories and experiences" in the form of poems. In between Maples' poems are excerpts from J. Marion Sims' autobiography and historical accounts of slavery—a choice that exemplifies the stock story vs. counterstory methodology. Situating Sims' stock stories next to Maple's counterstories directly confronts readers with the trauma produced by scientific racism, unethical physicians, and the cruelty of curiosity.

It is important, however, to recognize the potential to retraumatize BIPOC learners when only drawing from narratives that highlight the violent oppression of BIPOC communities. The possibility of evoking empathy in non-Black learners is not worth the additional trauma Black learners might endure through the process. Thus, it's crucial for educators to be clear with content warnings when assigning materials that highlight racial trauma, and also to make sure that BIPOC learners are given options for how to engage with the racialized subject material to avoid being further traumatized.

Claudia Rankine's *Citizen* may prove useful in this respect, as Rankine intentionally subverts voyeuristic appetites aimed at Black victimization by instead situating her focus on exposing white supremacy. One example from the mixed genre collection appears in a photoshopped image of the lynching of Thomas Shipp and Abram Smith where the men's bodies have been removed from the image, thus leaving only the unabashed—even smiling—faces of the white perpetrators of this terrorism. The text accompanying the image expertly implicates the reader through the use of second-person perspective ("you"), thereby inviting the (white) reader to adopt a form of double consciousness to "see themselves differently through the experiences of Black people and people of color" (Yancy, 2008, p. 12). Such an orientation may invite learners to not just cultivate empathy concerning BIPOC experiences but may situate learners as change agents who can remain complicit with systems of oppression or become proactive in ending it.

Learners might critically examine counterstories and stock stories using the set of questions outlined by Lee Anne Bell (2020):

- What are the stock stories about race and racism that operate in U.S. society to justify and perpetuate an unequal status quo? How do we learn these stories? Who benefits from stock stories and who pays?
- What are the stories about race and racism that we don't hear? Why don't we hear them? How do we recover these stories? What do these stories teach us about racism that stock stories do not?
- What stories exist that serve as examples of resistance? What can we learn about antiracist action by looking at these stories? How can we create new stories where differences are valued?

These questions can also be used to guide discussions or prompt reflective writing.

There are several sources for contemporary place-based counterstories about health, particularly concerning the pandemic. One example is the COVID-19 Oral History Project, housed at IUPUI's Arts & Humanities Institute. These oral histories, in particular, highlight the varied dimensions that impact health and wellness—with storytellers weaving intersectional narratives that situate the pandemic alongside racial violence and police brutality, gendered violence in the wake of Trump's presidency, and socioeconomic violence pertaining to poor working conditions during lockdown. These textured stock and counter-narratives attest to the real experiences of those living and dying through COVID-19.

Another potential source for contemporary stock and counter-narratives includes commentaries from major medical publications, such as the "A Piece of My Mind" column in *JAMA* (see Fayanju, 2019; Brooks, 2015; Vince, 2020) and the commentaries section of the Hastings Report (see Wilson, 2022; Thomas, 2022). But perhaps most importantly, educators should encourage learners to follow Richard Delgado, Aja Martinez and other CRT scholars who listen to and create their own stock and counterstories through real or composite experiences. As Ray reminds us: "Using testimonies from Black people gives them an authority over their own stories in health care, which too often either doesn't trust Black people to be narrators of their own stories or removes their voice from those stories" (2021, p. 727). As such, practitioners interested in practicing narrative medicine through counterstorytelling should listen closely to BIPOC patients and their experiences and bring those stories and their tellers into critical reflections, using Bell's (2020) aforementioned questions as a guide.

Conclusion

The potential implications of intentionally incorporating CRT's counterstorytelling into the training of current and future healthcare practitioners could be wide sweeping, enriching not just the clinical encounter but also research, education, and policy interventions. I don't stand alone in this belief. Others have advocated for the inclusion and proliferation of minoritized voices in healthcare research, education, and policy (Russell, 2022; Jones et al., 2022; Barnett et al., 2022; Ray, 2021). As Kierra Barnett and colleagues point out, healthcare that attends to *contextualized* patient stories "has the capacity to elevate the voices of traditionally marginalized groups and help ensure that research informing policy and practice affords a seat at the table to those most deeply affected by the study topic" (2022, p. 2). Importantly, counterstorytelling offers a way for narrative medicine practitioners to more ethically encounter patients through an anti-racist framework that prioritizes *listening* to the experiences of marginalized groups while also *recognizing* the role that (racial) trauma and whiteness play in the unequal power dynamics present in the clinical encounter.

Reference List

Association of American Medical Colleges (AAMC) (2019) *Diversity in medicine: facts and figures 2019.* Available at: https://www.aamc.org/data-reports/workforce/interactive-data/figure-18-percentage-all-active-physicians-race/ethnicity-2018 (Accessed: 28 August 2023).

Barnett, K.S. et al. (2022) "I just want us to be heard': A qualitative study of perinatal experiences among women of color,' *Women's Health*, 18, pp. 1-12. doi: https://doi.org/10.1177/17455057221123439

Bell, L.A. (2020) *Storytelling for social justice.* New York: Routledge.

Brooks, K.C. (2015) 'A silent curriculum,' *JAMA: Journal of the American Medical Association*, 313(19), pp. 1909-1910. doi: https://doi.org/10.1001/jama.2015.1676

Caruth, C. (1996) *Unclaimed experience: trauma, narrative, and history*. Baltimore: John Hopkins University Press.

Charon, R. (2005) 'Narrative medicine: attention, representation, affiliation,' *Narrative*, 13(3), pp. 261-270. doi: https://doi.org/10.1353/nar.2005.0017

Charon, R. (2006) *Narrative medicine: honoring the stories of illness*. New York: Oxford University Press.

Comas-Díaz, L., Hall, G.N. and Neville, H.A. (2019) 'Racial trauma: theory, research, and healing: introduction to the special issue,' *American Psychologist*, 74(1), pp. 1-5. doi: https://doi.org/10.1037/amp0000442

Crenshaw, K. et al. (eds.) (1996) *Critical race theory: the key writings that formed the movement*. New York: New Press.

DasGupta, S. (2008) 'Narrative humility,' *Lancet*, 371(9617), pp. 980-981.

Delgado, R. (1989) 'Storytelling for oppositionists and others: a plea for narrative,' *Michigan Law Review*, 87(8) pp. 2411-2441. doi: https://doi.org/10.2307/128 9308

Fallot, R.D. and Harris, M. (2009) *Creating cultures of trauma-informed care (CCTIC): a self-assessment and planning protocol*. Washington, D.C.: Community Connections.

Fayanju, O.M. (2019) 'Hiding in plain sight,' *JAMA: Journal of the American Medical Association*, 322(22), pp. 2173-2174. PMID: 31821434. PMCID: PMC7 049073. doi: https://doi.org/10.1001/jama.2019.19326

Gaston, S. (2021) 'Historical racist violence and intergenerational harms: accounts from descendants of lynching victims,' *AAPSS: The Annals of the American Academy of Political and Social Science*, 694 (1), pp. 78-91. doi: https://doi.org/10.1177/00027162211016317

Grooms, J. et al. (2022) 'Racial and ethnic disparities: essential workers, mental health, and the coronavirus pandemic,' *Review of Black Political Economy*, 49(4), pp. 363-380. doi: https://doi.org/10.1177%2F00346446211034226

Hall, W.J. et al. (2015) 'Implicit racial/ethnic bias among health care professionals and its influence on health care outcomes: a systematic review,' *American Journal of Public Health*, 105(12), pp. e60-e76. doi: https://doi.org/10.2105% 2FAJPH.2015.302903

Jones, K.F. et al. (2022) 'Top ten tips palliative care clinicians should know about delivering antiracist care to black Americans,' *Journal of Palliative Medicine*, 25(3), pp. 479-487. doi: https://doi.org/10.1089/jpm.2021.0502

Maples, K.F. (2018) *Mend*. Lexington: University Press of Kentucky.

Martinez, A.Y. (2020) *Counterstory: the rhetoric and writing of critical race theory*. Illinois: CCCC/NCTE.

Morrison, T. (2022) *Recitatif: a story*. New York: Knopf.

Quiros, L., Varghese, R. and Vanidestine, T. (2020) 'Disrupting the single story: challenging dominant trauma narratives through a critical race lens,' *Traumatology*, 26(2), pp. 160-168. doi: https://doi.org/10.1037/trm0000223

Ray, K.S. (2021) 'Going beyond the data: using testimonies to humanize pedagogy on black health,' *Journal of Medical Humanities*, 42(4), pp. 725-735. doi: https://doi.org/10.1007%2Fs10912-021-09681-7

Russell, C. (2022) 'Meeting the moment: bioethics in the time of black lives latter,' *American Journal of Bioethics*, 22(3), pp. 9-21. doi: https://doi.org/10.1080/15265161.2021.2001093

Solórzano, D.G., and Yosso, T.J. (2002) 'Critical race methodology: counter-storytelling as ananalytical framework for education research,' *Qualitative Inquiry*, 8(1) pp. 23-44., doi: https://doi.org/10.1177/107780040200800103

Thomas, S.P. (2022) 'Trust also means centering black women's reproductive health narratives,' *Hastings Center Report*, 52, suppl. 1, pp. 18-21. PMID: 35470876. doi: https://doi.org/10.1002/hast.1362

Vince Jr, R.A. (2020) 'Eradicating racial injustice in medicine-if not now, when?,' *JAMA: Journal of the American Medical Association*, 324(5), pp. 451-452. PMID: 32644105, PMCID: PMC7484353. doi: https://doi.org/10.1001/jama.2020.12432

Wear, D. and Aultman, J.M. (2005) 'The limits of narrative: medical student resistance to confronting inequality and oppression in literature and beyond,' *Medical Education*, 39(10), pp. 1056-1065. PMID: 16178833. doi: https://doi.org/10.1111/j.1365-2929.2005.02270.x

Williams, D.R. and Mohammed, S.A. (2013) 'Racism and health I: pathways and scientific evidence,' *American Behavioral Scientist*, 57(8), pp. 1152-1173. PMID: 24347666. doi: https://doi.org/10.1177%2F0002764213487340

Wilson, Y. (2022) 'Is trust enough? Anti-black racism and the perception of black vaccine "Hesitancy,"' *Hastings Center Report*, 52, pp. 12-17. doi: https://doi.org/10.1002/hast.1361

Yancy, C.W. (2020) 'COVID-19 and African Americans,' *JAMA: Journal of the American Medical Association*, 323(19), pp. 1891-1892. PMID: 32293639. doi: https://doi.org/10.1001/jama.2020.6548

Yancy, G. (2008) *Black bodies, white gazes: the continuing significance of race.* Washington, D.C.: Rowman & Littlefield.

3.2.3

Trauma and Healing: Finding Meaning, Identity, and Transformation Through Self-Reflection and Self-Expression

Victoria Simpson

University of Texas at San Antonio, US

Abstract

May 4, 1970, will forever be etched in my memory. The date is significant in my memory because it is the last day I saw my father. Who would have thought it would be his last when he left home that spring day? My father died suddenly at fifty-four on the hospital floor where he had been employed for over two decades. I was eleven years old at the time and could not make sense of his unexpected death. This tragedy would be my first, but not my last, encounter with traumatic events. Five years later, two weeks before my sixteenth birthday, my mother, a registered nurse, died suddenly at age fifty-four, the same age as my father. As an eleven-year-old, I could not articulate the pain I was feeling. Nor navigate through the impact that the trauma had left in the blind spot of my life. So, I began to journal in hopes of processing the trauma. At the onset of Trauma, I first experienced a rupture, leaving me with a vast hole, a complex void to fill. Left with tiny fragments of myself, I had hoped journaling would allow me to begin the healing process, and gain a sense of safety and find my way out of the suffering I was experiencing. At the time of the event, I did not know that my encounter with Trauma would not cease with the death of my parents. I would lose eight siblings before death stopped knocking on my door.

A loss of this magnitude attempted to render me silent. But instead, I found solace in self-reflective writing. Journaling allowed me to embrace the process of healing through self-reflection and self-expression. This transformative process gives the individual the power to heal. For Black people, the interpersonal storytelling works within the transformative process of healing to enable the individual to highlight their experiences of Trauma, oppression, and resistance through writing and sharing their stories. How do Trauma and illness shape our perceptions of self and identity? How can storytelling lend clarity and power when performed in the context of illness? This chapter will examine the effects of story-making and storytelling as praxis for negotiating meaning and identity. Additionally, I will interrogate the role that the story and its telling play in the liberation of those voices of the storytellers.

***

The use of storytelling is nothing new. In fact, it is one of the most basic forms of communication when it expresses matters of the self. Scholars have conducted discourse analysis of storytelling and the performance of narrative language for years, researching their effects on the human mind and body. What *is* new is the integrated use of the less conventional methods employed in conjunction with traditional methods as an alternative for healing. In the case of Trauma and illness, stories can give us a sense of control of the narrative. We can emphasize the self through the embodiment of stories. Christina Sharpe refers to this as "wake work" and demonstrates how we can thrive and create im/possible futures from traumatic events through art, resistance, attention, and imagining. (2016).

In her text, *Counterstory: The Rhetoric and Writing of Critical Race Theor,* Aja Y. Martinez defines counterstory as "a methodology that functions through methods that empower the minoritized through the formation of stories that disrupt the erasures embedded in standardized majoritarian methodologies" (2020, p. 3). Martinez's methodological practice of gathering and shaping data that draws on the theoretical specifications of counterstory includes its histories, tenets, key figures, methods/genres, and pedagogical implications. Black people have experiential knowledge from having lived under such systems of racism and oppression. Due to this knowledge, they "have developed methods and methodologies that serve as coping mechanisms and navigation strategies, while also serving as ways to raise awareness of issues affecting them that are overlooked, not considered, or otherwise invisible to whites" (ibid., p. 10).

Black Feminist Thought

This essay relies on a Black feminist decolonial theory, which, addresses Black Trauma and connects it to the legacy of chattel slavery. The principles formed by Black feminist thinkers are to advocate for emancipatory freedom and reconceptualized liberation by utilizing theoretical traditions such as Black feminist theory, antiracist politics, critical race theory, and the praxis of protest and liberation to create a more meaningful and authentic depiction of Black women truths, which are vital to interpret and understand the role and value of Black feminist thought in past, present, and future. Historian Saidiya Hartman, in her text, *Lose Your Mother: A Journey Along the Slave Route,* points out that the present state of Black people's oppression in America is connected to the afterlife of slavery,

> … black lives are still imperiled and devalued by a racial calculus and a political arithmetic that were entrenched centuries ago. This is the afterlife of slavery—skewed life chances, limited to health and education, premature death, incarceration, and impoverishment (Hartman, 2007, p. 6).

Christina Sharpe's *In the Wake: On Blackness and Being*, in which Sharpe lays bare not only what it means to be Black in America but what that Blackness actually means *to* America, builds upon Hartman's analysis of the afterlife of slavery. In the text, Sharpe argues that "the past that is not the past reappears, always, to rupture the present" (2016, p. 9). Sharpe traces how the aftershock of chattel slavery still animates daily representations of Black life. What, then, is the effect of Black people's inherent ability and *necessity* to shift between public and private personas based on their sub-status as Black people in America? This double consciousness aptly describes the struggle that is being Black in America; generally, however, it does not fully capture the simultaneous oppressions that Black women experience. However, expressing this intimate ability, Fannie Lou Hammer, Angela Davis, Deborah King, bell hooks, Kimberle Crenshaw, Patricia Hill Collins, the Combahee River Collective, and other Black feminists have written about the intersectional nature that burdens forced upon Black women. In *The Combahee River Collective Statement*, the authors wrote, "our politics initially sprang from the shared belief that Black women are inherently valuable, that our liberation is a necessity not as an adjunct to somebody else's may because of our need as human persons for autonomy" (1986, p. 4). Further,

> We also often find it difficult to separate race from class from sex oppression because, in our lives, they are most often experienced simultaneously… If Black women were free, it would mean that everyone else would have to be free since our freedom would necessitate the destruction of all the systems of oppression (ibid., p. 5-7).

Storytelling and Counter-Storytelling

In *The Cancer Journals* (2020), Audre Lorde narrates her breast cancer and mastectomy. Audre Lorde's method of writing may be considered unconventional by academic standards. However, Black women's life writing can be seen as its own genre as it contests the long-held assumptions about the self and the body. Lorde's writing, like many Black feminist writers, pushes back on masculine stronghold on identity. Instead, Lorde undermines the social desire for the old forms of stable subjectivity as she demonstrates her autobiographical practice that promotes endless fragmentations throughout her text that encapsulate the multiplicity of Blackness and being.

Lord maintains that "survival is only part of the task. The other is teaching" (Lorde, p. 40). She clarifies that the lessons she's learned throughout her ordeal have been painful. However, her primary concern is that her pain will not be in vain as a writer and activist for justice. Both serve as essential tools in the struggle for a more human world. She interrogates the silence and pain Black women experience when confronted with breast cancer and how we can transform that silence into healing narration. As Lorde examines her own illness, she asks, "is this pain and despair that surrounds me a result of cancer, or has it just been released by cancer?" (Lorde, 2020, p. 9). Lorde speaks to the enormity of our task to turn the world around and suggests that her task feels like turning life around inside out.

In *The Cancer Journals*, Lorde responds to interrogating the limits of medical discourse by reclaiming the voice of illness narratives and responding by making the personal political. She breaks the silence and redoes the metaphoric dimension of struggling with breast cancer. Lorde deconstructs the triumph narrative of the cure for cancer to bear her experience from the disease. From the moment she discovered the symptoms, receiving the diagnosis, making decisions concerning treatment, confronting death, and continuing life after treatment. Lorde put into words what, even today, few women can dare say. Through self-expression and self-reflection, Lorde is able to humanize her illness narrative while at the same time shining light on the limitations of traditional medical discourse.

Like Audre Lorde, Gloria Anzaldúa's *autohistoria-teoría* (Anzaldúa and Keating, 2015) has given voice to women of color by acknowledging the importance of self-expression, which allows others to seek transformative change through writing as they highlight their experiences of Trauma, oppression, and resistance in their everyday lives. Self-writing enables you to interrogate your feelings as a means of understanding the self. *Autohistoria-teoria* allows us not only to demonstrate self-knowledge but also to put this knowledge into practice.

In *Light in the Dark*, the editor Ana Louise Keating refers to this Anzaldúian state of awareness as "Coyolxauhqui consciousness," defined as "both the process of emotional, psychical dismemberment, splitting body/mind/spirit/soul, and the creative work of putting all the pieces together in a new form" (ibid., 2015, p. xxi). It is through this fragmented pain and self-expression that we find transformative healing. Keating defines healing:

I define healing as taking back the scattered energy and soul loss wrought by woundings. Healing means using the life force and strength that comes with el ánimo to act positively on one's own behalf and on others. Often, a wound provokes an urgent yearning for wholeness and provides the ground to achieve it. In shadow work, the problem is part of the cure – you don't heal the wound; the wound heals you. (ibid., p. 89).

Trauma and Resilience

The discourse surrounding breast cancer and other illnesses has been a significant factor in dehumanizing medical narratives. However, the scholarship of Black feminists and scholars intervenes by examining illness from an interdisciplinary approach. Employing rhetorical studies as a means for studying languages and their purposes at large allows us to humanize illness narratives further to dismiss the tropes of breast cancer and other illnesses. Research has led to ways to think of humanizing work Black feminists create to illuminate alternative worlds for Black people while drawing on Black scholars' disruptive work. I argue that storytelling and counterstorytelling offer new ways of humanizing patient stories of illness. Narrative medicine as an intervention opens a magnitude of possibilities for promoting health and healing, allowing patients' agency in making decisions regarding their health care and coming to terms with their illness.

Audre Lorde's *The Cancer Journal* is not just a journal; it is a manifesto for survival, a guide to survival for the twenty-first century "body and soul" (2020, p. xii). Reading Lorde's journal caused me to reflect on my personal experiences of loss, grief, and Trauma. Stories of illness and Trauma are told through fatigue, uncertainty, and pain. I have lost both parents and eight siblings, and I try to speak to the Trauma that tries to ravage my body, mind, and spirit. What was meant to destroy me has, in fact, made me stronger. I have emerged from the fire unsinged. Black people have weathered storms since our ancestors; we carry within us generational Trauma. In *The Cancer Journals,* Lorde asks, "How do we muster the faith, courage, and will to keep living and fighting? What does it mean to claim for ourselves a sense of wholeness and visibility when the world insists on us being hidden or disguised?" (ibid., p. xiii). As a collective, we rise from the ashes, overcoming grief, pain, and oppression ignited by society's fires, celebrating our resilience.

Lorde's first journal entry, dated December 1978, asks, "What is there possibly left for us to be afraid of after we have dealt face to face with death and not embraced it? Once I accepted the existence of dying, as a life process, who can ever have power over me again?" (ibid., p. xii). Tracy K. Smith describes Lorde's state of being as a "survivor's mind" as Lorde interrogates her illness and its implications while at the same time aligning herself with a collective *us,* Black people, as we confronted the violent struggle of Black being and invisibility.

In the forward of Audre Lorde's *The Cancer Journals*, Tracy K. Smith describes the compelling text as an "invitation to compassion, fury, reflection, and action for all of us living in a world ravaged by myriad forms of violence, shot through by so many reminders of mortality" (ibid., p. iix). Smith acknowledges that the physical and psychic violence against Black bodies, female, queer, and otherwise marginalized, have not been vanquished. The attack against Black bodies is meant to render us invisible and voiceless. Therefore, Smith regards *The Cancer Journals* as a guide to survival for the twenty-first century "body and soul."

Smith admits she is not sure how many writers or human psyche could make the leap from personal survival to the survival and flourishing of the collective if confronted with the stakes of life and death. However, she credits Lorde for doing just that. She believes questions and urgencies driving Lorde's work before her diagnosis – "How do we muster the faith, courage, and will to keep living and fighting? What does it mean to claim for ourselves a sense of wholeness and visibility when the world insists on us being hidden or disguised?—are catalyzed by Lorde's private, subjective journey through illness and recovery" (ibid., p. xiii).

Black Creatives as Spaces of Liberation

The purpose of Lorde's work is to draw attention to how creative work such as storytelling and counterstorytelling can create concepts in innovative and humanizing ways, attentive to racism while at the same time creating a space for narrative medicine as a way to define Black life. Her journals give Black women a text about Black livingness and ways of knowing. Furthermore, within the journals are ways of seeking liberation and reinventing the terms of Black life regarding negative conceptions of Blackness. This method of counterstorytelling allows Black people to bring together radical ways of knowing, thinking, writing, and imagining, bringing together various sources, texts, and narratives to challenge racism. Lorde's motivation comes from a deep love for Black people and Blackness. Her work feels urgent, both because she is trying to honor and save Black lives and because she is conscious of her own mortality. Lorde describes the motivation driving her work as "the anger of exclusion, of unquestioned privilege, of racial distortions, of silence, ill-use, stereotyping, defensiveness, misnaming, betrayal, and co-option" (ibid., p. xiv), Lorde's work is to argue and to convince people, that anger can be a productive, a source of growth and change.

Lorde admits that she writes so much about fear because in shaping *The Cancer Journals*, she was in the midst of fear, confronted with the disease and the mastectomy. She did not want to rejoice in her survival at the time for fear of the disease returning. However, Lorde reminded herself that she had already lived through it. She had known the pain, and she survived it. She then knew she had to name it and give it voice, “to share it for use” so that her pain would not be in vain. So that the pain was not wasted. (ibid., p. 9). She came to terms with death and realized she and the notion of death must co-exist.

As early as the late 1970s, medical narratives have, and continue to perpetuate, a dominant narrative that views Black bodies in opposition to their white counterparts, seeing them as less human. Sylvia Wynter argues, "We must now collectively undertake a rewriting of knowledge as we know it. This rewriting in which, inter alia, I want the West to recognize the dimensions of what it has brought into the world—this with respect to, inter alia, our now purely naturalized modes of genres, of humanness. Because the West *did* change the world, *totally*” (Wynter, 2015, p.18); Wynter's work examines ways to decolonize white Western modes of the human to argue for other Black modes of being and of the human.

Dehumanizing Medical Narratives

The use of storytelling and narrative language is nothing new. In fact, it is one of the most basic forms of communication when it expresses matters of the self. Scholars have conducted discourse analysis of storytelling and the performance of narrative language for years, researching their effect on the human mind and body. In order to recenter the narrative, counterstory and critical race theory (CRT) allow us to revise the stories of dehumanizing narratives of breast cancer and other illnesses. Black feminists and scholars wish that people in the medical field would take Black illnesses more seriously. From invisibility, many are left trying to answer W.E.B. Du Bois’ poignant query, “How does it feel to be a problem? And yet, being a problem is a strange experience—peculiar even for one who has never been anything else” (Robvais, 2020, p. 2).

To bridge the gap between studying science and studying ways of knowing, we must include a medical narrative beyond scientific knowledge. Moya Bailey and Whitney Peoples’ research on Black women and dehumanizing medical narratives focuses on “how, if at all, can biomedicine and Black auto/biography produce just and ethical narratives of Black lives and Black futures?” (2021, p. 177). Their study examines the role of biomedicine in twentieth-and twenty-first-century African American life narratives. Bailey and Peoples’s findings suggest “while the biomedicalized narrative is positioned as truer, more scientific than the traditional life narrative, it neglects the questions of justice and the realities of interpersonal relationships as well as the feelings at the heart of life narrative in the first place” (ibid., p. 188). The use of storytelling and narrative language is nothing new. In fact, it is one of the most basic forms of communication when it expresses matters of the self. Scholars have conducted discourse analysis of storytelling and the performance of narrative language for years, researching their effect on the human mind and body. Black feminists and scholars' critical interventions felt an emerging sense of the need to intervene in theorizing Blackness and ways to recreate humanizing medical narratives of Black bodies related to breast cancer and other illnesses.

Bailey examined the concept of "*palimpsestic memorialization,*" a form of narrative they describe as one that attends to the "messiness of human existence in the midst of structures of both inequality and innovation" (ibid., p.187). She argues that formulation, *palimpsestic memorialization,* is a way to tell Black life because it allows for nonlinear storytelling and does not claim to know all the answers.

Bailey's concept of *palimpsestic memorialization* also provides an ethical framework that addresses both the limits and the possibilities of biomedicine for mapping Black lives as she examines the interconnections between histories and memories. The cultural memories of otherness from our past travel with us to become a part of our present, allowing Black people to curate and embody the memories of the past for a contemporary present. This process complicates Western conceptions of time as linear and fixed.

Bailey and Peoples examine Rebecca Skloot's book *The Immortal Life of Henrietta Lacks* (2010) and Henry Louis Gates, Jr.'s work on genetic ancestry testing as vehicles to past stories and how they rely on biomedicine to tell their narratives. "Using Black feminist theories of the body and feminist techno/science studies as primary frameworks, we highlight the impact of biomedicalization on Black life, complicating the value of genetic testing of knowing Black lives" (Bailey and Peoples, 2021, p. 177). They offer the autobiographical work of "black lesbian warrior poet" Audre Lorde in *The Cancer Journals* as a model of a narrative "informed by biomedical intervention but remain critical of its role in the story of her life and the ways she constructed it" (ibid., p. 177).

Bailey explains that where Gates sees a cross-racial love, "we see a historical reality in which Black women have a few options for survival" (2010, p. 188). Bailey sees the medical racism in *The Immortal Life of Henrietta Lacks* as an "unintentional profit by well-meaning scientists; we see legacies of scientific racism and continued racial health disparities unhampered by biomedical revolution built on the cancerous cells of a working-class Black woman" (Bailey and Peoples, 2021, p. 188). We cannot give rise to complicated and fascinating stories until we disrupt the idea that all narratives of time and space are layered in nicely aesthetic tiers. Black life (narratives) embraces the messiness of time and memory to produce a rich and complex narrative that includes a racialized history of Black people.

Through her complex narrative, Lorde chronicles her treatment as a breast cancer patient and her feelings about the disease in a world "devoid of the kind of personal narratives she wanted to read about the experience." She asks,

"Where are the models for what I am supposed to be in this situation?" (ibid., p. 186). Lorde, as an autobiographer, Bailey states, "masterfully wields the power of words and writes deliberately to address the realities for women with breast cancer" (ibid., p. 186). Lorde's *The Cancer Journals* gives us critical insight into how biomedical intervention plays a role in Black American counter-narrative of life writing. Her counterstory advocates for Black women's voice and visibility as she addresses the maltreatment regularly received by breast cancer and argues for those in their death sentences, those who suffer from perpetual pain, those who are marginalized, and those rendered invisible and maltreated because they are considered and called a problem.

Through her poetry collection titled *Patient* (2014), Bettina Judd gives a riveting account of the current US healthcare system and the history of Black women in American (gynecologic) medicine. She was a patient and spoke of her own "bodily vulnerability as a Black patient," stating, "I had an ordeal with medicine and was found innocent or guilty, it feels the same because I live in a haunted house. A house can be a dynasty, a bloodline, a body" (ibid., p. 179). Bettina describes the dehumanizing ways Black women are traumatized as they face US healthcare. Bailey and Peoples argue, "for Black people, American biomedicine has always been a haunted house, filled with the ghosts of Black lives lost in the name of racist science and scientific racism" (ibid., p.176). How do we begin to address Black humanity and the vulnerability of Black women patients? Historically, Black women have been rendered silent and invisible and denied the most basic medical care.

Bailey believes biological science is the sole basis for medical practice and was instrumental in shifting medical education from an apprenticeship model to one of institutional education. Stating, "'Biomedicine' encapsulates the biological and related sciences that are integral to the clinical practice of medicine" (ibid., p.176). The focus becomes the Patient by shifting from studying science to studying science as a clinical practice of medicine. This patient-centered practice presents the Patient in a more humanistic way and changes to a patient/physician dynamic to include a more collaborative model for patient care.

Lorde complicates the narrative of biomedicalization as she questions Black lives and Black futures as she reconstructs the role of biomedical intervention in her life story in *The Cancer Journals*. She challenges the structures of both inequality and innovation. To bridge the gap between studying science and studying ways of knowing, we must include a medical narrative beyond scientific knowledge.

Lorde's counterstory advocates for Black women's voice and visibility as she addresses the maltreatment regularly received by breast cancer and argues for those in their death sentences, those who suffer from perpetual pain, those who are marginalized, and those rendered invisible and maltreated because they are considered and called a problem. She understood the enormity of the task to change the "barbarity of the forces aligned against us," which meant teaching, surviving, and fighting with every resource of every inch of her being. For her, that meant also recognizing the enemy outside and the enemy within, "and knowing that my work is part of a continuum of women's work, of reclaiming this earth and our power, and knowing that this work did not begin with my birth, nor will it end with my death" (2020, p. 10). She believes her life, love, and work have a particular power and meaning relative to others.

Illness Narratives as a Tool for Healing

Arthur Kleinman, a professor of medicine at Harvard University, stresses to his colleagues and students the importance of allocating time to attend to the stories of their patients as they attempt to uncover and reveal possible meanings in their suffering. Kleinman emphasizes the importance of acknowledging the stories of the profoundly ill and asserts that “a powerful therapeutic alternative is at hand.” He argues:

> Evidence indicates that examining the particular significance of a person’s illness makes it possible to break the vicious cycles that amplify distress. The interpretation of illness meanings can also contribute to the provision of more effective care ... This key clinical task may even liberate sufferers and practitioners from the oppressive iron cage imposed by a too intensely morbid preoccupation with painful bodily processes and a too technically narrow and therefore, dehumanizing vision of treatment, respectively. (1988, p. 41)

Self-Reflection and Self-Expression of Black Livingness

Healing is connected to wholeness, and wholeness is experienced in connection to others. Through her curiosities, Katherine McKittrick was interested in how race is attended to as she worked through the “thorny racial privileges and biases” of Black livingness (2021, p. 1). She wanted to bring attention to how Black creatives (poets, musicians, visual artists) worked to find ways to humanize and define Black life. She states, “I imperfectly draw attention to how seeking liberation, and reinventing the terms of black life outside normatively negative conceptions of Blackness, in onerous, joyful, and difficult, yet unmeasured and unmeasurable. Mnemonic black livingness. My heart makes my head swim" (ibid., p. 3). McKittrick calls for a mode of recognition that does not itemize-commodify Black liberation, and Black embodied knowledge.

Storytelling is a mode of Black creatives that embodies Black knowledge, allowing space for self-expression and self-reflection for transformative healing.

McKittrick defines story, telling, sharing, listening to, and hearing stories as "rational and interdisciplinary acts that are animated by all sorts of people, places, narrative devices, theoretical queries, plots" (ibid., p. 6). She suggests the process is sustained by invention and wonder and argues, "the stories offer an aesthetic relationality that relies on dynamics of creating-narrating-listening-hearing-reading-and sometimes-unhearing. The stories do not offer lucid tales or answers; rather, they signal ways of living in a world that denies black humanity (or, more aptly, the stories signal ways of black livingness)" (ibid., p. 7). She believes the stories do not simply describe; they demand representation outside themselves. Furthermore, she argues the stories are a way to hold on to the rebellious methodological work of sharing ideas in an unkind world.

Critical Race Theory (CRT)

Critical race theory plays a crucial role in the ethical framework of storytelling by authenticating the stories as they relate to multiple systems of oppression. Erin Atwood and Gerardo R. López argue that "critical race theory does not aim to tell a 'truer' account of reality, but a more honest one. Therefore, critical race scholars need not ask permission – nor seek forgiveness – for their counterstories but hold themselves to communicate stories and narratives that are not only honestly critical but critically honest" (2014, p. 1134).

Through the reconstruction of Black narratives, Black people can speak truth to their stories, naming their own realities and experiences. Counterstorytelling creates a space for resistance against dominant narratives that create and uphold existing power dynamics. "Counterstories seek to challenge the assumptions of power and Eurocentric notions of normativity" (ibid., p. 1135)—Atwood and López credit critical race theory for promoting clinical activism to achieve racial justice.

Conclusion

Richard Delgado and Jean Stefancic describe critical race theory (CRT) as a movement that consists of a "collection of activists and scholars engaged in studying and transforming the relationship among race, racism, and power" (2012, p. 3). CRT is used to deconstruct the power structures that surround racism. Some of the characteristics used to create counterstorytelling are the reexamination of history to include the narrative of Black people's struggles, voices, and invisibility in dominant culture. Counterstorytelling emphasizes stories, experiences, narratives, and truths of marginalized people.

I offer storytelling and counterstorytelling as new ways of humanizing patient stories of Trauma and illness. Narratives of illness and Trauma can serve as an intervention for discovering a magnitude of possibilities for promoting health and healing, allowing patients' agency in making decisions regarding their health care and coming to terms with their illness.

Employing rhetorical studies as a means for studying languages and their purposes allows us to examine discourse surrounding breast cancer and other illnesses as it pertains to Black people and Black bodies. The foundation for addressing dehumanizing medical narrative must be examined from an interdisciplinary approach. Black feminists and scholars such as Audre Lorde, Bailey, Moya, and Raquel Robvais illuminate alternative worlds for Black people while at the same time drawing on the disruptive work of promoting health and healing. The use of narrative medicine foregrounds the limits scientific methods possess in advancing patient care in the areas of performance and healing.

Reference List

Anzaldúa, G. (2015) *Light in the dark/luz en lo oscuro: rewriting identity, spirituality, reality.* Durham: Duke University Press. doi: https://doi.org/10.2307/j.ctv1220hmq

Atwood, E. and Lopez, G. (2014) 'Let's be critically honest: towards a messier counterstory in critical race theory,' *International Journal of Qualitative Studies in Education,* 27(9), pp. 1134-1154. doi: http://dx.doi.org/10.1080/09518398.2014.916011

Bailey, M. and Peoples, W. (2021) 'The biomedicalization of black life narratives,' in Moody, J. (ed.) *A history of African American autobiography.* Cambridge: Cambridge University Press, pp. 176-190. doi: https://doi.org/10.1017/9781108890946.011

Delgado, R. and Stefancic, J. (2012) *Critical race theory: an introduction.* Critical America, 59. 2nd edn. New York: New York University Press.

Kleinman, A. (1988) *The illness narratives: suffering, healing, and the human condition.* New York: Basic Books.

Hartman, S. (2007) *Lose your mother: a journey along the slave route.* New York: Farrar, Straus, and Giroux. Print.

Judd, B. (2014) *Patient.* Black Lawrence Press.

Lorde, A. and Smith, T.K. (2020 [1980]) *The cancer journals.* New York: Penguin Books.

Martinez, Aja Y. (2020) *Counterstory: the rhetoric and writing of critical race theory.* Champaign, IL: National Council of Teachers of English.

McKittrick, K. (2021) 'Curiosities (my heart makes my head swim),' in *Dear Science and other stories,* New York: Duke University Press, pp. 1-13. doi: https://doi.org/10.1515/9781478012573-002

Robvais, R.M. (2020) 'We are no longer invisible,' *Poroi,* 15(1). doi: https://doi.org/10.13008/2151-2957.1296

Smith, T.K. (2020) 'Foreword,' in Lorde, A. and Smith, T.K. *The cancer journals.* New York: Penguin Books.

Sharpe, C. (2016) *In the Wake: On Blackness and Being*. Durham: Duke University. Print.

The Combahee River Collective (1986) *The Combhee River Statement: Black Feminist Organizing in the Seventies and Eighties*. Albany: Kitchen Table: Women of Color Press. Print.

Wynter, S. (2015) 'On being human as praxis,' in McKittrick, K. (ed.). Durham: Duke University Press, pp. 18.

3.2.4

Watchmen: Nostalgia and Bearing Witness to Intergenerational Racial Trauma

Margaux Danby

University of Kentucky College of Medicine, US

Abstract

HBO's miniseries *Watchmen*, which takes place in Tulsa, Oklahoma in 2019, follows protagonist Angela Abar, a police officer who moonlights as a masked vigilante, and fellow characters while they experience and investigate a series of violent, racially-charged events. One narrative arc involves Angela's encounters with her 105-year-old estranged paternal grandfather, Will Reeves. Will is a survivor of numerous traumatic events, including Tulsa's Black Wall Street Massacre of 1921, a real event that has been almost entirely whitewashed out of American history. In the sixth episode of *Watchmen*, Angela bears witness to a lifetime of her grandfather's trauma after she swallows a bottle-full of his Nostalgia, a personalized medication that delivers concentrated memories to the taker. By taking Will's Nostalgia pills, Angela witnesses his trauma through the testimony of his memories as she literally metabolizes them. Angela's experience both exemplifies the reality of witnessing as described by the psychoanalytic trauma theory of Dori Laub and extends beyond its boundaries as a fully embodied, albeit fictional, witnessing experience. Moreover, the series as a whole exemplifies how artistic narratives such as *Watchmen* serve as a kind of Nostalgia pill for society to witness and metaphorically metabolize traumas both in historical context and as they perpetuate in current times.

***

HBO's Emmy Award-winning 2019 miniseries *Watchmen* depicts a contemporary cinematic universe derived from Alan Moore's graphic novel and comic book series of the same name, originally published by DC Comics in 1986-87. The show, which takes place in Tulsa, Oklahoma in 2019, follows protagonist Angela Abar, a police officer who moonlights as masked vigilante Sister Night, and fellow characters while they experience and investigate a series of violent, racially-charged events. One major narrative arc involves Angela's encounters with her 105-year-old estranged paternal grandfather, Will Reeves. Will is a survivor of numerous traumatic events, including Tulsa's Black Wall Street Massacre of 1921, a real event which has been almost entirely whitewashed out of American history. In "This Extraordinary Being," the sixth episode of *Watchmen*, Angela bears witness to a lifetime of her grandfather's trauma after she swallows a bottle-full of his Nostalgia, a personalized medication that delivers concentrated memories to the taker. By taking Will's Nostalgia pills, Angela witnesses his trauma through the testimony of his memories as she literally metabolizes them. Angela's experience both exemplifies the reality of witnessing as described by the psychoanalytic trauma theory of Dori Laub and extends beyond its boundaries as a fully embodied, albeit fictional, witnessing experience. Moreover, artistic narratives such as *Watchmen*, and the film and television depicted within the series, serve as a kind of Nostalgia for society to witness and metaphorically metabolize traumas both in historical context and as they perpetuate in current times.

Nostalgia as Testimony

In "Bearing Witness or the Vicissitudes of Listening," the second chapter of *Testimony: Crises of Witnessing in Literature, Psychoanalysis, and History*, Dori Laub uses his own experience as a witness to the testimonies of Holocaust survivors to describe a psychoanalytic understanding of the act of witnessing, or listening to the trauma of others. Laub suggests that a trauma, "in spite of the overwhelming and compelling nature of the reality of its occurrence," does not come into existence "as a known event and not simply as an overwhelming shock" until it is heard, listened to, witnessed (1992, p. 57). He posits that trauma cannot be known or understood until there is a witness to the narrative of its occurrence, a person with whom the victim can share his testimony. Laub explains that "the testimony to the trauma thus includes its hearer, who is, so to speak, the blank screen on which the event comes to be inscribed for the first time" (ibid.). As such, the listener is a vital component of and participant in the testimony. Laub elaborates:

> The listener to trauma comes to be a participant and a co-owner of the traumatic event: through his very listening, he comes to ... feel the bewilderment, injury, confusion, dread, and conflicts that the trauma victim feels ... The listener has to feel the victim's victories, defeats and silences, know them from within, so that they can assume the form of testimony. (1992, p. 57-58)

Therefore, for a trauma to become known to the victim, it must not only be told to the listener, but also partially experienced and felt by that listener. Only through such a dyadic experience can the trauma come into existence as a known event.

In this way, Angela bears witness to Will's testimony in *Watchmen*, though her witnessing takes the experiencing and feeling of trauma to a new, embodied extreme. After Angela swallows the Nostalgia, fellow detective Laurie Blake explains that the medication, containing harvested memories to be reexperienced upon ingestion, was developed for patients with Alzheimer's Disease and Dementia. *"You're not supposed to take someone else's Nostalgia,"* Laurie says as Angela staggers under the influence ("This Extraordinary Being," 2019). She succumbs to the effects of the Nostalgia and begins to witness.

The rest of the episode follows Angela through Will's black-and-white memories, a stark contrast to Angela's reality depicted in color. The camera consistently pans away from young adult Will and returns to find Angela in his place, wearing his clothes and speaking his words (ibid.). She is completely immersed in his memories, which Laub describes as an active participant in and co-owner of his trauma. Not only does she feel his emotions, she undergoes his bodily experience as well. The concept of Nostalgia, edible embodied memories, thus allows Angela's witnessing to both fulfill and extend beyond Laub's understanding of witnessing.

The memory sequence begins with Will's graduation from the NYC Police Academy in 1938 as the only Black cadet in his class. He is warned by the only other Black officer to "beware of the Cyclops," a white supremacist organization (ibid.). As he investigates hate crimes against Jewish businesses and Black movie theater patrons, and identifies a leniency of the law toward white perpetrators, Will becomes a target of his white colleagues. Eventually, a group of three white police officers corner Will in a dark alley and beat him unconscious. He wakes with his hands tied as the white officers drag him towards a tree, where they put a noose around his neck and a black hood over his head. The camera shows Will's perspective, a glimpse of Angela's witnessing experience; the image is dark and blurry under the hood as they hoist him into the tree. The sounds of Will's gasps and the creaking rope are audible as the image loses focus. Before the lynching is complete, the white officers cut the rope, letting Will fall to the ground as he gasps for air, and threaten: "keep your Black nose out of white folks' business, n*****, or next time we won't cut you down" (ibid.). When the camera returns to an external perspective on Will, it finds Angela, coughing and bloodied, on the ground at the base of the tree. The expression on her face shows his fear and his anger as well as her own. More than Laub's metaphorical blank screen, Angela's body becomes physically inscribed with this traumatic event through her act of witnessing.

After the near-lynching, Will walks through the city with the cut noose around his neck, carrying the black hood. When he hears screams, he pokes eye holes in the hood and comes to the rescue of the victims of a robbery. From this moment on, Will maintains a secret identity as the masked vigilante Hooded Justice (ibid.). To appeal to the racist masses, he paints his eyelids to make himself appear white under the hood, an action reminiscent of Angela's own transformation into Sister Night, though she notably uses black paint rather than white ("If You Don't Like My Story, Write Your Own," 2019).

Even though Angela participates in Will's testimony by experiencing the trauma in her own body, she also remains herself. While she experiences the trauma of the victim, "[s]he nonetheless does not become the victim – [s]he preserves [her] own separate place, position and perspective" (Laub, 1992, p. 58). While the exchange of young adult Will for Angela emphasizes how close Angela's experience of Will's trauma is, she remains connected to herself and her body as it exists in her reality outside the Nostalgia testimony. This becomes obvious to the viewer when Angela's experience of Will's memory suddenly freezes as Will crashes through a window. Angela is suspended in midair, surrounded by floating shards of broken glass, as if the action of the memory is paused ("This Extraordinary Being," 2019). Detective Laurie Blake approaches and asks, *"Angela, can you hear me?"* in an echoing voice. Angela has consumed a lethal dose of Nostalgia and is now in a coma. *"You may be confused as to who you are right now,"* Laurie tells her. *"If you can hear what I'm saying … I need you to blink"* (ibid.). With some effort, Angela blinks. Twice Angela confirms that she can hear Laurie. In this scene, Angela proves that she has preserved her own subjective experience despite being submersed in Will's memories. Though Angela's witnessing experience is vivid and even embodied, she knows she is experiencing Will's particular trauma and not her own. Likewise, the viewers watching the episode remain intact as they witness the testimony on screen.

However, even though Angela maintains her own identity, she is still at risk during the Nostalgia testimony, as any witness to trauma is. Laub writes: "for the listener who enters the contract of the testimony, a journey fraught with dangers lies ahead. There are hazards to listening to trauma. Trauma – and its impact on the hearer – leaves, indeed, no hiding place intact" (1992, p. 72). For Angela, these dangers are both mental and physical. The extreme, embodied nature of her witnessing experience is traumatizing in itself, and taking the Nostalgia has put her life at risk as her body struggles to literally metabolize the overdose of Will's traumatic memories. Here again, *Watchmen*'s depiction of Angela's witnessing both upholds Laub's conception of witnessing and extends beyond its boundaries, expanded by fictional possibilities.

And yet, the components of Angela's witnessing expanded by fictional possibilities are grounded in the realities of intergenerational trauma. In *Watchmen*, Angela metabolizes Will's trauma with the Nostalgia medication. In reality, trauma is not literally "metabolized," but it is genetically encoded via epigenetic mechanisms such as (de)methylation, cellular processes which turn gene expression on and off; the altered expression of genes can cause both behavioral and neuroanatomical changes which can be passed through generations (Dias and Ressler, 2014). Thus, trauma can become intergenerational via both testimony and genetics, and Nostalgia is both a physical manifestation of testimony and an analogy for intergenerational trauma. While most witnesses, including Laub, are not related to the victims of trauma offering them their testimony, Angela is Will's granddaughter, and therefore carries his trauma in her body, genetically, even before ingesting his Nostalgia.

Film and Television as Societal Nostalgia

It is fitting that Laub describes a witness as "the blank screen on which the event comes to be inscribed for the first time" (1992, p. 57), given that film and television have become the chosen media through which society witnesses historical and collective trauma testimonies. Like Nostalgia, works of film and television deliver concentrated memories to audience witnesses, and the artistic styles available in cinematography lend themselves to testimony by creating a dyadic relationship between the viewer and the narrative. For example, the eyewitness perspective used during the lynching scene in episode six and the Massacre scene in episode one allows the audience to become immersed in the testimony along with the characters, and the paused crash through the window reminds audiences as well as Angela that we remain ourselves as we witness, just as Laub posits. As a testimony, *Watchmen* allows us to remember our historical traumas and reimagine how we might continue to metabolize them. Moreover, *Watchmen* both depicts reality, recreating real people, places, and events, and alters reality, revising history to consider alternative outcomes and exploring possibilities that do not, yet, exist in our world.

For example, *Watchmen*'s depiction of the Tulsa Black Wall Street Massacre is one of the first in popular cinematic history. The event was whitewashed out of American history for most of the century since its occurrence, and widespread attention has only recently focused on the facts of the tragedy that forever changed the economic and racial landscape of Tulsa. *Watchmen*'s creator Damon Lindelof was inspired to center the show around the Massacre after reading Ta-Nehisi Coates' "The Case for Reparations," which provides a historical overview of the Tulsa Massacre and other racist American phenomena while making the case for reparations as a means of reconciling America's racist history (Coates, 2014). *Watchmen*'s scenes of the Massacre allow viewers, especially Americans, to bear witness to this historical and enduring trauma, to remember and metabolize our past, reckon with its aftermath, and consider our future. No longer whitewashed out of history, the Massacre becomes a known event – a reality inflicted upon real people and real places.

One of those real places, which becomes a symbol of the impacts of the Massacre throughout the *Watchmen* series, is, poignantly, a cinema: the Williams Dreamland Theater. In addition to the appearance of the theater's marquee in images, murals, videos, and displays incorporated into many scenes across multiple episodes, the theater also bookends the series as a physical refuge for 7-year-old Will during the Massacre in the opening scene ("It's Summer and We're Running Out of Ice," 2019) and for 105-year-old Will, along with Angela's children, during the season's climactic finale ("See How They Fly," 2019). Both in the show and in reality, it serves as a haven for Black art, culture, and joy. The theater, a real Black-owned business (Gardullo, 2021), represents the Black economic prosperity of Tulsa's Greenwood district that was destroyed by the Massacre, altering the futures of thousands of Black Americans and underscoring the case for reparations. Furthermore, the Dreamland, as a cinema, upholds the conceptual importance of film and television, in addition to other forms of artistic narrative, in offering historical testimony and creating opportunities for society to bear witness.

In addition to the opportunity to witness representations of historical events, film and television also enable audiences to explore possibilities only available in fictionalized, alternate, or revisionist versions of reality. *Watchmen* plays out the case for reparations, imagining how the enactment of such a policy might impact American life, culture, and politics. A fictional reparations policy called the "Victims of Racial Violence Act" serves as a major impetus for much of the racialized action of the series. The Act establishes the Greenwood Center for Cultural Heritage and provides monetary reparations to Americans who can trace their ancestry back to survivors of the Tulsa Massacre. The Center operates as both a history museum and a DNA collection point where citizens can check their eligibility. When Angela brings in Will's DNA in episode two, she walks past a group of protestors outside the Center and approaches an interactive digital kiosk where a recording of the US Treasury Secretary explains the history of the Tulsa Massacre and the reparations policy before asking permission to process the visitor's DNA for eligibility. It says:

> For far too long this horrific chapter in our nation's history went untold and unacknowledged. On behalf of the entire United States government, [the President] offers his sincerest condolences for the trauma you or your family may have suffered ... Our country appreciates the opportunity to right the wrongs of a dark past so that we may all share a bright future. ("Martial Feats of Comanche Horsemanship," 2019)

Toward the end of the recording, the "Battle Hymn of the Republic," an American abolitionist anthem, begins to play. However, the series doesn't only play out the case for reparations by imagining how such a policy might be created and executed, it also anticipates the stark opposition that would likely arise and envisions the dangers such an opposition might pose. In addition to the protestors outside the Center chanting "[repar]ations are abominations" and hoisting signs with similar slogans (ibid.), the reparations policy has ignited the formation of the 7th Kavalry, a white supremacist organization described as "the Klan with different masks" ("She Was Killed by Space Junk," 2019). The Kavalry is responsible for much of the civil unrest depicted throughout the show, providing an extreme example of how twenty-first-century racism might manifest in America, especially if it becomes exacerbated by anti-racist policy such as reparations.

In addition to the *Watchmen* series as a whole, the fictional film and television content viewed by characters within the *Watchmen* universe reflects that of the real world, serving a similar purpose as a form of societal Nostalgia for fictional audiences. For example, an attendee at a group therapy session explains the significance of film in processing her experience of the central traumatic event of the *Watchmen* universe: the teleportation of a massive alien squid onto New York City in 1985, which killed over 3 million people and created a psychic blast zone that wounded and traumatized millions more ("Little Fear of Lightning," 2019). She describes the fictional movie *Pale Horse*, which in the *Watchmen* universe is an Academy Award-winning Spielberg film released in 1992. She says:

> There's this one scene with this little girl in a red coat. The movie's black-and-white, so the red really pops, you know? And the girl's stumbling around Herald Square, walking under the tentacles through all the dead bodies. And she's scared. And she's calling out for her mom. It just really stuck with me, you know? I mean I know it's stupid, being obsessed with a movie, but watching it just makes me feel better. Face-your-fears thing. Cause I'm scared all the time. (ibid.)

This fictional film alludes to *Schindler's List*, a real Academy Award-winning Spielberg film released in 1993 which allows viewers to collectively witness another historical trauma, the Holocaust, and famously includes a girl in a red coat which stands out against the rest of the black-and-white film (Spielberg, 1993). Both the real and fictional versions of this film offer a cinematic testimony to be witnessed by a broad audience, turning a collective trauma into a known event.

Similarly, *American Hero Story* (AHS), a television show within *Watchmen*, serves as a form of societal Nostalgia directly juxtaposed with Will's Nostalgia testimony. The show has a wide audience, as evidenced in episode two when *AHS* appears during primetime hour on the televisions of various characters: Angela's son Topher watches in the Abar's living room; Angela's colleague Wade sits down to dinner in front of his TV; members of the 7th Kavalry watch as they continue their nefarious tasks ("Martial Feats of Comanche Horsemanship," 2019). As the opening credits conclude, the camera closes in on the television and the *AHS* episode takes over the screen. Both real and fictional audiences watch as the show introduces the origin story of its narrator, Hooded Justice. However, while there are parallels and hints of Will's experience as the real Hooded Justice in *AHS*, the show takes massive creative liberties in the representation of his story and his trauma.

In *AHS*, Hooded Justice is purported to be Ralph Mueller, a circus strongman who fakes his own death and lives under the guise of the masked vigilante. The first action sequence in *AHS* depicts the robbery of a grocery store – the same store that later appears in Will's memories in episode six. The *AHS* Hooded Justice bursts into the store to intervene through the same window that Will/Angela crashes out of during the Nostalgia testimony. In *AHS*, the store appears in bright colors rather than black-and-white like Angela's experience of Will's memories. The storekeeper asks Hooded Justice, "*Who are you?*" A voiceover responds:

> Who am I? When I was little, every time I looked in the mirror I saw a stranger staring back at me, and he was very, very angry ... I never felt comfortable in my own skin, so I made a new one, and when I slipped it on, he and I became one. His anger became mine, as did his thirst for justice. So, who am I? If I knew the answer to that I wouldn't be wearing a fucking mask. ("Martial Feats of Comanche Horsemanship," 2019)

Even the character himself admits that no one telling this story really knows who Hooded Justice is. The irony of slipping into a second skin is lost on the fictional show's writers and audience, who have no idea that the man under the hood is Black, not white. The noose around his neck is purported to be a prop for "sex stuff" rather than the remnants of a racist attack ("This Extraordinary Being," 2019). Hooded Justice may be the main character and narrator of *American Hero Story*, but the fictional show is clearly not an accurate representation of Will's testimony. What *AHS* gets wrong is a necessary reminder of the myriad ways representation can distort reality, history, and collective memory, and raises important questions of narrative ethics: How do we tell stories of past trauma? Whose stories get told, and by whom? How do we do them justice, and remember them accurately? Who decides when justice is done and what memory is accurate? And, perhaps most importantly, what happens when we get them wrong?

Whether misrepresentation is accidental or purposeful, it creates an ethical problem. By depicting this ethical problem directly, *Watchmen* and its viewers are able to acknowledge and grapple with it in a fictional context. Only by intentionally and self-referentially raising questions of narrative ethics can *Watchmen* uphold these ethics as it provides societal Nostalgia to real viewers. Like patients prescribed new medication, these viewers must be made aware of the potential adverse effects of cinematic Nostalgia. As a show about historical trauma that also explores the consequences of representing such a testimony, *Watchmen* exemplifies how film and television provide a powerful, effective mechanism through which to offer testimony while simultaneously warning that the potential dangers accompanying such a powerful tool are just as great.

Conclusion

In episode seven, Lady Trieu, the inventor of Nostalgia, identifies the drug as her greatest failure. Intended to provide a means for people to "visit the past so they could learn from it, so they could evolve and transform and better themselves," Nostalgia instead enabled takers to fixate on their most painful memories and thus avoid moving "gloriously into the future" ("An Almost Religious Awe," 2019). For individuals reliving their own memories rather than offering their testimonies to others, fixation may indeed be burdensome since, according to Laub, trauma cannot become known until it is witnessed. However, in a societal context, can we ever move gloriously into the future without remembering the most painful memories of our collective past? Which memories, and to what extent, are we obligated to remember?

In *Regarding the Pain of Others,* Susan Sontag explores these types of questions vis-à-vis viewing photographs of war, death, and suffering. On the subject of obligated looking, she explores two distinct scenarios. The simpler of the two is an obligation to look at atrocious photos because there is "something to be done, right now, about what they depic[t]" (2003, p. 91). Obligation becomes more complicated when "we are invited to respond to a dossier of hitherto unknown pictures of horrors long past" (ibid.). This obligation, as Sontag argues, is questionable:

> What is the point of exhibiting these pictures? To awaken indignation? To make us feel 'bad'; that is, to appall and sadden? To help us mourn? Is looking at such pictures really necessary, given that these horrors lie in a past remote enough to be beyond punishment? Are we the better for seeing these images? Do they actually teach us anything? (2003, p. 91-92)

There are certainly moral downfalls associated with looking, such as "cater[ing] to voyeuristic appetites and perpetuat[ing] black victimization" in the case of lynching photographs (ibid., p. 92), though these downfalls may not outweigh the obligation to look. Thus, the question is: "Which atrocities from the incurable past do we think we are obligated to revisit?" Then, once we decide we must look, it becomes: "Whom do we wish to blame? More precisely, whom do we believe we have the right to blame?" (ibid., p. 93).

Watchmen, perhaps, takes this line of questioning one step further: What if we accept blame ourselves? Sontag points out: "to remember is, more and more, not to recall a story but to be able to call up a picture ... Harrowing photographs do not inevitably lose their power to shock. But they are not much help if the task is to understand. Narratives can make us understand" (2003, p. 89). As a narrative representation of America's traumatic racial history and an exploration of American responses to that history, *Watchmen* aims to help viewers in the US and beyond better understand our collective past and how we, as individuals, relate to it. The series is both an invitation to respond to horrors long past and a call to action to do something, right now.

What if we accept blame for ourselves?

Reference List

'An almost religious awe' (2019) *Watchmen*, Season 1, episode 7. Warner Bros. Television. Available at: HBO Max (Accessed: 8 January 2023).

Coates, T. (2014) 'The case for reparations,' *The Atlantic*. Available at: https://www.theatlantic.com/magazine/archive/2014/06/the-case-for-reparations/361631/ (Accessed: 8 January 2023)

Dias, B.G. and Ressler, K.J. (2014) 'Parental olfactory experience influences behavior and neural structure in subsequent generations,' *Nature Neuroscience*, 17(1), 89-96. doi: https://doi.org/10.1038/nn.3594

Gardullo, P. (2021) 'Artifacts from the Tulsa Race Massacre,' *Smithsonian Magazine*. Available at: https://www.smithsonianmag.com/smithsonian-institution/reflections-artifacts-left-behind-tulsa-race-massacre-180977779/ (Accessed: 8 January 2023).

Hansen, H.P. 'If you don't like my story, write your own' (2019) *Watchmen*, Season 1, episode 4. Warner Bros. Television. Available at: HBO Max (Accessed: 8 January 2023).

'It's summer and we're running out of ice' (2019) *Watchmen*, Season 1, episode 1. Warner Bros. Television. Available at: HBO Max (Accessed: 8 January 2023).

Laub, D. (1992) 'Bearing witness or the vicissitudes of listening,' *Testimony: crises of witnessing in literature, psychoanalysis, and history*. New York: Routledge, pp. 57-74. doi: https://doi.org/10.4324/9780203700327

'Little fear of lightning' (2019) *Watchmen*, Season 1, episode 5. Warner Bros. Television. Available at: HBO Max (Accessed: 8 January 2023).

Moore, A. (1986-87) *Watchmen*. New York: DC Comics.

'Martial feats of Comanche horsemanship' (2019) *Watchmen*, Season 1, episode 2. Warner Bros. Television. Available at: HBO Max (Accessed: 8 January 2023).

Rankine, C. (2014). Citizen. Minneapolis, MN: Graywolf Press.

Schindler's List (1993). Directed by S. Spielberg. Available at: Peacock (Accessed: 8 January 2023).

'See how they fly' (2019) *Watchmen*, Season 1, episode 9. Warner Bros. Television. Available at: HBO Max (Accessed: 8 January 2023).

'She was killed by space junk' (2019) *Watchmen*, Season 1, episode 3. Warner Bros. Television. Available at: HBO Max (Accessed: 8 January 2023).

Sontag, S. (2003) *Regarding the pain of others*. New York: Picador.

'This extraordinary being' (2019) *Watchmen*, Season 1, episode 6. Warner Bros. Television. Available at: HBO Max (Accessed: 8 January 2023).

3.2.5

Traumatic Family Memories, Questions of Care, and the Role of Next of Kin in Contemporary Norwegian Fiction

Nora Simonhjell

University of Agder, Norway

Abstract

All families have secrets. What is told and retold can vary from one family member to another. An episode that seems harmless to one may have had a traumatic effect on another. Cathy Caruth argues, "If Freud turns to literature to describe traumatic experience, it is because literature, like psychoanalysis, is interested in the complex relation between knowing and not knowing" (1996, p. 3). Narrative medicine has focused chiefly on patient stories (Frank, 1995, 2010; Charon, 2006) and the patient as text (Aaslestad, 1997), but a "growing importance of caregiving is also seen in arts" (Berman, 2020, p. 4).

The role of next of kin is complex. Care relations and care practices are both socially and culturally constructed. Care-related experiences have become an increasingly thematic topic in Scandinavian fiction. In Norway, a white paper on the role of next of kin was published and launched in 2020, and several contemporary novels deal with the complexity of this relational situation (Nilssen, 2017, 2020; Knausgård, 2009; Ørstavik, 2021; Knausgård, 2016; Dåsnes, 2021). As Amelia DeFalco argues, "Narrative fiction is an ideal form for the study of care. In fact, one could argue that fiction has the most to contribute to ethics of care debates in its representation of particular scenarios of dependence, responsibility, compassion, and care" (2012, p. 378).

In this chapter, I will analyze Sandra Lillebø's novel *Tingenes tilstand* [The State of Things] (2020),[1] which thematizes how a mother's mental illness affects and partially controls her adult daughter's life. She must free herself from her

---

[1] The novel has not been translated into English yet. A rough translation of the title is *The State of Things*. The use of direct quotations is reduced to a minimum.

mother's invisible power. The novel addresses questions of traumatic childhood memories, the role of next of kin, and gendered implications of care relations and care ethics.

***

No story stands alone. Different stories "continue in other stories," Arthur Frank argues in his Walter Benjamin-inspired understanding of the storyteller (2013, p. 220). Different stories weave through a person's life experiences and carry "the *resonance* from previous stories" (ibid.). Lillebø's nameless first-person narrator is in her mid-thirties, a mother herself, and an author. She stands at the crisscross in her life. She had a difficult childhood. The narration starts when she experiences anxiety, restlessness, and several vague physical symptoms. She is afraid that she has inherited her mother's illness. Her body becomes a placeholder for memory and trauma.

The novel is structured as a writing process. It might become a way out of her traumatic experience. During her writing process, she explains and finds arguments for why she must distance herself from her mother. The text is organized into short fragments and dominated by small glimpses into some present situations or memories. They vary from one sentence up to two or three pages. Some of them function as traumatic flashbacks. Others are philosophical reflections, and still others are disruptive emotional outbursts. It is impossible for her to create a coherent narrative. The first-person narrator tries to come to terms with her childhood memories. She has broken all contact with her mother, and a sub-theme in her reflection is to find an argument for herself, why this is crucial for her existence. Her mother has an undiagnosed condition with both physical and mental symptoms. She has not understood her daughter's need for distance and constantly tries to contact her. The narrator's memories and experiences make it impossible for her to live up to the cultural and gendered norms for how to be a good daughter. As the closest next of kin to her mother, she has a constant inner struggle: What is she supposed to do, and what is she able to do in case of having to care for her mother—and at the same time be able to care for herself and her own family?

Caruth pinpoints the conflicting aspects of trauma and sees it as "a response, sometimes delayed, to an overwhelming event or events" (1995, p. 4). Trauma, then, is understood as "a wound inflicted not upon the body but upon the mind" (ibid., p. 3). The protagonist in Lillebø's novel experiences this. As Roger Luckhurst argues, "Trauma disrupts memory" (2008, p. 1). The narrator tries to organize her memories. She struggles to remember and to understand what really happened and to understand the relationship with her mother. "I am trying to remember her, but I only see myself" (Lillebø, p. 12). Why does she experience her childhood in the way that she does? How come no one understood that she grew up in a dysfunctional family? The question of what is seen out in public and what is not seen or is hidden behind the walls is crucial. No sudden traumatic event, like a car crash, haunts the protagonist, but her childhood, in general, was very unstable. She grew up to realize that her mother's feelings and needs were more important than her own. "When children are ignored, chastised or dismissed, or trained to meet the parent's needs and ignore their own, when adults are overly controlling and critical, constantly overriding the child's opinions, this will probably have a long-term and profound impact on the child's sense of self and identity" (Etherington, 2003, p. 24).

The writing process functions as a recognition of her trauma. It is through the verbalization of her anger and memories she can accept her experiences and trauma. The writing process functions as a confidant. She is creating the manuscript as an emphatic witness to her struggles. According to Dori Laub, "Testimony is, therefore, the process by which the narrator (the survivor) reclaims his position as a witness" (1992, p. 85). Even though this novel has an autobiographical and therapeutic level, it is important to underline that it is not a self-help book but a work of fiction. The narrative form is an aesthetic investigation of the theme in question. "Caregiving stories or films, unlike self-help books, dramatize problems and may be wary of solutions" (Berman, 2020, p. 12). Lillebø examines how the narrator tries to understand her mother's neglect and its effects.

Verbalizing her loss and traumatic childhood experiences is necessary for her recovery. Articulating her ugly feelings (Ngai, 2005) toward her mother raises complex emotions like anger, irritation, sadness, but also grief. She mourns the lost possibility of reconciliation with her mother. She grieves that her children would not have a relationship with their grandmother. "Working through one's grief is both an individual and collaborative process" (Berman, 2010, p. 2). Family structure implies a dependency on each other. Emotional feeling is relational, intertwined in the muddy family history. They transfer power according to whose pain and suffering have the inner value to be regarded as the most important. This inner conflict over emotions is also bound to the question of care and who is to care for the other, and as DeFalco argues, "Care comes to resemble a battle between giver and receiver" (2012, p. 386).

The absence of "adequate loving, the failure to support the child's self-esteem effort, failure to supply adequate sensory and cognitive stimuli, and other failures" (Schreiber, 2010, p. 8) can, from a psychiatric point of view, also be understood as traumatic. This disruption of home destroys the "home" as a safe place and puts the question of care and support in the spotlight. Who is to care for the child when the mother cannot create a caring environment for her children? The adult daughter still suffers from these experiences. Kim Etherington discusses the possibility of transforming trauma and underlines that transformation implies more than recovery or healing because it implies a fundamental shift "at the core of being. Transforming trauma requires a willingness to challenge our basic beliefs about ourselves and the world around us and enough faith to accept and trust what we cannot fully understand" (Etherington, 2003, p. 31). This is also part of a healing process for the daughter in Lillebø's novel. She is transforming trauma through the writing process.

> As we begin to tell our stories, we might find out things about ourselves that we didn't know before, discover strengths and resources within that we did not know existed, enjoy feelings that we no longer have to deny or feel controlled by, acknowledge and welcome thoughts we might probably have feared, and behave in ways we now understand and can put to good use. (ibid., p. 34)

Today, the mother is physically absent but still constantly present in her daughter's thoughts. It is as if she were even more present now than she ever was. The experiences of this haunting presence are almost retraumatizing: "Then she turns up from nowhere. It's when I forget her, when I forget to be on my guard. Then she's standing in front of me with staring eyes and open mouth showing all her teeth" (Lillebø, 2020, p. 14).

Reversal of Care Relations

The novel draws our attention to the concepts of "mother," "home," and "family." The protagonist has never experienced these as stable structures. However, she has a clear understanding of the importance of structure. "But things have always been in order around my mother. The order of things has protected her. And the order of things has protected me" (Lillebø, 2020, p. 18). Structure equals normality and care. During her childhood, they moved around from different places and flats; her mother had several boyfriends, and her own father was not around. Neither home nor family provided any protection for the narrator as a child. In contrast, "home," "family," and "mother" became the base for the unsafe and dangerous. Their mother-child relationship has been disrupted and almost turned around, making the daughter care for her mother—and act as a parent for herself. "A mother who displaces her emotional distress onto physical pain teaches her child an important lesson about how to elicit care: the child might learn that attention given to an illness or physical pain will not be forthcoming in response to heartache or sadness" (Etherington 2003, p. 30). As a child, she was constantly focused on her mother's emotions, neglecting her own.

> I realise that I need to protect her and become obsessed by rules, procedures, by morality. I need to know all the codes to be on top of all conventions. I pretend that I'm a grownup who has to pretend that I'm a child. The child I am is a mask, and the grownups let themselves be captivated by it, by the maturity it exudes [...] I'm the one who makes sure that traditions are kept up, and at Christmas, it's me who's Father Christmas. (Lillebø, pp. 19-20).

Retelling the traumatic events is an important part of the healing process of trauma. "The task then is to render body memoirs tellable, which means to order and arrange them in the form of a story, linking emotion with event, event with event, and so on" (Culbertson, 1995, p. 179). Past and present events blur into each other for the narrator. It is as if all things happened at the same time since one sentence might start in recent time, for then suddenly the narrator falls into a memoir for a short time, and then back again to the thing she began to tell. This eruptive narrative style creates a kaleidoscopic portrait of the past. The narrator is both part of and tries to distance herself from what is retold. "Telling, in short, is a process of disembodying memory, demystifying it, a process which can begin after memories have been re-membered and the mystical touched by a buried self-seeking in own healing" (ibid.). The novel is structured as a survivor narrative. Despite her childhood and mother's demands and emotional pressure, the narrator put words to her traumatic experiences. "It's a puzzle that falls apart when you try to put the pieces together. Nothing is left other than a vague notion of a mother's impaired mental faculties, and how unusual is that?" (Lillebø p. 18).

The writing process becomes a possible way out of the traumatic experience. "Memory is always at the end subjected to those conventions which define the believable" (ibid.). She experienced her childhood as threatening and disturbing. Now, she is trying to gain recognition for her traumatic memories. They haunt her as constant thoughts and as unclear bodily pain. "Thus, for the memoirs of a child's trauma to become 'memory,' in any socially recognized, narrative sense, the leap from the known to the said is large, and the chance of missing the other side of the divide, great" (ibid., p. 181). The uncertainty related to what the daughter experienced as a child remains throughout the novel. The choice of a first-person narrator also means that we, as readers, never get an insight into the other side of the story. Again, the question of the narrator's credibility is raised. She can only tell her version of what happened. Culbertson argues, "The question is not only 'what is there to say,' but 'who is there to talk'" (1995, p. 191). A person who has a traumatic experience and lives to tell about it, is from her perspective, a survivor who *survives twice.* If the protagonist should be able to continue to be a writer, this story must be told. However, what version of the childhood experiences is to be expressed? There is always the possibility of telling a story from another point of view. This is reflected in the first-person narrator's perspective: "All stories could be different; they can always be something else. The characters and props change place, the stage revolves, the plots change shape. Not this one" (Lillebø, p. 15).

From Marianne Hirsch's perspective, the family gaze is important. "Family life, even in its most intimate moments, is entrenched in a collective imaginary shaped by a shared archive of stories and images that inflect the transmission of individual and family remembrance" (Hirsch, 2008, p. 114). The family is an "affiliative group" (ibid., p. 110). Hirsch is especially interested in family photographs. I will argue that her point is relevant to the understanding of family memoirs as such. A family is a place where memories are created, told, and retold. However, how memories are shared and transferred from one generation to another is not a simple process. Who decides over a family's memories and history? Different family members can all have different perceptions of what has happened in a situation, and thus, they will also have different memories. This can create conflicts within the family, and "transgenerational haunting" (Raskin, 1992) might occur: A secret from the past might affect a person's behavior in later generations. "It holds the individual within a group dynamic constituted by a specific familial topography that prevents the individual from living life as her or his own" (ibid., p. 27). The family dynamic that unfolds in the novel is an example of how a person tries to act against and challenge this transgressional haunting. The narrator tries to find a voice to utter her wounds to gain recognition for her history: "It may be the case that all I need from her, all anyone ever needs from a mother, is a justification; a certificate of one's own calamity, ready signed, waiting to be written out" (Lillebø, p. 55).

Joan Tronto (1993) argues that the relationship between the caregiver and the receiver of care is asymmetrical. This is the case both on a personal and a general level. The person in need of care can often feel powerless toward these care relation structures. The role of next of kin is a fundamental relational and situated-based identity. The emotional or familiar closeness to the other defines the role, and this identity category is thereby not based on an individual fundament. The nearness to another person's suffering and pain creates the base for this identity category. Both social and juridical factors decide what it means to be close to the other person. How literary fiction can address questions on the role of next of kin is a question asked by Amelia DeFalco (2016) and David Morris (2017). "Care describes an approach to personal and social morality that shifts ethical considerations to context, relationships, and affective knowledge in a manner that can only be fully understood if its embodied [and performative] dimension is recognized. Care is committed to the flourishing and growth of individuals, yet acknowledges our interconnectedness and interdependence" (Hamington and Rosenow, 2019, p. 10). Based on this understanding, care is a relational approach to ethics.

As a child, the narrator constantly had to find her survival strategies herself. As an adult woman, her explicit distancing from her mother leads her into a series of self-examining thoughts about whether she can actually make the choices to distance herself from her mother in the way she has now chosen. To be able to care for herself and her own family, she must distance herself from her mother, her demands, and several attempts to stay in touch with her. Both require a care the other is unable to provide. The novel can be read as a documentation of how and why the daughter has ended up making this choice and why she must maintain this distance. The meta-narrative layer creates a space for the narrator to deal with the haunting transgenerational emotional wound. This pinpoints ambivalence in family and care relations. "To start writing is not about sloughing off your skin, it's about replacing your core. It's about throwing out everything that is to be hidden and protected. It's to annihilate through display" (Lillebø, p. 173).

By opposing the role of caregiver for her mother, she breaks out of a normative, gendered pattern. This is a choice with practical, emotional, political, and ethical implications. Even though the narrator's mother was physically present in the narrator's childhood, her illness made her distant from her daughter. This has made the narrator extra vulnerable. She is afraid she might become a "bad mother" herself; she scrutinizes the relationship with her mother—trying to find a way to cope with her experiences, memories, and trauma. At the same time, she wonders about the consequences her text might have: "This text is her greatest terror. It may have been me who made her sick" (Lillebø, p. 177).

Questions of Care and Responsibility

The novel poses questions of responsibility and what it means to care for another person. "Responsibility for the other involves assuming the other's need, being willing to be called to account for the other, surrendering one's goals and desires in defense of the other's" (Attridge 1999, p. 27). The novel is an example where a daughter is unwilling to take on this responsibility, even though the person in need of care is her mother. How can her mother demand her daughter's attention now when she was not able to see her needs as a child? What kind of social or moral obligation has the neglected child to care for her mother despite all that has happened in the past? Is it possible for her to forgive her mother's actions?

A subtheme in the novel is the first-person narrator's struggle to find herself and claim her identity. The role of the mother is ambivalent even though it seems like the narrator has an understanding of the difficulties of her mother's situation, but her lack of real ability to act as a loving and supporting mother made it necessary for the child to act as the caregiver. "And I know that if my mother should now be parted from her illness, her illness can never be parted from the mother I had" (Lillebø, p. 177). This shift in roles throws the entire fragile family dynamic out of balance. There is no verbal confrontation between them. Instead, the narrator gives her mother the silent treatment. This chosen wordlessness prevents her from getting close to her mother. The mother's powerlessness is manifested in the things she did not do or did not say. In contrast, the first-person narrator's investigation of this relationship manifests in the power structures intertwined in the writing process. By doing this, they oppose the social and emotional codes for care and the role of the next of kin. The meta-narrative reflections uttered by the first-person narrator thereby hold the role of both a trauma-healing process and a process of self-care, almost like therapeutic writing. The mother as a speaking subject is missing. The first-person narrator's task is to create a powerful self-narrative, making her write through her traumatic relationship with her mother. She wants to become a better mother for her children. This act of abandonment is twofold and, thereby, an act of care: It creates distance from her mother, and at the same time, she creates a space for herself. Saying no to her mother's demands is a self-protective action. According to DeFalco, compassion is a term "denoting privilege: the suffering is *over there*" (2012, p. 381). It is a doubling of the suffering position in this novel. The suffering is both over there and present here at the same time. Is the suffering in question the same suffering she experienced in childhood, or is it another pain? Could it be that "the very mechanisms that have helped the child survive may then become the problem" (Etherington, 2003, p. 29)? Lillebø's narrator pinpoints this urgent dilemma.

Conclusion

"Care is a human trouble" (Bellacasa, 2017, p. 2). As I have argued, Lillebø's novel creates a multi-layered investigation of childhood traumas and questions of care. The traumatic childhood experiences haunt the protagonist's present life. The emotional distress caused by her mother functions as a black hole for the narrator's voice. How can she get recognition for her memories and actions toward her mother? Lillebø draws our attention toward ethical questions of storytelling family memories, and how this also involves questions of care. To tell a story has a caring dimension since it involves an awareness of the other's situation and feelings. To be excluded from a family story or a person's memory work might have a traumatic effect. One might ask, is the narrator, by telling the story of her traumatic childhood, causing a new trauma for her mother? When the daughter breaks the norms and conventions of how she should act in relation to her sick mother, she emerges as a literary character who becomes someone to whom it is difficult to relate. To what extent can we trust her perspective? Was the mother, in fact, as demanding and unsympathetic as the daughter portrays her?

"If literary works and our responses to them could be programmed in advance, innovative literature and creative criticism-literature, and criticism, as we understand them, would, cease to be" (Attridge, 1999, p. 30). This novel raises questions about the power of language: "The story's power struggle between caregiver and care-receiver demonstrates the potency of knowledge and secrets" DeFalco (2012, p. 389). Lillebø investigates how care is always a question of relational power and how the question of individual suffering and the impossibility of shared pain is manifested through family dynamics and is a concrete work with ethical and affective implications. Care can turn into moral pressure, as seen in this novel. "The possibility of knowing history ... is thus also raised as a deeply ethical dilemma: the unremitting problem of *how not to betray the past,*" Caruth argues (1996, p. 27). *Tingenes tilstand* is a complex literary text that opens ambiguous understandings of trauma, ethics, and caring relationships.

Reference List

Attridge, D. (1999) 'Innovation, literature, ethics: relating to the other,' *PMLA: Publications of the Modern Language Association of America,* 144(1), pp. 20-31. doi: https://doi.org/10.2307/463424

Bellacasa, M.P. de la (2017) *Matters of care: speculative ethics in more than human worlds.* Series: Posthumanities, 41. Minneapolis and London: University of Minnesota Press.

Berman, J. (2010) *Companionship in grief: love and loss in memoirs of C.S. Lewis, John Bayley, Donald Hall, Joan Didion and Calvin Trillin.* Amherst: University of Massachusetts Press.

Berman, J. (2020) *The art of caregiving in fiction, film, and memoir.* London: Bloomsbury Academic.

Caruth, C. (ed.) (1995) *Trauma: explorations in memory.* Baltimore: Johns Hopkins University Press.

Caruth, C. (1996) *Unclaimed experience: trauma, narrative and history.* Baltimore: Johns Hopkins University Press.

Charon, R. (2006) *Narrative medicine: honoring the stories of illness.* New York: Oxford University Press.

Culbertson, R. (1995) 'Embodied memory, transcendence and telling: recounting trauma, re-establishing the self,' *New Literary History,* 26(1), pp. 169-195. doi: https://doi.org/10.1353/nlh.1995.0007

DeFalco, A. (2012) 'Caretakers/caregivers: economic of affection in Alice Munro,' *Twentieth Century Literature,* 58(3), pp. 377-398. doi: https://doi.org/10.1215/0041462X-2012-4001

DeFalco, A. (2016) *Imaging care: responsibility, dependency and Canadian literature*. Toronto, Buffalo and London: University of Toronto Press.

Dåsnes, N. (2021) *Ubesvart anrop* [Missed call]. Oslo: Aschehoug.

Etherington, K. (2003) 'Trauma, the body ad transformation,' in Etherington, K. (ed.) *Trauma, the body and transformation: a narrative inquiry*. Philadelphia: Jessica Kingsley Publishers, pp. 22-38.

Frank, A.W. (1995) *The wounded storyteller: body, illness, and ethics*. Chicago: University of Chicago Press.

Frank, A.W. (2010) *Letting stories breathe: a socio-narratology*. Chicago: University of Chicago Press.

Frank, A.W. [1995 (2013)] *The wounded storyteller: body, illness and ethics*. 2nd edn. Chicago and London: University of Chicago Press.

Hamington, M. and Rosenow, C. (2019) *Care ethics and poetry*. London: Palgrave Macmillan.

Hirsch, M. (2008) 'The generation of postmemory,' *Poetics Today*, 29(1), pp. 103-128. doi: https://doi.org/10.1215/03335372-2007-019

Knausgård, K.O. (2009) *Min kamp 1* [My struggle 1]. Oslo: Forlaget Oktober.

Knausgård, K.O. (2016) *Om våren* [In the springtime]. Oslo: Forlaget Oktober.

Laub, D. (1992) 'An event wihtout a witness: truth, testimony and survival,' in Felman, S. and Laub, D. (eds.) *Testimony: crices of witnessing in literature, psychoanalysis, and history*. New York: Routledge, pp. 75-92.

Lillebø, S. (2020) *Tingenes tilstand* [The State of Things]. Oslo: Forlaget Oktober.

Luckhurst, R. (2008) *The trauma question*. New York: Routledge.

Morris, D.B. (2017) *Eros and illness*. Cambridge, Massachusetts and London, England: Harvard University Press.

Ngai, S. (2005) *Ugly feelings*. Cambridge and London: Harvard University Press.

Nilssen, O. (2017) *Tung tids tale* [Speaking in times of adversity]. Oslo: Samlaget.

Nilssen, O. (2020) *Yt etter evne, få etter behov* [Contribute as you can, receive as you need]. Oslo: Samlaget.

Raskin, E. (1992) *Family secrets and the psychoanalysis of narrative*. Princeton: Princeton University Press.

Schreiber, E.J. (2010) 'Introduction: trauma, memory and subjectivity. The healing power of home,' in *Race, trauma, and home in the novels of Toni Morrison*, Los Angeles: Barton Rouge, pp. 1-31.

Tronto, J. (1993) *Moral boundaries: a political argument for an ethic of care*. London: Routledge.

Ørstavik, H. (2021) *Ti amo* [I love you]. Oslo: Forlaget Oktober.

Aaslestad, P. (1997) *Pasienten som tekst. Fortellerollen i psykiatriske journaler. Gaustad 1890-1990* [The patient as text. The narrative role in psychiatric journals. Gaustad 1890-1990]. Oslo: Universitetsforlaget.

3.2.6

Narratives of Healing and Healers: Malay Muslim Identity in Southeast Asia

Hannah Ming Yit Ho

University of Brunei Darussalam, Brunei

Abstract

This chapter explores narrative medicine to examine intersubjective dynamics between those who suffer from and treat illnesses in a contemporary Anglophone Bruneian novel. In Kathrina Daud's *The Witch Doctor's Daughter* (2022), identity issues are addressed by a young family member who becomes disillusioned with her parents' traditional medicinal practices. This female protagonist's declining relationship with her Muslim parents causes her to leave home to learn about traditional healing in her mother's longhouse community. Her encounters with indigenous healers, a linguistic researcher and an orphan see her bearing witness to traumatic suffering. Importantly, her narrative becomes an act of decolonization as she works to heal communal and personal traumas. The cognitive, symbolic, and affective energies of her narrative and other storytellers are highlighted too. Such curative impulses offer productive ways to understand traditional medicinal use in the Malay Muslim nation of Brunei Darussalam. In its critique of post/colonial hegemonic discourses, this novel addresses intricate relations between healing agents and recipients that resonate with the rest of the Malay world in Southeast Asia.

***

Within Southeast Asia, the practice of healing is a contentious field due to competing philosophies derived from colonial influences on medicinal practices, on the one hand, and locally informed cultural therapies to alleviate physical and psychical illnesses, on the other hand. Steeped in oppositional ideas of modern or Western and traditional or Eastern modes of cure, Southeast Asian communities share a common history of European colonization that has resulted in nation-building along the lines of Benedict Anderson's (1983, p. 6) "imagined political community" and Partha Chatterjee's (1986, p. 66) "spiritual" domain, which positions cultural differentiation as an act of decolonization in postcolonial nations. The horizontal comradeship or fraternity established between individual members within the collective community is reinforced by culture, subsuming language, religious belief, and nation-state's political policies that are determined by intricate aspects of cultural identity. For many Southeast Asian postcolonial nations, a discourse of national identity is often rooted in ethnoreligious tenets that assert core differences from the European colonizer. For Malaysia, Indonesia, and Brunei Darussalam, a Malay Muslim configuration has been ideologically established as the dominant marker of state-promulgated identity.

This chapter deals with the ethics of healing, but also politics of identity. Malay Muslim hegemonic power structures within Southeast Asia, including the post-protectorate nation of Brunei Darussalam, influence identity politics that govern therapeutic and medicinal services sought by cultural communities within the nation and wider regional realm. Through a literary analysis of a contemporary Bruneian novel, two main areas of inquiry are opened up. Firstly, the act of decolonizing identity by re-centering traditional healing practices to undo oriental myths of the indigenous other, while also exploring the limitations of traditional medicine and their practitioners. Secondly, the act of Islamic conversion to legitimize traditional therapies carries great import in Southeast Asia, especially within Malay Muslim nations that espouse state-ascribed orthodox Islam and promote a reconfiguration of traditional healing according to state regulations.

In examining Bruneian author Kathrina Mohd Daud's contemporary novel entitled *The Witch Doctor's Daughter* (2022), this study interrogates the roles and responsibilities of healers as well as the community that become recipients of traditional medicine in the Malay world. Through a personal crisis over an Islamic conversion in support of the "business" (ibid., p. 144) of traditional therapy, an ideological conflict between contending practices of modern and traditional medicine unfolds. Growing up with her parents' craft of indigenous healing, the female protagonist Safiyya confronts her discomfort with her parents' exploitation of their patients seeking to ease the heterogeneous traumas of heartbreak, terminal illnesses, and vitamin deficiencies – various sites contending with the way trauma may a category that transcends these differences. Through a critical discussion of the narrative representations of modern and traditional medicine, this chapter aims to illuminate ethical dilemmas in trauma management in a narration that prompts a decolonizing agenda at global and local levels. In Daud's fictional work, Muslim identity in the Malay world is thus analyzed to offer a commentary of local culture through narratives of healers, which simultaneously reveal inherent contradictions of religious identity and traditional healing cultures within a Malay Muslim nation even while decolonizing narrative medicine is performed.

In this study, a dual conceptual lens is adopted to address the complexities of medicinal practices that are informed by sociocultural hegemonic structures—for one, postcolonial ideological powers; and for another, state-dictated legitimate Muslim identity. Along this line, a postcolonial lens is first employed to deconstruct healing from prescriptive colonial hegemonies. Second, a poststructuralist approach demystifies local medicinal practices to promote an understanding of narrative medicine that elicits fluid meanings of identity which challenge boundaries between local and national, as well as healers and those seeking to be healed. Through blurred identities and flexible engagements with state-Islam for legitimizing traditional healing, narratives dealing with ethical dimensions of therapy and political constructs of a healer's identity are foregrounded here.

The Malay World

Malay Muslim identity in Southeast Asia is a fundamental constituent of the Malay world – a geographical region known as Nusantara and whose nation-state membership encompasses Malaysia, Singapore, Brunei Darussalam and Indonesia (Evans, 2016). Malay communities in Southeast Asia also subsume the Orient (Boomgaard, 2001). In fact, the orientalization of Malay Muslim people and their lands provided justification for the project of European colonization (Said, 1978; Alatas, 1977). Binary oppositions between modern and traditional, male and female, as well as civil and savage promulgated stereotypes that disparaged non-European identity. As "a political concept," Nusantara is crucial to the anticolonial struggle in Malay Muslim nation-states (Evans, 2016, p. 5).

Apart from their Malay ethnicity, the Malay people within the Malay world identify with the Malay language and Muslim identity. An intertwining of Malay and Muslim identities is a rudimentary constituent of state-sanctioned discourses, such as in Brunei Darussalam, Malaysia and Indonesia with a Malay Muslim dominant population. While the Islamization of Malay identity is entrenched in the national practices and identity policies of the latter, Brunei Darussalam adopts a more fluid approach to define the Malay people or "puak jati," who comprise the Brunei Malay, Murut, Dusun, Tutong, Belait, Bisaya, and Kedayan (Ho, 2019; Deterding and Ho, 2021). Bruneian Malays are thus not necessarily Muslims. The native languages and religious affiliations of these people are heterogeneous and do not conform to a coherent Malay Muslim identity discourse.

Traditional Healing Practices

The communal agents and individual actors of traditional healing are increasingly subjected to a "bureaucratization of Islam" (Müller, 2018a, p. 212), as they engage in practices involving supernatural spirits in ways that deviate from Islamic teachings. Writing on the criminalization of supernatural healers in Brunei Darussalam, Dominick Müller explicates that "exorcism" has "long been the domain of Malay supernatural specialists whose once-normalized practices have become bureaucratically categorized as deviant" (Müller, 2018b, p. 147). As "Islam forbids trances" (Farrer, 2008, p. 35), spiritual healing practices dealing with *jinn,* spirits or ghosts (Müller, 2018b, p. 167) are regarded as unethical. As part of the Malay Muslim world, spirits are often featured in Bruneian Anglophone fiction, which deals with the relations between earthly and ethereal figures that evoke a struggle with hegemonic power structures embedded in the independent nation-state (Ho, 2020).

Nonetheless, healing practices involving jinns that are fended off through exorcisms are used to mitigate psychic disturbances, known as *gangguan* in the Malay world. Supernatural healers may also employ traditional herbs and natural remedies to cure spiritual possessions or *kerasukan* and *histeria* in Malay-speaking communities. Hysteria as a mental illness is prominently conceptualized in Sigmund Freud's (2001) work that identifies it as a disorder due to physical and psychical traumas affecting women with a "hystera" (uterus in Greek). Even as Freud's gendered configuration of this illness can be applied to its manifestations in the Malay world, hysteria lacks cultural nuances and local contexts of psychological disorders. Daud's novel advances a narrative about *histeria* handled by local people through local methods of understanding and therapies, in spite of inherent tensions, which posits trauma as a category that transcends heterogeneous sites.

Consequently, there continues to be great traction for "local and indigenous medical systems [that] still provide a real health service of the great majority of people in Southeast Asia" (Yoshida, 1985, p. 232). A currency for services of the *bomoh* or witch doctor, whose healing practices when aligned with Islamic codes is dubbed as *orang pandai* (or clever people), remains. The socio-cultural dimension of indigenous therapy appeals to those seeking trauma management. The cultural economy of traditional healing can be explicated as "[i]ndigenous healers provid[ing] culturally meaningful explanation and interpretation of the illness experience and culturally sanctioned treatment" (Yoshida, 1985, p. 232). While Sufi mysticism connects to a spiritual world, Sunni Islam prescribed in the Malay world focuses on conventional codes of life in the Quran (Holy Book of Islam). Nevertheless, a simultaneous recourse to traditional healing and modern medicine is also not uncommon, as they are not mutually exclusive and can be conterminously consulted to address trauma's heterogeneous psychic, physical and physiological sites as demonstrated in Daud's novel.

Despite their ostensible polarization, modern medicine may be derived from traditional medicine. Hugo J. de Boer and Crystle Cotingting clarify that "a large percentage of modern pharmaceuticals have been derived from [traditional] medicinal plants" (2014, p. 747). A clear distinction between the two kinds of medicine is thus elusive. Nevertheless, traditional healing continues to be regarded dubiously as it is historically viewed as subpar to modern or Western medicine. The further criminalization of spiritual and indigenous healers is also evidence of a bureaucratization of Islam within independent Muslim nation-states in post/neocolonial times.

Analysis: Ethics and Politics of Trauma Therapy in *The Witch Doctor's Daughter*

Unlike the national endorsement of Malay literature (Ho, 2022a), Anglophone literary writings on Brunei are in their nascent stage. Anglophone writings are mostly self-published or printed by international presses (Daud, Chin and Jukim, 2016). Their readership includes a local audience, and a regional readership in Southeast Asia and the global realm. With the colonial history of Southeast Asia, the anticolonial dimensions of the Anglophone writings cannot go unnoticed. Bruneian fiction is no exception as it engages with local and national discourses of identity and culture in response to British administrative rule and colonial legacies. Significantly, narrative practices become decolonizing acts through integrating this political impulse, especially via discursive tensions within healing practices, when narrating the ethics of trauma management through characters.

The Witch Doctor's Daughter is one such narrative that performs this act. Bruneian Anglophone novel that deals with healers, with a focus on their ethics and politics. Familial, cultural and national affiliations are forged through the protagonist and her mother who both "like the idea of helping people" (Daud, 2022, p. 18). A narrative about trauma and grief is presented through the female protagonist's lens. As a Muslim convert, Safiyya raises ethical questions about her Muslim parents' healing practices. Amongst those patronizing their services are women who "grieve and long and desire" (ibid., p. 38). Some "don't trust" (ibid., p. 66) medicine dispensed through Dr Rafidah and other doctors in a governmental hospital. Safiyya's subsequent adoption of an orphan named Adam is her means of dealing with traumatic loss. Adam represents cognitive, symbolic, and affective affiliations to healing. On a cognitive level, she grieves his physical loss of his mother. Symbolically, Adam reminds her that she is also a child in need of hope ["*I don't know what I'm doing. I am my only hope*" (ibid.,

p. 13, original emphasis)]. Affectively, she connects her father's past with Adam's history as both have been "*adopted as a baby*" (ibid., p. 84, original emphasis).

While Safiyya displays "narrative competence" (Charon, 2001, p. 1897) as a first-person narrator witnessing loss, there are multiple narratives of healing featuring the voices of other healers, such as her father Haji Umar, her mother Khadijah, and Mak Soton who is a traditional healer in the Kalangang community. Their rationales for, and gravitation towards, traditional healing are framed through Safiyya's narration. Notwithstanding this, traditional healing encounters skepticism from a villager named Mak Timinah, who expresses her antipathy due to her conviction that Khadijah treats her patients as mere "customers" (ibid., p. 21). Consequently, curative story-telling in Safiyya's narration articulates losses, but also signals an urgent need for trauma therapy.

The Witch Doctor's Daughter is a postcolonial fiction that writes back to the historical marginalization of indigenous identities, cultures and traditional practices in Southeast Asia. With a central narrative of healing told through a Bruneian female protagonist-cum-narrator, indigenous and local identities are redefined and reconfigured in "herstories" (Ho, 2013, p. 153). This kind of anti-colonial writing, evident through the following analyses of narratives of death and language loss that are featured in this section, is offered without romanticizing Safiyya and her local community. Even while healing others, Safiyya possesses insecurities that warrant her own need of therapy that leads her back to her maternal community of traditional healers. This study discusses healing practices to render further insights into Malay Muslim identity in the nation-state. The analysis proceeds in two strands: a mitigation of physical and spiritual death, and the cultural economy of Islam as a political means to validate identities of traditional healers in a Malay world.

In this Bruneian novel, death is a formidable source of trauma and grief that is dealt with through both modern and traditional medicine, which blur the heterogeneous sites of trauma to challenge hegemonic interpretations and treatments of illnesses. A simultaneous solicitation of modern and traditional healing forms reinforces trauma as a category transcending differences. The narrative force of characters' discussions on traumatic loss highlights comparative approaches to frame and contextualize local illnesses and their therapies. For one, both physical and psychological illnesses are confronted through Safiyya's narrative. Crucially, the story of her grandmother's death catalyzes her return to her mother's longhouse, a location that is replete with knowledge and resources on traditional medicine. Even while it is a political move, Safiyya's homecoming to learn more about her maternal community and Mak Soton's traditional medicinal resources is filled with ethical dilemmas. In fact, Safiyya is no stranger to traditional healing to mitigate illnesses in the Water Village where she resides with her parents. Ever since she was a child, she has witnessed her mother prescribing natural plants, such as "akar pahit" (Daud, 2022, p. 59), to relieve bodily aches and treat vitamin deficiencies of her clients. Furthermore, heartbreak in failing relationships (ibid., p. 12) is assuaged by prescribing "[b]ag[s] of bark, flowers, herbs and words" (ibid., p. 13). In a world where "[d]eath happens" (ibid., p. 25), Safiyya's mother narrates her unfailing determination to "see if there is a genuine way she could help" (ibid., p. 144)—a curative impulse to offset death and its precursors. As her mother recounts, "I have never used what I can see to do anything but help people" (ibid., p. 26). This is her immediate rejoinder to Mak Timinah who questions Khadijah's ethics in her healing practices. A young client called Dora who has leukemia seeks recourse to Khadijah's traditional medicine within the wards of the government hospital. Safiyya's grief when observing her mother's actions in vain is articulated when she narrates: "Even if I did not know where learning these things would lead me, I knew that at least they would not take me back to that hospital room, to that grief, to that heartbreak. To that guilt." (40) While traditional healing is meant to ease a patient's pain, they can also cause a healer's guilt during a failure "to help people to live" (Daud, 2022, p. 26). In this ethical dilemma, traditional healers rise to the challenge to contest the notion of their alternative modes as a "threatening Otherness" (Said, 1978, p. 29). In particular, Khadijah's and Safiyya's narration about healing provide insights into indigenous people's traditional medicine as a mode to deal with heterogeneous sites of trauma ranging from physical illnesses to psychological disturbances and physiological deficiencies. Despite traditional healers being oft perceived as "irrational, depraved (fallen), childlike, [and] 'different'" (Said, 1978, p. 48), they shift knowledge production away from hegemonic institutions that are represented in the government hospital. Exemplifying Michel Foucault's concept of biopolitics (2008), the hospital underpins a governmentality over a nation's population. While demystifying traditional healing, Khadijah's and Safiyya's intent to mitigate the effects of illnesses, which is aligned with attenuating trauma, is underscored in a healing beyond, and not necessarily within, the hospital's remits. Although death is associated with loss, it is not defined by it. While presented with physical illnesses, Safiyya is adamant to seek her mother's narrative of embracing her traditional heritage by revisiting her Kalangang community of healers.

In terms of discourses that speak to language losses, narrative practices become acts of decolonization through probing hegemonic systems that have embedded a colonial mentality. Discursive acts become political while confronting processes of neocolonization—in this case, a linguistic imperialism that is foregrounded in Safiyya's narrative. Conversations of language loss shape narratives that open up dialogs about identity loss due to language demise. A narrator's medium determines stories that are (re)told, which feeds into practice and action. As an ardent researcher and advocate of indigenous languages named Dr Jonah narrates to Safiyya, "Everything dies, [b]ut not everything that dies is lost" (Daud, 2022, p. 53). This idea of recovery is central to a rejection and reclamation of that which has been suppressed, which include cultural stories conventionally narrated in the mother tongue that inform identity. Safiyya's interactions with Dr Jonah, who studies indigenous languages in the Kalangang community, reveal a threat to the Jiku language as a result of "[w]ars, colonisation, exile. Politics" (ibid., p. 53). Jiku's essence that encapsulates "the spiritual greatness of Eastern culture" (Chatterjee, 1993, p. 73) dies because "the most dominant being Pawan or Malay" (Daud, 2022, p. 57) pushes this language to the fringes.

Consequently, indigenous communities' bolstering of their cultural identity pushes back against being "punished for using [their native] language and made to learn a new one—the dominant one—if they want to socialize or assimilate or find employment" (Daud, 2022, p. 53). Healing from this cultural erasure indicates an effort to recover from the linguistic losses inflicted by post- and neocolonial hegemonic powers. As an urgent mission, narrative acts mitigate the effect of "allowing an entire culture, an entire people, an entire history to die" (ibid., p. 53). In line with language as a battleground of identity, state-sanctioned Islam is an impetus for conversion into the spiritual dimension of national identity. Viewing her father "is a charlatan, a consummate performer and a compulsive liar" (ibid., p. 14)—a disingenuous witch doctor whom "people look for when both religion and God fail them" (ibid., p. 147), Safiyya reveals her frustrations with unethical medicinal practices. In questioning his Islamic conversion, Safiyya recounts her father's justification of "We are safer as Muslims" (ibid., p. 144). His rationale that "[p]eople will accept from Khadijah Abdullah things they will be angry with Bulan [now Khadijah] for" (ibid., p. 144) heightens ethical and identity issues around healing. In spite of her father's shoring up his medicinal practice through an Islamization that fulfills national cultural goals (Ho, 2022b), Safiyya undermines his authority as the leader in the family. She questions his patriarchal leadership in exposing him for monetizing their newly embraced Muslim identity. In deriding his "charlatan tricks" (Daud, 2022, p. 13), she narrates that his healing acts are "sorrowful piece[s] of performance art" (ibid., p. 12). In stark contrast to his lackadaisical attempts at traditional ecological knowledge, her mother's efforts prompt Safiyya's affinity for her maternal community. Even though spiritual traditions are validated by a Muslim patriarchal system that demarcates between ethical and unethical healing practices, Safiyya's disappointment in her father's "lies" and "tricks" (ibid., p. 13) despite his "powerful vocabulary of legitimation" (Müller, 2018b, p. 174) becomes highly evident.

Consequently, the spiritual world is a significant avenue for overturning the governmentality of medical institutions. Recalling Jacques Derrida's (1981, p.

41) deconstruction that focuses on incoherence rather than stability, the challenges to state-Islamic discourses elicit complex local identities through their difference from state rhetoric. With cultural and national economies of Islam, Muslim practitioners are regarded as stable and legitimate figures. For instance, Dr Rafidah who works in a government hospital is ranked highly by the authoritative state. In terms of Foucault's governmentality (2009), medical institutions transform citizens into targets of state objectification and power. As a counter-response, local Muslim communities teach "everything about jamu [natural herbs] and [spiritual] protection" (Daud, 2022, p. 16) to subvert the hierarchy of state-approved Muslim therapeutic practices. While healing is legitimized via Islam, there are also "hybrid pathways to orthodoxy" (Müller, 2018b, p. 141) that are demonstrated within her mother's traditional village located away from medical institutions which are situated near the Water Village.

Relevant to this discussion of a religious legitimization of traditional healing practices is Gilles Deleuze and Félix Gauttari's idea of deterritorialization, which may be understood as a delocalization (Tomlinson, 1999, p. 199). As Arjun Appadurai explicates, deterritorialization is "one of the central forces of the modern world" (1990, p. 301), which "create[s] a complicated network of finances and religious identifications" (ibid., p. 302) that entails fluidity and connectedness. Coupled with globalization in Southeast Asia (Ullah and Ho, 2020), deterritorialization underscores the untenable boundaries between the local and national as well as the East and West binary. In relation to jinns permeating the Malay Muslim world, Khadijah's reminder that the "veil is there for a reason" (Daud, 2022, p. 21) evokes a tenuous delineation between earthly and spiritual figures that reflects interconnected or delocalized worlds. As demonstrated in Dora and Tini, another young girl who is physically poorly, jinns that inhabit their bodies denote "thin and translucent" (ibid., p. 22) thresholds that invoke a problematic discourse related to hierarchical structures and dichotomies of East and West, traditional and modern, as well as Muslim and non-Muslim. A recourse to Western medicine to alleviate Dora's suffering from leukemia and Tini's illness of rickets (ibid., p. 37) signals their attempts at physical healing. Alternatively, traditional therapy via their soliciting of Khadijah's services articulates efforts to heal their psychic traumas. These Malay girls exhibit symptoms of spiritual vulnerability manifested in their display of hysteria. Their subscriptions to psychosomatic and physical therapies indicate "brain-body-world entanglements" (Blackman, 2012, p. 1), which accentuate linkages between corporeal and cognitive trauma that warrant a resolve for concurrent modern and traditional therapies resonating with deterritorialization.

Conclusion

This chapter has discussed the ethics of healing and identity that are entangled in decolonizing self, community and nation. In view of historical legacies, linguistic losses and personal experiences of trauma, *The Witch Doctor's Daughter* delineates characters who suffer from physical and spiritual ailments that are symptomatic of their traumas, but also reiterates an urgency to reclaim narratives of cultural erasure rooted in entrenched binary structures. In Malay Muslim nations, hierarchical structures shaping spiritual practices produce an economy of Islamization, which is a metanarrative that undermines narratives of spiritual healing that may be disregarded as unethical. Relations between healing agents and recipients have been interrogated to offer a critique of the practices in Brunei Darussalam and, by extension, the Malay world in Southeast Asia.

Reference List

Alatas (Syed), H. (1977) *The myth of the lazy native: a study of the image of the Malays, Filipinos and Javanese from the 16th to the 20th century and its function in the ideology of colonial capitalism.* London: Frank Cass.

Anderson, B. (1983) *Imagined communities: reflections on the origin and spread of nationalism.* London: Verso.

Appadurai, A. (1990) 'Disjuncture and difference in the global cultural economy,' *Theory, Culture and Society*, 7(2), pp. 295-310. doi: https://doi.org/10.1177/026327690007002017

Blackman, L. (2012) *Immaterial bodies: affect, embodiment, mediation.* Singapore: Sage.

Boomgaard, P. (2001) *Frontiers of fear: tigers and people in the Malay world, 1600-1950.* New Haven: Yale University Press.

Charon, R. (2001) 'Narrative medicine: a model for empathy, reflection, profession, and trust,' *JAMA: Journal of the American Medical Association*, 286(15), pp. 1897-1902. doi: https://doi.org/10.1001/jama.286.15.1897

Chatterjee, P. [1993 (1986)] *Nationalist thought and the colonial world: a derivative discourse.* Minnesota: University of Minnesota Press.

Daud, K.M. (2022) *The witch doctor's daughter.* Singapore: Epigram.

Daud, K.M., Chin, G.V.S. and Jukim, M. (2016) 'Contemporary English and Malay literature in Brunei: a comparison,' in Haji-Othman, N.A., McLellan, J. and Deterding, D. (eds.) *The use and status of language in Brunei Darussalam.* Singapore: Springer, pp. 241-251.

De Boer, H.J. and Cotingting, C. (2014) 'Medicinal plants for women's healthcare in Southeast Asia: a meta-analysis of their traditional use, chemical constituents, and pharmacology,' *Journal of Ethnopharmacology*, 151(2), pp. 747-767. PMID: 24269772. doi: https://doi.org/10.1016/j.jep.2013.11.030

Derrida, J. (1981) *Positions.* London: The Athlone Press.

Deterding, D. and Ho, H.M.Y. (2021) 'Overview of language, literature and culture,' in Ho, H.M.Y. and Deterding, D. (eds.) *Engaging modern Brunei: research on language, literature and culture.* Singapore: Springer, pp. 1-17.

Evans, H.D. (2016) 'Nusantara: history of a concept,' *Journal of the Malaysian Branch of the Royal Asiatic Society,* 89(1), pp. 3-14. doi: https://doi.org/10.1353/ras.2016.0004

Farrer, Ds (2008) 'The healing arts of the Malay mystic,' *Anthropology Review,* 24(1), pp. 29-46. doi: https://doi.org/10.1111/j.1548-7458.2008.00003.x

Foucault, M. [2008 (1978-79)] *The birth of biopolitics: lectures at the Collège de France, 1978-1979.* Senellart, M. (ed.). Translated from the French by Graham Burchell. Hampshire: Palgrave Macmillan.

Foucault, M. [2009 (1977-79)] *Security, territory, population: lectures at the Collège de France, 1977-78.* Senellart, M. (ed.). Translated from the French by Graham Burchell. Hampshire: Palgrave Macmillan.

Freud, S. [2001 (1901)] 'Fragment of an analysis of a case of hysteria,' in *The standard edition of the complete psychological works of Sigmund Freud, Volume VII (1901-1905): a case of hysteria, three essays on sexuality and other Works.* London: Hogarth Press, pp. 1-122.

Ho, H.M.Y. (2013) 'Depathologising racial melancholia in intergenerational Herstories,' in Andermahr, S. and Pellicer-Ortin, S. (eds.) *Trauma narratives and Herstory.* London: Palgrave Macmillan, pp. 153-168.

Ho, H.M.Y (2019) 'Women doing Malayness in Brunei Darussalam,' *SARE: Southeast Asian Review of English,* 56(2), pp. 147-165. doi: https://doi.org/10.22452/sare.vol56no2.14

Ho, H.M.Y. (2020) 'The violence of othering and (non)indigenous revival: Aammton Alias' The Bastion of Ingei as postcolonial speculative fiction of Brunei Darussalam,' *Southeast Asian Review of English,* 57(1), pp. 55-79. doi: https://doi.org/10.22452/sare.vol57no1.6

Ho, H.M.Y. (2022a) 'Beyond intractability: muslim women negotiating identities in Brunei Darussalam,' in Jussawalla, F. and Omran, D. (eds.) *Muslim women's writings from across South and Southeast Asia.* London: Routledge, pp. 240-251.

Ho, H.M.Y. (2022b) 'Localisation of Malay Muslim identity in Brunei Darussalam: a modern nation's cultural and economic goals,' in Ho, H.M.Y. and Deterding, D. (eds.) *Engaging modern Brunei: research on language, literature and culture.* Singapore: Springer, pp. 127-143.

Müller, D.M. (2018a) 'Bureaucratic Islam compared: classificatory power and state-ified religious meaning-making in Brunei and Singapore,' *Journal of Law and Religion,* 33(2), pp. 212-247. doi: https://doi.org/10.1017/jlr.2018.29

Müller, D.M. (2018b) 'Hybrid pathways to orthodoxy in Brunei Darussalam: bureaucratised exorcism, scientisation and the mainstreaming of deviant declared practices,' *Journal of Current Southeast Asian Affairs,* 37(1), pp. 141-183. doi: https://doi.org/10.1177/186810341803700106

Said, E. (1978) *Orientalism.* London: Verso.

Tomlinson, J. (1999) *Globalization and culture.* Cambridge: Polity Press.

Ullah, A.K.M.A. and Ho, H.M.Y (2020) 'Globalisation and cultures in Southeast Asia: demise, fragmentation, transformation,' *Global Society, 35*(2), pp. 191-206. doi: https://doi.org/10.1080/13600826.2020.1747992

Yoshida, M. (1985) 'Indigenous healers and healing: their persistence and vitality in Southeast Asia,' *Journal of Asian and African Studies,* 29, pp. 232-24.

Afterword: Narrative Medicine as Resistance

Arthur W. Frank

University of Calgary, Canada

As soon as the word *trauma* refers to more than injuries to bones and tissues, it challenges institutional biomedicine. The biomedical response is to specify problems, effect a treatment intervention, and if that does not fix the problem, then either reassess the diagnosis or move to the next level of treatment. Most of the traumas described in this volume do not fit that model. Problems are diffuse, often involving long, complicated histories that are difficult for anyone to sort out, even with the best of intentions. Specifying what was injured is another difficulty: beyond bodily injury, we struggle to make words like psyche, soul, and memory describe what has been hurt. Perhaps most importantly, the chapters in this book demonstrate the range of responses that different traumas call for. In response to some traumas, clinicians can only demonstrate a willingness to hear the story, often repeatedly – to be the victim's witness. But a recurring theme of these chapters is that telling the story of a trauma is more than difficult; it can itself be traumatizing.

Of particular relevance to this book's title, these chapters also raise questions about which traumas are usefully addressed by responses that are *medical*; in responses to trauma, the boundaries of what counts as medicine stretch thin. Thus I reach my main concern in this afterword: what counts as *medicine* in the term *narrative medicine*? I take the position that narrative medicine begins in a critique of fundamental habits of thought in institutional medicine. At the core of this critique are questions about forms of power, including power to define types of persons, power to decide which of life's problems will receive how much institutional assistance, and power to make money: who will make how much money from doing what, and what will be low paid or not paid at all.

With this focus on power, a dilemma takes shape. Not all but most of what these chapters call trauma results from power being inflicted on bodies in order to increase that power. When narrative medicine seeks to respond to trauma, it must acknowledge that institutional medicine is itself a structuring of power; in diverse acts of defining and allocating, institutional medicine reaffirms its fundamental power to say *which troubles count*: what is understood to be the cause different problems and what solutions can be imagined; who gets what kind of help, from whom, for which troubles, at whose cost, and who is left outside, literally. Thus we confront a potentially vicious circle: can institutionalized mechanisms of power respond to traumas that were caused by institutionalized mechanisms of power? I do not present that as a question to answer, but rather as a dilemma to return to as the background of other considerations.

To support my contention that narrative medicine is fundamentally a work of resistance, I propose three habits of thought that are pervasive in institutional biomedicine but create contradictions when they work their way into narrative medicine practice. That these habits of thought have been frequently noted does not lessen the need for continuing attention to them, because that attention has not loosened their grip on how people expect themselves to do their work, and what they are accountable to in that work.

The first is the split between a knowing subject – the professional – and an object-to-be-known, the patient. This split, so ingrained that it defines medical thought, shows up in the unreflective usage of the term *patient*; who is the patient, and more importantly, what kind of relationship is presupposed by assimilating someone's identity to being a patient? People become patients when they are attended by healthcare professionals; taking that further, patients are *available* to healthcare professionals: available to questioning and testing, available to assessment, evaluation, and judgments of multiple kinds, available to treatment interventions, and available to be kept waiting – this last is not least important, as it sets a tone for other forms of availability. Thus, a "patient narrative" is a story told by someone available to healthcare professionals, and by implication it's a story for professionals to use for their purposes, not unlike a patient's blood or urine sample. I don't think I'm being overly sensitive on this point: narrative practice presupposes that language matters, and what we call things affects our relationship to them. By calling people's stories *patient narratives*, a split is sustained between the teller and the receiver/interpreter.

Subject/object splits become most distorting when clinicians do what narrative medicine begins and sometimes ends by doing: inviting people to tell stories about their lives, with those lives including illness but not defined by illness. On the contrary: a narrative medicine practitioner listens for how the rest of a person's life defines their illness. Eliciting such stories seems, to me at least, to promise a relationship of partners in dialog. This dialog is not an equality of whose stories get most air time, but it rejects any presumption of one party to the dialog having epistemological privilege in interpreting what the other says; each is always interpreting the other. Thus I get nervous when colleagues in narrative medicine align themselves with predominate professional assumptions by promising to teach interpretive *skills* honed through training techniques. Presenting narrative medicine as a specialized skill set reinforces the presumption that clinicians are the privileged knowing subjects who confront patients whose stories are a means of knowing them.

That is my understanding of what medical history taking does. History taking is a necessary component of clinical care, but it is not dialog. It's an exercise in beneficent power, and foregrounding trauma keeps us worrying about how beneficent power ever can be.

A second pervasive habit of thought in institutional medicine can be called metrification: the assumption that anything can be subject to measuring that produces a rank order, whether that refers to degree of arterial blockage, cognitive decline, lung capacity, or intensity of pain. As I read the stories of trauma that are told in these chapters, my recurring thought is that what has happened is immeasurable, and any attempt to measure risks becomes a way of evading the embodied horror that makes what happened worth calling traumatic.

What deserves to be called traumatic is terrifying: one primary terror is realizing what some human beings can do to other human beings and then keep on doing in systematic, organized ways that include planning, building and devising, and always *calculating*. Many of the traumas in these chapters describe the calculated infliction of pain that will permanently affect memory. Here we return to the vicious circle I suggested earlier: can a medical system structured around calculations, whether of disease or clinical efficacy, address traumas that people were organized to inflict in calculated ways?

The narrative medicine I want to participate in includes a continual questioning of the limits of metrification: it asks what can be usefully measured, and when does measurement become an act of reduction through which a subject distances itself from an object by reducing that object to a quantitative score, ironically but significantly called a *value*? I question, for example, medical school narrative medicine programs scoring student writing—that seems to be how narrative medicine should be teaching students *not* to respond to their patients' stories. What is the message when students – who are smart enough to get the latent message—are trained by using techniques that the training is supposedly teaching those students to move beyond?

Medical education and practice need to be clear: metrification is a technique of power. It accustoms people to being *ordered*, both in the sense of being given commands and also in accepting being known according to rank orderings of value, significance, or priority. In clinics and hospitals, metrics are attached to clinical performance as much as to disease and patient status. People who know themselves to be divided between those who do the ordering and others who are being ordered cannot engage together in narrative medicine. But, narrative medicine can tell stories that reveal clinical ordering practices to be what they are.

The third habit of thought, which depends on the previous two, is the imperative of productivity, usually defined by metrics, whether those measure patient recovery or professional output. To count as being productive, something must have measurable effects, and doing the measuring implements a split between the subject-who-measures and the object-to-be-measured, although someone who does the measuring one moment may be what is measured the next; it's fluid. Productivity also means staying on schedule and on budget, neither of which is bad, but to paraphrase Michel Foucault (1997, p. 256), both are dangerous. Narrative medicine requires constant attention to those dangers, repeatedly asking an old question: What are people *for*? Which practices serve whom, at what cost to who else?

If critiques of these three habits of thought – and refusal of uncritical participation in them—are the negative, oppositional aspect of narrative medicine, what does it affirm? My simplest account is that narrative medicine affirms *people's ability to know themselves through dialog with others*, when those others seek to know them because they are worth knowing. For me, narrative medicine begins and ends in listening that enables speaking. We might talk more about *tactful* listening, in the sense of listening that knows when to just listen, rather than responding too quickly and showing the listening to be instrumental to the listener's purpose.

Among the many difficulties of listening to stories of trauma, especially relevant for narrative medicine is the difficulty professionals have listening to troubles that they have no capacity to do anything about; that leads to difficulty acknowledging the reality of those inaccessible troubles. Such listening is difficult for any of us, but it especially challenges those who believe it is not only their job but their responsibility to *do something* about what they hear, and if they cannot do something, then their defensive instinct is either to reframe the problem as what they can act upon or else move on. To a traumatized person, both those responses can seem like forms of dismissal.

The listening I idealize does not hold itself accountable to producing measurable clinical value in doing what it does. Nor is there any particular technique to such listening; it requires only practice in asking questions that encourage finer-grained descriptions, up to a point when the teller may not be ready to say more. These chapters refer to the need that people living with trauma have to tell their stories and have their telling witnessed, but balancing that is respect for what people are not yet ready to hear themselves say out loud. For some of the traumas discussed in these chapters, that readiness to tell is a major issue, and for others it is hardly an issue at all. A goal of narrative medicine is to make all stories, but especially trauma stories, less shameful to tell. Many traumas are inflicted as they are precisely to induce shame; that part of how they exercise power.

Listening understands itself as a practice of *respect*, and narrative medicine is nothing if it does not constantly question how to be more respectful to people. These chapters risk making that question seem easier than it is, because those who are written about probably meet most readers' criteria for being worthy of respect. We all have such criteria and should admit it. A question for narrative medicine is how to respect those people from whom we most want to set ourselves apart. How to find terms to honor their stories calls for another book.[1]

As three very preliminary guidelines to practicing respectful clinical care, I recommend the points of critique I have proposed. First, by what practices am I positioning myself as a knowing subject and the other person as the object of my knowledge and action? Second, how am I reducing the other person to what is measurable, susceptible to ranking, categorizable? What is denied in assuming all that counts is measurable? And third, how are demands of productivity affecting the relationship I might have with this person? How does my institution define my productivity, and how far does that overlap with what I expect, or once expected, of myself?

None of these questions denies either that people come to medical settings in order to get help, or that helping often involves doing things. But stories of trauma remind us of the limits of what can be helped – the limits of what *doing* can do – and the need for humility when confronted with what demands the most honest recognition of our own limits, both personal and professional.

Institutional medicine does not routinely – in its routine practices – respect people, however much it claims to. Institutional medicine often serves people well, but it does so by processing them, and many professionals believe that may be as far as the work can go. Processing works by dividing subjects from objects, by treating anything worth knowing as measurable, and by making productivity a paramount value. Narrative medicine begins in refusal of processing; it moves toward affirmation of persons' capacity for respectful dialog. That affirmation can only ever be mutual, asymmetrical in content but still mutual. These chapters help us in the continuing – never ending – work of thinking through the fine balancing of mutuality in clinical care.

First-person stories of trauma challenge institutional medicine, and these stories challenge narrative medicine to ask on what terms it participates in institutional medicine. The great risk of any movement that starts out as seeming radical is assimilation, as the assumptions that it once questioned work their way into its own practices. Attention to the needs of traumatized

---

[1] One example of such narrative practice is the work of the narrative therapist Michael White with abusive men, indicatively titled: "The Responsibilities: Working with Men Who Have Perpetrated Violence." (White, 2011, pp. 98-117).

people is not the only way of keeping narrative medicine true to its founding intentions, but it is one crucial way.

Reference List

Foucault, M. (1997) *Ethics: subjectivity and truth.* New York: The New Press.

White, M. (2011) *Narrative practice: continuing the conversations.* New York: Norton.

Biographies

Mona Baie

Medical degree and PhD student, University of Heidelberg, Deutschland

Mona Baie, MD, is research associate at the Chair of Medical Humanities at the University of Fribourg, Switzerland. She studied medicine, health humanities, and literature in Heidelberg, London, and Fribourg. In her PhD project in Comparative Literature she explores the semantics of clinical spaces in German and English pathographies (1950-present). Her research interests include medical humanities and spatial studies, German and English literature of the twentieth and twenty-first centuries, history of medicine and the hospital from the nineteenth to the twenty-first century, illness metaphors, and medical didactics.

Ssanyu Birigwa

Adjunct Professor, Columbia University, US

Ssanyu Birigwa is a Narrative Medicine Clinician, Indigenous Bone Healer and Adjunct Professor for the Master of Science Narrative Medicine program at Columbia University. A nonprofit executive with 17+ years of experience building healthier communities, she is now the co-founder of Narrative Bridge, an innovative communications & culture firm that brings sustainable Narrative Medicine training to education, healthcare, and other mission-driven organizations.

Hilde Bondevik

Professor, University of Oslo, Norway

Hilde Bondevik is Professor of Medical and Health Humanities at the Department of Health Sciences, Institute of Health and Society, University of Oslo, Norway. Bondevik holds a master's degree in history of ideas and a PhD in Medical History and works with applying perspectives from the humanities and gender studies to health sciences. Her key areas of interest include feminist theories, gender and health, phenomenology and embodiment, medical history, creative writing in health care settings (e.g., in cancer care and mental health care), literary representations of illness and social epistemology.

Mark Celinscak

Professor, University of Nebraska Omaha, US

Dr. Mark Celinscak is the Louis and Frances Blumkin Professor of Holocaust and Genocide Studies and the Executive Director of the Sam and Frances Fried Holocaust and Genocide Academy at the University of Nebraska at Omaha. He is the author of *Distance from the Belsen Heap: Allied Forces and the Liberation of a Nazi Concentration Camp*, winner of a Vine Award for Non-Fiction, and *Kingdom of Night: Witnesses to the Holocaust*, winner of a Canadian Jewish Literary Award for Holocaust literature. He is the co-editor of *Artistic Representations of Suffering: Rights, Resistance, and Remembrance* and the forthcoming International *Approaches to the Holocaust* (University of Nebraska Press). He currently serves as co-chair of the Consortium of Higher Education Centers for Holocaust, Genocide, and Human Rights Studies and is the Editor-in-Chief of the *Journal of History.*

Brooke Covington

Assistant Professor, Christopher Newport University, US

Dr. Brooke Covington is Assistant Professor of English at Christopher Newport University, where she teaches courses in rhetoric and composition, professional writing, medical humanities, and civic engagement and social justice. As the academic director of the university's Center for Community Engagement, Brooke aims to integrate community-engaged learning into the curriculum by fostering deep, reciprocal, and sustainable connections between community partners, faculty, and students. She holds a PhD in Rhetoric & Writing from Virginia Tech, and her research interests include rhetorics of public memory, anti-oppressive forms of community engagement, and narrative medicine. Her work has appeared in *Journal of Medical Humanities, Community Literacy Journal, Western Journal of Communication, Journal of Curriculum and Pedagogy*, and *Campus Compact.*

Margaux Danby

Narrative Medicine Scholar, University of Kentucky College of Medicine, US

Margaux Danby is a narrative medicine scholar, writer, and medical student. She holds a Master of Science in Narrative Medicine from Columbia University, where she also taught as a Faculty Associate. She continues to work as a freelance narrative medicine educator and workshop facilitator. A graduate of Vanderbilt University, Margaux is currently completing a Doctor of Medicine at the University of Kentucky College of Medicine.

Georgia Fagan

Lecturer, University of Sydney, Australia

Georgia Fagan has an academic and professional background in applied ethics and feminism. They teach philosophical ethics at the University of Sydney and the Australian Catholic University in addition to working as both an ethical counsellor and Primary Ethics teacher in Australia.

Arthur W. Frank

Professor Emeritus, University of Calgary, Canada

BA in English Literature from Princeton University. MA in Communications from the University of Pennsylvania. PhD in Sociology from Yale University. Professor Emeritus at the Department of Sociology, University of Calgary. Author of The Wounded Storyteller: Body, Illness, and Ethics (1995), Letting Stories Breathe: A Socio-Narratology (2010) and King Lear. Shakespeare's Dark Consolations (2022).

Rishi Goyal

Director, Associate Professor and attending physician, Columbia University, US

MD, PhD in English Literature. Associate Professor at Columbia University Medical Center and head of the master's program in Medical Humanities at that university's Institute for Comparative Literature. Attending physician in the Emergency Department at Columbia University Medical Center. Head of the steering group of *CHCI Medical and Health Humanities Network*. Adjunct associate professor at the Department of Humanities, University of Southern Denmark. First editor of *Culture and Medicine. Critical Readings in Health and Medical Humanities* (2022), and author of several articles and book chapters on narrative medicine.

Hannah Ming Yit Ho

Assistant Professor, University of Brunei Darussalam, Brunei

She read her PhD in English at the University of York (UK). She has been a research fellow at the Asia Research Institute, National University of Singapore. Her postdoctoral fellowships were completed at King's College London and the University of California, Berkeley. She has received numerous local and international grants to conduct research in Southeast Asian literary studies. In addition to publishing book chapters, her journal articles appear in *Asiatic, Kritika Kultura, Southeast Asian Review of English, The Wenshan Review of Literature* and *Culture, Global Society* and *International Journal of Asia Pacific Studies*. She co-edited the seminal volume entitled *Engaging Modern Brunei: Research on Language, Literature and Culture* (Springer, 2021).

Sue Joseph

Associate Professor, Central Queensland University, Australia

A journalist for more than forty years, working in Australia and the UK, Sue Joseph (PhD) began working as an academic, teaching print journalism at the University of Technology Sydney in 1997. As a Senior Lecturer, she taught in journalism and creative writing, particularly creative non-fiction writing. Now as Associate Professor, she works as a supervisor and trainer at Central Queensland University, holds an Adjunct position at Avondale University, is a Senior Research Fellow at the University of South Australia and is a doctoral supervisor at the University of Sydney, and the University of Technology Sydney. She is currently Joint Editor of *Ethical Space: The International Journal of Communication Ethics* and co-editor with Willa McDonald and Matthew Ricketson of the *Palgrave Studies in Literary Journalism* book series.

Astrid Joutseno

PhD, University of Turku, Finland

Astrid Joutseno/Swan currently conducts her post-doctoral research on grief of the dying and grief as an effect in intergenerational cultural memory. Her research interests lie in the crossroads of gender studies, literary and cultural studies as well as medical humanities. Joutseno's award-winning PhD dissertation Life Writing from Birth to Death: How M/others Know examined maternal life writing online. In 2023-2024 she is the Fellow in Arts at the Helsinki Collegium of Advanced Study, University of Helsinki. Joutseno is also affiliated with SELMA, Centre for the Study of Storytelling, Experientiality and Memory, at Turku University. She is a researcher in the Academy of Finland project "Counter-Narratives of Cancer: Shaping Narrative Agency" (2023–2027). With the artist's name Astrid Swan, the author has published seven albums internationally between 2005 and 2021. Swan won the prestigious Teosto Award in 2018. The same year, her music was nominated for the Scandinavian Music Prize. In 2019 Swan published a memoir, *Viimeinen kirjani (Nemo)*. In 2024 she published her first novel (*S&S Kustannus*).

T.S. Kavitha

Assistant Professor, Banaras Hindu University, India

She is the Assistant professor of French at Banaras Hindu University, Varanasi, India. She has earned a PhD from The English and Foreign Languages University, Hyderabad, on the subject of the Representations of the Arab Spring in Media and Francophone Novels. She has published extensively in the area of multiculturalism, the Arab Spring, francophone postcolonial writing and ecocriticism. Her recent research project is on the notion of Memory and

Trauma Studies in context to communities like harki, pieds-noirs, rapatriés, and appelés.

Elizabeth Lanphier

Assistant Professor, University of Cincinnati College of Medicine, US

PhD, MS, HEC-C, is Assistant Professor in the Ethics Center at Cincinnati Children's Hospital Medical Center and in the Department of Pediatrics at the University of Cincinnati College of Medicine with affiliations in the University of Cincinnati Departments of Philosophy and Women, Gender, and Sexuality Studies and the Center for Public Engagement with Science. Dr. Lanphier is also a non-resident research fellow in the Institute for Philosophy and Public Policy, and an elected board member of the Bioethics Network of Ohio. Dr. Lanphier received a master's degree in Narrative Medicine from Columbia University and completed a PhD in Philosophy and a clinical ethics fellowship at Vanderbilt University. Her scholarship in feminist bioethics and social and political philosophy engages and theorizes narrative and trauma informed practices in healthcare and ethics. Her work has appeared in journals including *Hastings Center Report, American Journal of Bioethics, Cambridge Quarterly Health Care Ethics, Pediatrics, Social Philosophy Today, Perspectives in Biology and Medicine*, as well as in several edited books and public-facing media outlets.

John Launer

Lecturer, University College London, England

John Launer is a family physician, family therapist, educator and writer. He is an honorary associate professor at University College London, UK and an honorary consultant at the Tavistock Clinic, London UK.

Molly Lindberg

PhD, Columbia University, US

She is a French teacher at Friends Academy, a Quaker school. Molly holds a PhD from the Department of French at Columbia University. Her dissertation focused on depictions of trauma in English and French novels and films about the conscription of soldiers in West African and the memorialization of the Rwandan genocide. She uses a health-humanities approach to stories, guided by an ethics of care and the goal of maintaining the dignity of real and fictional people represented.

Emma McKenzie

Team leader at Converge, York St John University, England

Emma is a practicing occupational therapist and has spent her career specializing in mental health rehabilitation and recovery. Over the last ten years Emma, has focused on innovative work bringing together health services with education providers at York St John University in York, for a project called *Converge.* Emma is currently studying for a practice led PhD in Humanities (creative writing) to re-tell stories of mental health care as a way of instigating compassion and empathy towards both patients and staff working within the mental health system, with the aim of highlighting the need for humanity to be placed at the forefront of care.

Colleen McMillan

Scientific Co-Director and Associate Professor, University of Waterloo, Canada

Colleen McMillan is a clinical health care provider, academic and researcher in the health care field for four decades. As a qualitative health researcher, her research interests focus on the intersection of gender, stigma, disability and use of the self. She teaches family practice residents the benefits of narrative medicine, including reflectivity, self-care and avoidance of burnout. She recently concluded a national study on trauma and trauma informed care. She maintains a clinical practice focused on mental health at a family health team. Colleen recently accepted the position of Scientific Co-Director at a CIHR and PHAC funded research hub with a mandate to promote mental health promotion across Canada.

Sarah Pini

Associate Professor, University of Southern Denmark, Denmark

Sarah works at the intersection of cultural and medical anthropology, arts and health, dance and performance studies, and phenomenology of the body and illness. Her research explores experiences of illness, presence, agency, and healing across different mindful bodies, dance practices, environments, and cultural contexts. Sarah's research has been published in *The Oxford Handbook of Contemporary Ballet, Synthese, Performance Research, Collaborative Embodied Performance: Ecologies of Skill* (Bloomsbury), and *The Australian Journal of Anthropology*, among others.

Preeti Puri

Assistant Professor, National Institute of Technology Hamirpur, India

Dr Preeti Puri is Assistant Professor in the Department of Humanities and Social Sciences at National Institute of Technology Hamirpur, Himachal Pradesh, India. She is the Senate Member of Indian Institute of Information Technology (IIIT) Una, Himachal Pradesh, India. Her forte is Literary Theory and Criticism, and her research concentrates on Deleuze and Guattarian Studies, Psychoanalysis and Popular Culture, and Health Humanities.

Anders Juhl Rasmussen

Associate Professor, University of Copenhagen, Denmark

MA in Danish and Philosophy, and PhD in Danish literature. Associate professor in Danish literature with research obligations in narrative medicine at Department of Nordic Studies and Linguistics, University of Copenhagen. Member of the steering committee for *Nordic Network for Narratives in Medicine* and *CHCI Medical and Health Humanities Network*. First editor of the anthology *Narrative Medicine in Education, Practice, and Interventions* (Anthem Press, 2022), and author of several articles and chapters on narrative medicine.

Ricardo Rato Rodrigues

Assistant Professor, Uniwersytet Marii Curie-Skłodowskiej w Lublinie, Poland

Ricardo Rato Rodrigues is currently Assistant Professor of Portuguese Studies at UMCS (Uniwersytet Marii Curie-Skłodowskiej w Lublinie), Poland. In 2016, he obtained his PhD in Lusophone Studies from the University of Nottingham, with a thesis entitled *A Silent Scream: Madness and Trauma in the early works of António Lobo Antunes*. His research interests are varied, from trauma and madness in literature and the arts, health humanities, comparative literature (especially in between the lusophone and anglophone contexts), psychiatry, suicide studies, politics in literature, applied drama and gender studies (with a special focus on masculinities).

Mahesh Sharma

Assistant Professor, Central Institute at Higher Tibetan Studies, Sarnath, India

As Assistant Professor of English, he has been teaching in the Department of Classical and Modern Languages at CIHTS, Sarnath, Varanasi, India. He received his M.Phil. from the University of Rajasthan in the area of Rasa Theory and Indian Aesthetics. He earned PhD. from The English and Foreign Languages University, Hyderabad, from the Department of Indian and World Literatures with a specialization in Postcolonial Theory and Literature. As a creative writer, he has published various short stories in Hindi and English, bringing him various awards. He has published many seminal research articles in the area of postcolonialism, cosmopolitanism, literary theory, criticism, and sorry literature.

Shefali

Research Scholar, Dr B R Ambedkar National Institute of Technology, Jalandhar, India

Shefali is a Research Scholar in the Department of Humanities and Management at Dr B R Ambedkar National Institute of Technology Jalandhar, Punjab, India. Her research interests include Health Humanities, Narrative Medicine and Graphic Medicine. Her ongoing PhD dissertation focuses on the analysis of the experience of schizophrenia in comics.

Nora Simonhjell

Professor, University of Agder, Norway

PhD in Norwegian Literature and poet. Professor in Nordic literature at Department of Nordic and Media Studies, University of Agder, Kristiansand. Co-editor of the annual anthology of Norwegian Literature *Norsk litterær årbok* (Samlaget 2017-2023). Author of several articles and chapters on literary representations of illness, disability, care, and the role for next of kin.

Victoria Simpson

PhD Candidate, University of Texas at San Antonio, US

PhD Fellow in the English Department at University of Texas at San Antonio, Victoria currently has two published works, *El Mundo Zurdo 7 for the Selected Works From 2018 Meeting of The Society for the Study of Gloria Anzaldúa.* "Writing for Transformative Change Through Self-Expression and Self-Reflection" (Aunt Lute Publishers, 2018). *Voices Of Illness Negotiating Meaning and Identity,* "Narrative Medicine and Storytelling: An Alternative Method for Healing" (Brill Publishers, 2018).

Aaron Smith

Professor and Faculty Lead, Yorkville University, Canada

Aaron Smith has taught in social work, psychology, and psychotherapy programs at universities throughout Canada for more than ten years. He is a Registered Psychotherapist in the Province of Ontario and has worked for numerous health care and community-based organizations for more than fifteen years. Aaron is a sought-after speaker and has published and presented workshops across North America. Woven throughout his research is an emphasis on relational engagement and wellbeing.

Morten Sodemann

Clinical Professor, University of Southern Denmark, Denmark

MA, PhD, consultant physician in infectious diseases. Clinical professor in global health and immigrant medicine, Department of Clinical Medicine, University of Southern Denmark. Chief physician, Clinic for Immigrant Medicine, Odense University Hospital. Author of *What you don't know will hurt the patient* (Open Access, 2022) and several articles and chapters on narrative medicine.

Jacob Y. Stein

Senior Lecturer, College of Management, Israel

Dr. Jacob Y. Stein is a senior lecturer at the Department of Psychology in the College of Management Academic Studies, Israel. His fields of expertise include studies of loneliness and trauma, both separately and interactively. His studies include both longitudinal quantitative investigations and qualitative studies. He has co-authored several articles and book chapters in these interwoven domains.

Oddgeir Synnes

Professor, VID Specialized University, Norway

Oddgeir Synnes is Professor of Health Humanities at the Centre for Diaconia and Professional Practice, VID Specialized University, Oslo, Norway. Synnes has a master's degree in Nordic literature and a PhD in illness narratives and works with applying perspectives from the humanities to healthcare, both through practical projects and in research. His key areas of interest include cultural and narrative gerontology, creative writing in health care settings (e.g., in cancer care, palliative care, and dementia care), literary representations of illness, and narrative inquiry. His latest book is *A Poetic Language of Ageing* (with Olga V. Lehmann – Bloomsbury Academic, 2023).

Rivka Tuval-Mashiach

Professor, College of Management, Israel

Prof. Rivka Tuval-Mashiach is a clinical psychologist and full professor in the Department of Psychology at Bar-Ilan University, Israel. She serves as the chair of the steering committee of Natal, the Israel center for victims of trauma and terror, and served as the chair of the Gender graduate Program in Bar Ilan. Her fields of expertise include resilience, posttraumatic stress, and posttraumatic growth following terror and war, identity challenges and identity re-construction following traumatic events, gendered perspectives of trauma. Her research aims to bridge between theoretical models and applied as well as therapeutic approaches. Specifically, she focuses on the importance of constructing the trauma narrative, and on the power of bearing testimony in healing trauma. Prof. Rivka Tuval- Mashiach uses qualitative as well as mixed methods in her research, and is an expert in narrative and qualitative text analysis. She has published numerous papers and co-authored the books Narrative Research: Reading, Analysis and Interpretation (Sage, 1998, with Professor Amia Lieblich and Dr.Tammar Zilber) and Narrative Research: Theory, Interpretation and Creation, in Hebrew, with Dr. Gabriella Spector-Mersel.

Annmaree Watharow

PhD Candidate, University of Sydney, Australia

Dr. Annmaree Watharow is a clinician and academic who lives with disability. She is the author of *Improving the Experience of Health Care for People Living with Sensory Disability: Knowing What is Going On* (2023, Lived Places Publishing), and the playwright Harms Way. Annmaree is presently the Lived Experience Research Fellow at the Centre for Disability Research and Policy, University of Sydney.

Lillian Wilde

Research Associate, IU International University of Applied Sciences, England

Lillian completed her PhD on the phenomenology of intersubjectivity and post-traumatic experience at the University of York in 2022, with a focus on empathy, background feelings of belonging, and alienation Her research integrates work in phenomenology, psychopathology, philosophy of mind, philosophy of psychiatry, and trauma studies and has been published in *Phenomenology and the Cognitive Sciences, Psychopathology,* and *Medicine, Health Care, and Philosophy,* among others, https://philpeople.org/profiles/lillian-wilde

Author Index

S

T

V

W

Z

Subject Index

D

E

F

G

N

O

P

V

W

Z

www.ingramcontent.com/pod-product-compliance
Lightning Source LLC
LaVergne TN
LVHW020412220926
848484LV00016B/2542/J